MW00561383

# A PRACTICAL GUIDE TO
# CUPPING THERAPY

This book is edited and designed by the Editorial Committee of *Cultural China* series

Text by Wu Zhongchao
Translation by Cao Jianxin
Design by Wang Wei

Copy Editor: Susan Luu Xiang
Editors: Wu Yuezhou, Cao Yue
Editorial Director: Zhang Yicong

Senior Consultants: Sun Yong, Wu Ying, Yang Xinci
Managing Director and Publisher: Wang Youbu

ISBN: 978-1-60220-031-9

Address any comments about *A Practical Guide to Cupping Therapy: A Natural Approach to Heal through Traditional Chinese Medicine* to:

Better Link Press
99 Park Ave
New York, NY 10016
USA

or

Shanghai Press and Publishing Development Co., Ltd.
F 7 Donghu Road, Shanghai, China (200031)
Email: comments_betterlinkpress@hotmail.com

Printed in China by Shenzhen Donnelley Printing Co., Ltd.
3 5 7 9 10 8 6 4 2

The material in this book is provided for informational purposes only and is not intended as medical advice. The information contained in this book should not be used to diagnose or treat any illness, disorder, disease or health problem. Always consult your physician or health care provider before beginning any treatment of any illness, disorder or injury. Use of this book, advice, and information contained in this book is at the sole choice and risk of the reader.

Quanjing provides the images on pages 17 (fig. 5) and 38 (figs. 24–25) and on the front cover (bottom).

# A PRACTICAL GUIDE TO CUPPING THERAPY

## A Natural Approach to Heal through Traditional Chinese Medicine

By Wu Zhongchao

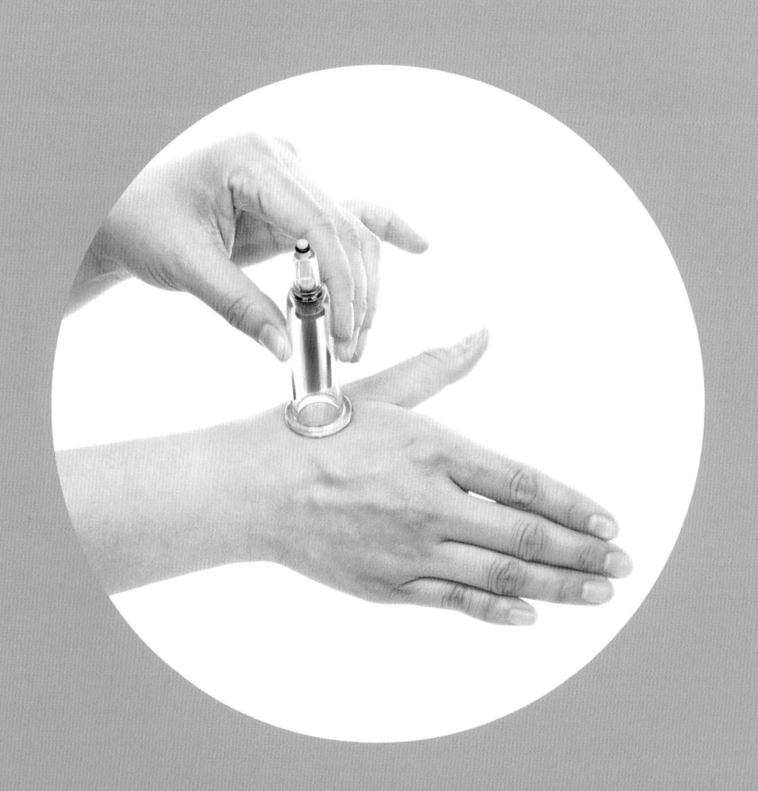

Better Link Press

# Contents



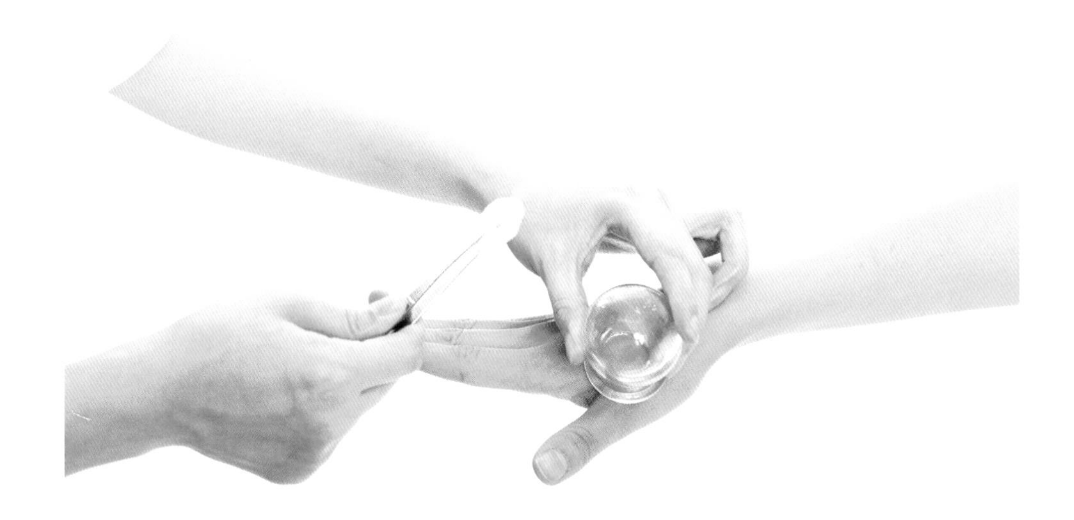

## Chapter Three
Meridians, Collaterals, and Acupoints 29



## Chapter Four
Sub-Health 35



## Chapter Five
Internal Diseases 55



## Chapter Six
Surgical Diseases 123



## Chapter Seven
Diseases of the Five Sense Organs 145

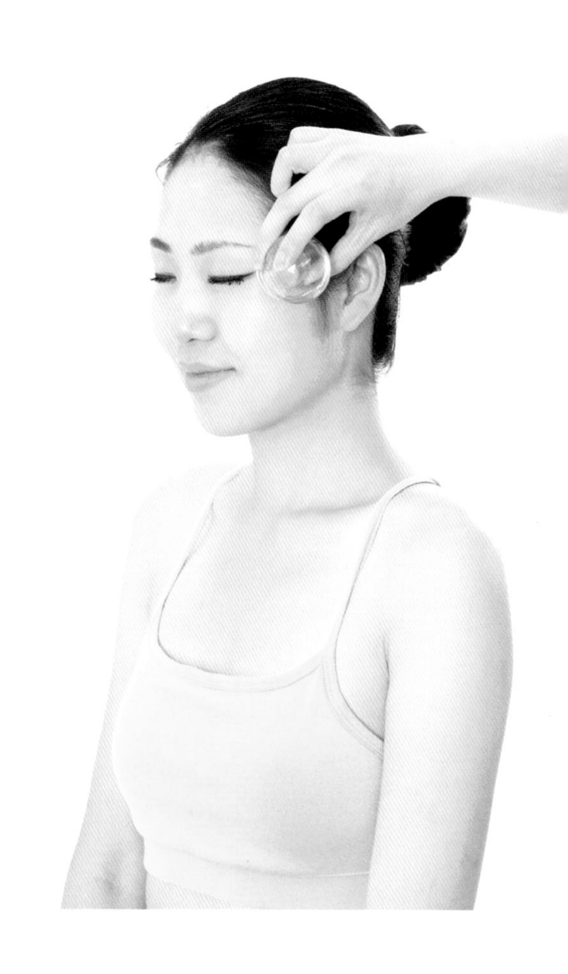

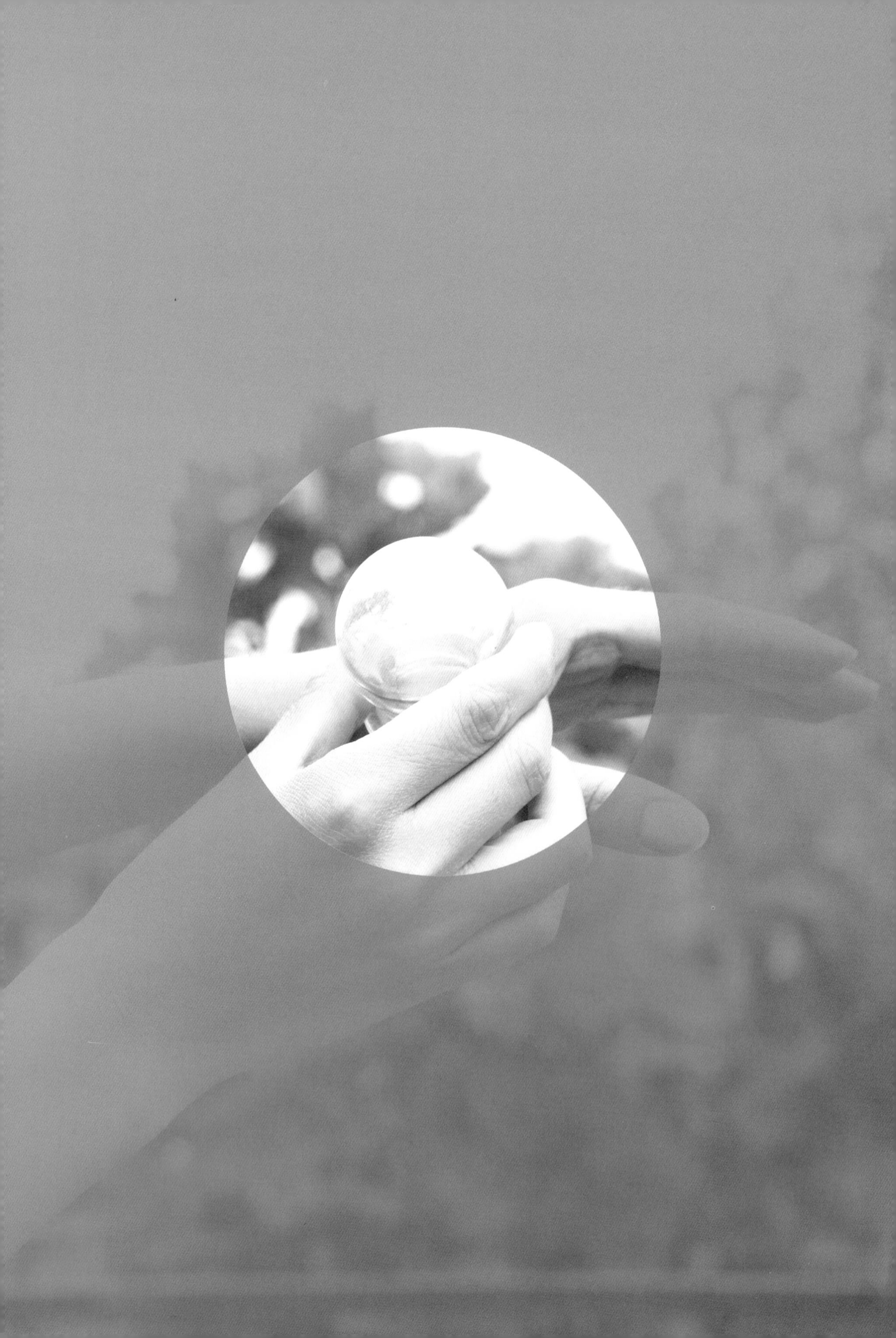

# Preface

Cupping, also known as cupping qi, or suction tube therapy, has a long history in China. As one of the Traditional Chinese Medicine (TCM) therapies, it is widely used as it is simple and practical with significant results. Developed from an ancient folk medicine, cupping therapy uses cups and jars as tools, suctioned to specific areas (affected parts or acupuncture points) of the body surface after the air in them is evacuated via heat to produce negative pressure, thereby creating warm stimulation to generate stagnation of blood in those areas. Today, this natural therapy is still popular among people.

People who have experienced cupping have found that if they have physical discomfort, they will feel much more comfortable after cupping, which is the magic of cupping therapy in Traditional Chinese Medicine. When you encounter a physical symptom, do you know how to relieve it through cupping? Other than professionals, how will self-learners perform cupping?

Cupping can be performed at home with safe and reliable tools as long as you have grasped the skills, and know specific information such as which acupoints should be cupped for certain symptoms, and how long the cupping should last. This book provides acupoint cupping techniques for nearly 100 diseases, and gives detailed description of cupping methods and cupping time for each acupoint, and the right way of cupping for different symptoms of each disease to achieve remarkable effects. Every cupping step in this book is accompanied with a picture, corresponding to bone-length measurement or anatomical location map, which can help you find the acupoints more easily. After reading this book, even beginners who are not familiar with acupoints can gradually learn to cup.

In addition to easing the symptoms of diseases, cupping therapy can also help you preserve your health and improve your looks. This book introduces cupping methods for 12 sub-health status and 8 common problems that affect your appearance. So even if you are not sick, you can use cupping to enhance your physical fitness and get rid of a variety of problems affecting your health and looks. As this book is very practical, professional readers can use it as a reference, while amateurs can acquire knowledge of cupping and try to learn simple cupping methods step-by-step. For the sake of safety, beginners who want to learn cupping may start with vacuum cupping to experience the fantastic feeling that results from this particular therapy.

Some operation charts in this book use cupping on clothes or hair for the need of photography. When operating at home, readers should cup directly on the skin without clothes and directly on the scalp after shaving off the hair instead of doing it on hair.

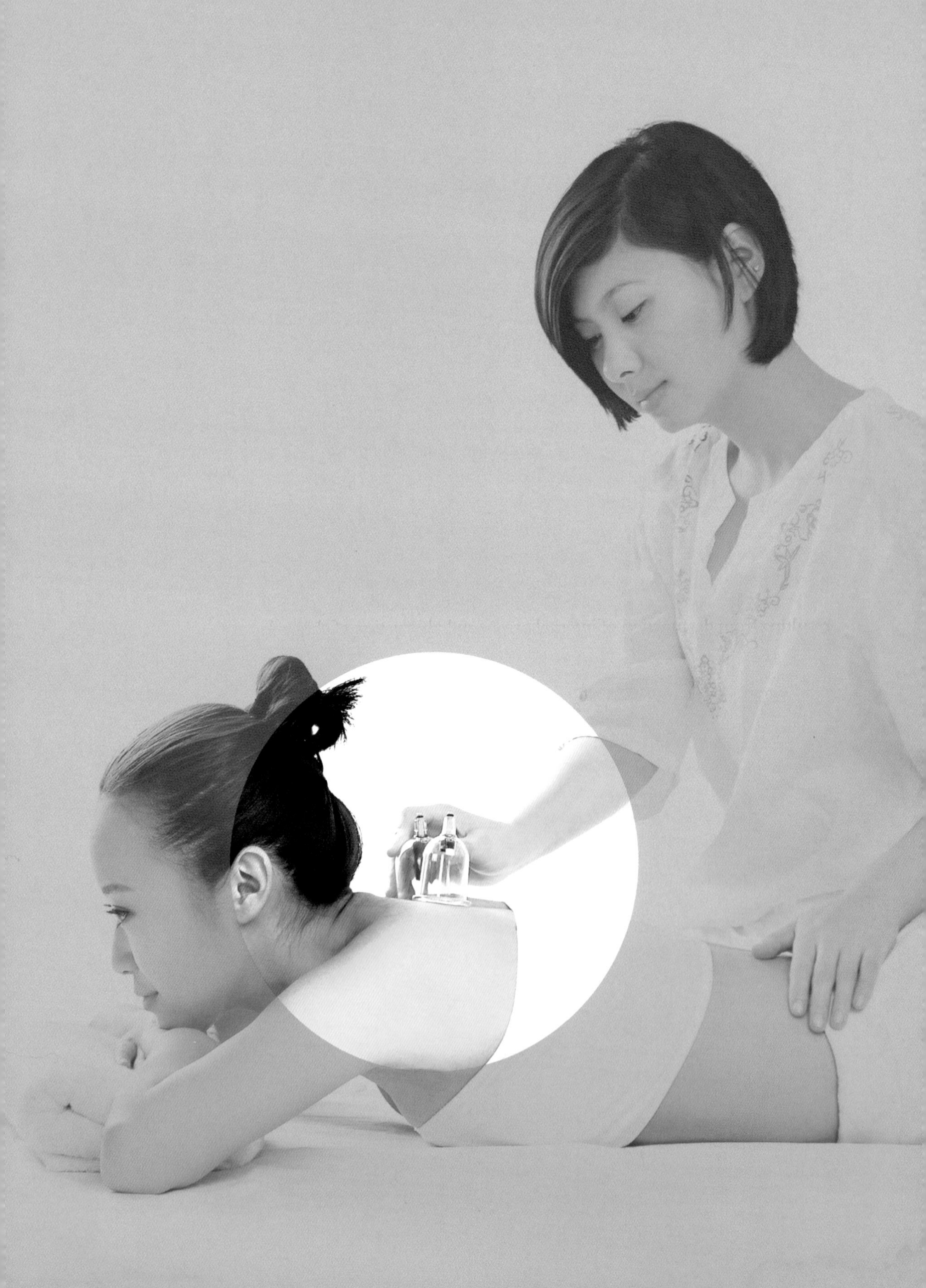

# Chapter One
# Benefits and Attentions of Cupping Therapy

With a history of thousands of years in China, cupping therapy is an important part of the Traditional Chinese Medicine, and is widely used in the medicine, surgery, gynecology, dermatology, ENT, and other departments through promotion by modern medicine, alleviating and even preventing and treating more than a hundred common diseases. However, cupping cannot be performed under all conditions. Techniques should be followed to take effect. Therefore, before cupping, one should not only understand its advantages and effects, but also know how to perform it in a scientific and effective manner, so that one can apply appropriate techniques to maximize the effects of cupping.

## 1. Benefits of Cupping Therapy

Cupping therapy is applicable to a wide range of symptoms, and has certain effects on a variety of diseases, which can be alleviated and treated by such methods as acupuncture, massage, traditional Chinese treatment, and Traditional Chinese Medicine. In particular, it has good effects on various painful diseases, soft tissue injuries, acute and chronic inflammations, syndrome of wind-cold dampness arthralgia, and symptoms resulting from dysfunction of internal organs and obstruction of channels.

Research has found that through the suction of the skin, pores, meridians, and acupoints, cupping can guide the transport and distribution of qi in the body, promote qi and blood in meridians, nourish viscera, organs, and tissues, warm the body, stimulate the functions of weak viscera, smoothen meridians, adjust the yin and yang balance of the organism, and also adjust qi and blood, thus achieving the purpose of improving health and warding off illness.

The negative pressure generated in the cup during cupping therapy can cause local capillary congestion and even rupture, rupture of red blood cells, epidermal blood stasis, and the phenomenon of hemolysis, and then produce a group of histamine and histamine-like substances which will flow all over the body with body fluid, stimulating organs, strengthening their functions and activities, and enhancing resistance of the body. Stimulation of negative pressure can cause dilation of local blood vessels, promote local blood circulation, improve the state of congestion, strengthen metabolism, change the status of local tissue nutrition, enhance permeability of vascular wall and leukocyte phagocytosis activities, and strengthen the body's physical fitness and immune capacity. According to modern medicine, the suction of pressure in the cup to local parts of the body can speed up blood and lymph circulation, promote gastrointestinal peristalsis, improve digestion functions, as well as promote and accelerate the muscles and viscera to excrete and eliminate metabolites.

After long-term practice, cupping therapy, which developed among common folks, has formed such characteristics as varied tools, varied techniques, and wide applicable parts of the body. Therefore, it can alleviate increasing number of diseases with the expansion of its scope of indications. Most diseases of the internal medicine, gynecology, traumatology, surgery, dermatology, ENT, and other departments can be alleviated by applying cupping therapy with good curative effects.

In summary, the cupping therapy has advantages as follows:

Mechanical stimulation: During cupping, the negative pressure in the cup can cause rupture of local capillaries to produce the phenomenon of autolysis, stimulate the body's microcirculation system, improve local blood circulation, and strengthen the body's protection and immune functions, thereby forming an optimal stimulation.

Warm stimulation: During cupping, the heating action of the cup can promote the expansion of local blood vessels, increase blood flow, and speed up blood circulation, thus improving the blood supply and nutrient supply to the skin, promoting metabolism, and improving the patient conditions and restoring their health.

Anti-inflammation and relieving pain: Cupping can promote local blood circulation. Strengthened local blood circulation can improve metabolism of inflammatory exudate and pain factors at local lesion, and further decrease or eliminate their stimulation to nerve endings, thereby eliminating inflammation, relieving pain and achieving the purpose of treatment.

Detoxification: During cupping, the negative pressure in the cup can cause rupture of local blood vessels, thus directly discharging local accumulation of metabolic wastes, and at the same time, improving respiration of the skin, which is conducive to the excretion and detoxification of sweat glands and sebaceous glands, and increasing metabolism in human bodies.

Regulating the immune function: Research has found that cupping can increase the total number of white blood cells, and at the same time, improve the phagocytic ability of white blood cells as the $\alpha$-globulin and $\beta$-globulin in blood increase obviously under the effect of mechanical stimulation, bleeding and congestion, thus greatly increasing the body's defense immunity.

Two-way optimal regulative effect: Cupping has the effect of a two-way optimal regulation. Take cupping at Zhongwan point as an example, when the stomach and intestine are inhibited, cupping can excite the functions of stomach and intestine. When they are excited, cupping can inhibit their functions. Another example is cupping at Tianshu point, when constipation occurs, cupping helps relieve constipation. When diarrhea occurs, cupping can stop diarrhea. The two-way optimal regulative effect of cupping therapy is consistent with the improvement of disease.

## 2. Considerations and Taboos of Cupping Therapy

During the cupping process, many aspects need to be considered, like cupping environment, correct cupping methods, cupping time, etc., which all influence the effects of cupping. Chapter Two will describe in detail the whole process from pre-cupping preparation to post-cupping observation of cupping marks, as well as the specific methods. While learning correct cupping methods, you should also be familiar with your own conditions, and clearly know the time when it is not suitable for cupping, so as to avoid adverse consequences. Below are the points of consideration and taboos of cupping, which will guide you to make full preparation before cupping.

### Attentions

- During cupping, keep the room warm, in case the patient catches cold.

- Do not practice cupping at the same area for a second time before the marks of the first cupping disappear.
- During cupping, the patient should try not to move so the cups will stay on.
- When several cups are used at the same time, the cups should not be placed too close to each other to prevent collision of cups or the stretching of the skin.
- Small cups and a small number of cups should be used for initial recipients and the weak and elderly people.
- Feeling warm, sore, tight, and sleepy during cupping is a normal phenomenon. Take off the cups if you feel obvious pain or discomfort, and perform cupping again after a short break depending on your situation.
- During cupping, be careful not to use too much alcohol, not to dip alcohol on the mouth of the cup to prevent the skin from being burned. Also pay attention to avoid the skin from being burned by boiling water and steam. For pricking cupping, disinfect the cupping tools strictly to prevent infection.

### Taboos

Before cupping, first understand your own status to avoid the conditions where cupping should be contraindicated. Cupping should be prohibited or applied with caution for those who have any of the following circumstances:

- Cupping should not be applied to patients during the outbreak of systemic severe convulsions or epilepsy.
- Cupping is contraindicated for those with mental disorder or during outbreak of mental illness, those who bleed easily, or suffer hemorrhagic diseases such as allergic purpura, thrombocytopenic purpura, hemophilia, leukemia, and positive results of capillary tests, and those with a large range of skin diseases, skin ulceration, or severe allergic skin.
- Cupping should not be applied to patients with malignant tumors, because it will promote tumor spread and metastasis.
- During pregnancy, to avoid miscarriage or discomfort, cupping should not be performed on lumbosacral region, lower abdomen and nipples.
- Cupping is contraindicated for patients with severe heart failure, those with kidney illness experiencing kidney functional failure, and those with liver illness experiencing ascites due to cirrhosis and general dropsy.
- Cupping should be performed on thickly muscled areas with thick subcutaneous fat and less hair. Cupping should not be applied to body surface with large blood vessels, position of apex beat, delicate skin, position with obvious blood vessels, scars, and nose, eyes, lips, bone protrusion, and loose skin or skin with large wrinkles.

However, the taboos and unsuitable areas of cupping therapy are not absolute. Those who have used this therapy to alleviate edema, mental illness, high fever, active tuberculosis and other diseases have not experienced adverse reactions, but have achieved very good results. No adverse reactions appear on some people when this therapy is performed on such areas as nipples, portion of apex beat, nose, ears, and external genitalia and anus. It should be determined depending on the actual case as application of cupping therapy in conjunction with other therapies also does good to appropriate indications, or can improve the curative effects. However, try to avoid cupping in case of the contraindications mentioned above during clinical applications. Be careful if the therapy must be performed.

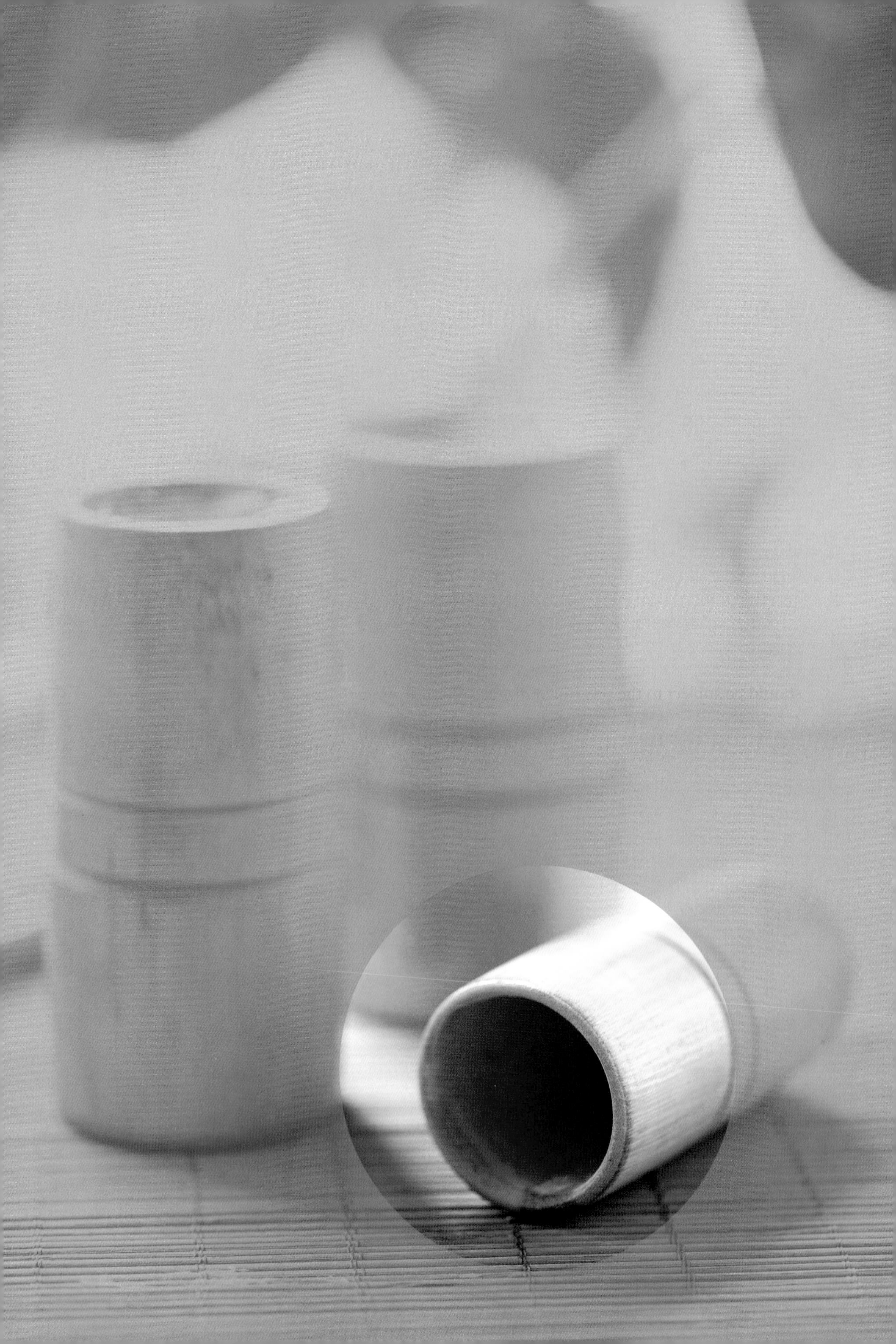

# Chapter Two
# Methods of Cupping Therapy

Cupping is easy to operate and you can complete it easily on your own as long as you have fully prepared all necessary tools and abide by the correct cupping techniques. In the order of before, during and after cupping, this chapter describes in detail from the cupping tools to each link of operation methods in the cupping process, and the treatment after cupping to help you operate efficiently in the whole process.

## 1. Process of Cupping Therapy

Before cupping, prepare all necessary tools such as cups, alcohol, cotton balls, pincers, and lighters per your own needs. In addition, appropriate tools should be prepared for some special cupping methods, for example, the kettle and the towel for water cupping, Chinese medicines, pot, etc., for herbal cupping.

Set out different cups for the different positions during cupping. In general principle, the position chosen should make the patient feel comfortable, also fully expose the cupping areas to facilitate the operation. The number and size of cups should be subject to the severity of disease, physical strength, size of the affected area, age, skin elasticity, etc. Cups should be placed on smooth parts of the skin. Avoid wrinkles and protrusions, especially those areas with prominent bones. The most suitable areas for cupping are those with thick muscle fat layers and fewer blood vessels. Large cups can be used on the flat and muscular areas with thick subcutaneous fat, while small cups can be used on those narrow areas with thinner muscles and less subcutaneous fat (fig. 1). Small rubber cups or suction cups can be applied to some special areas, for example, Sibai, Hegu, and Taichong points.

To remove cups, tilt the cup with one hand, and press the skin opposite to the cup with the other hand to form a gap, where the air will flow into the cup. Now, the cup will fall off because suction force disappears immediately.

Cupping generally lasts for 10–15 minutes. It can be adjusted based on the specific conditions of the patients. In general, it lasts preferably long in winter when it is dry, but short in summer when it is damp.

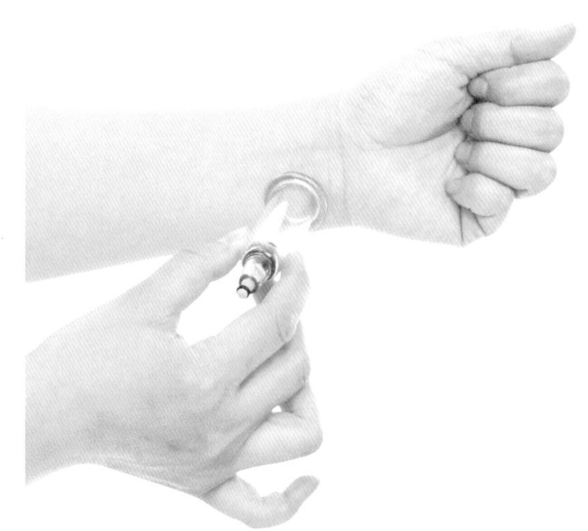

Fig. 1 A small-size cup should be used at hand joints.

Be aware of infection after cupping. Normal skin reactions after cupping generally do not need special treatment, but blisters and other conditions, if present, should be treated promptly to prevent infection. Use antibiotics in the event of infection. After cupping, cupping tools should be cleaned and disinfected in due time and kept properly. Bamboo cups should be placed in a cool and dry place and avoid exposure to sunshine.

## 2. Commonly Used Tools

The most important tools for cupping are cups. We can often see cupping therapists using different cups, for example, bamboo cups, glass cups, ceramic cups, metal cups, etc. Readers who are beginning to experiment with cupping may choose suction cups, and then gradually learn and practice the operation methods with other tools. When cupping at home, people may also use some daily necessities which can easily generate suction force. In addition, auxiliary tools are also essential, for example, combustion sources for fire cupping, carriers for burning such as alcohol and cotton. Below are brief introductions to commonly-used tools.

**Glass cup**, a more commonly used tool at present, is made of heat-resistant glass, and has a large cavity but a small mouth, and a slightly outward mouth edge. Glass cups can be divided into different models according to the mouth diameter and size of cavity. Their advantages include pleasant shape, clarity and transparency, being easy to observe the changes of skins, and easy to grasp the degree of congestion, blood stasis and bleeding, especially suitable for pricking-bloodletting cupping and moving cupping methods. Their disadvantages are marked by fragility, quick to heat, and low burn threshold (fig. 2).

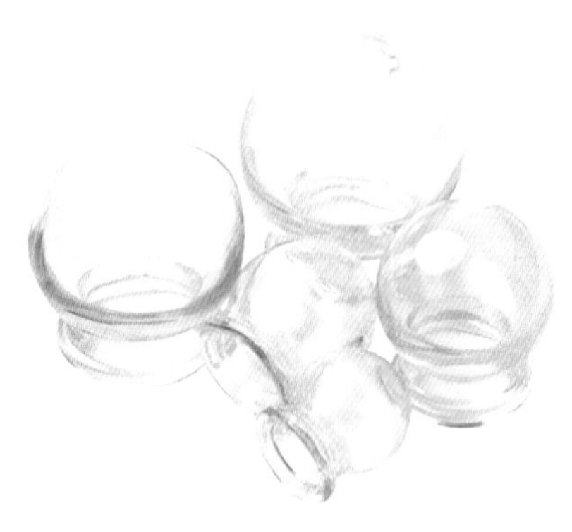

Fig. 2 Pleasant-looking glass cups are commenly used since they make it convenient for the operator to observe skin changes.

**Bamboo cups** are made of bamboo. Choose a solid and mature old bamboo, cut it at the joints, and use the end with joint as the bottom and the other end without joint as the mouth. Cut off the old skin, and make a cylindrical and waist-drum-shaped bamboo tube with slightly thick middle part and two slightly slim ends. The bottom and mouth of the bamboo tube should be flat, and its periphery should be smooth, 8–10 cm in length. Bamboo cups have advantages including lightness, durability, resistance to break, capability of absorbing liquid medicine, readily available materials, and convenience to produce. Their disadvantages mainly include proneness to dry, crack, leak, and opaque, and difficulty to observe the changes in skin color and bleeding (fig. 3).

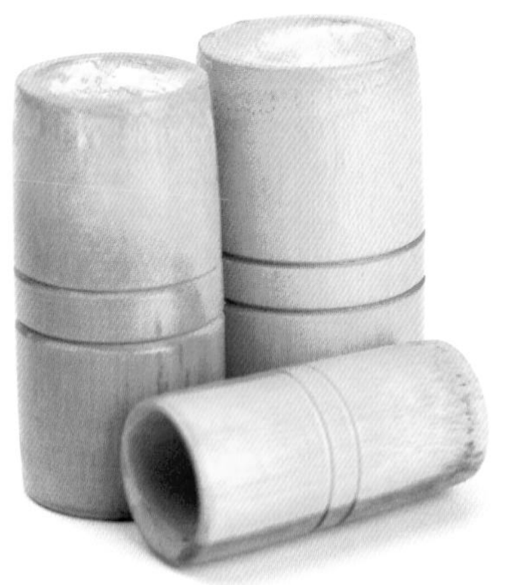

Fig. 3 Easily-made bamboo cups can absorb medicinal liquid.

**Ceramic cup** is a general term for pottery

cup and porcelain cup. The cups are more common in rural areas in northern China. Made of fired clay painted with black or yellow glaze, they are characterized by flat mouth and bottom, smooth inside and outside, slightly large middle, two slightly small ends, porcelain drum shape, appropriate thickness, and smooth mouth. Their advantages include low cost, big suction force, easy maintenance, and convenient to disinfect. Their disadvantages are marked by heaviness, fragility, difficult to carry, and inability to observe the changes of skin color within the cups (fig. 4).

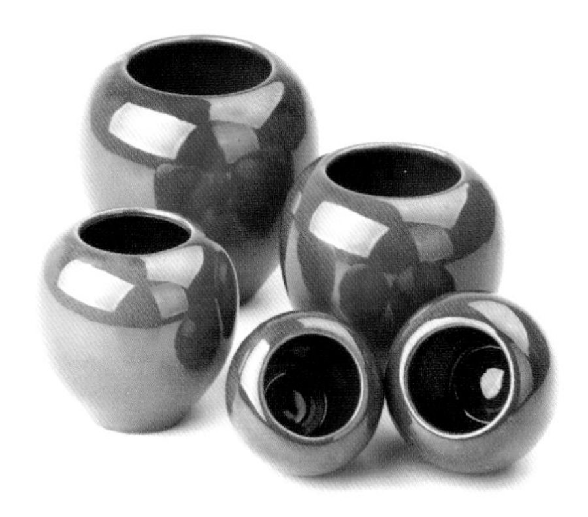

Fig. 4 It is not convenient to carry pottery cups and difficult to observe skin changes.

**Suction cup** is a relatively modern cupping set consisting of vacuum cups, pistol grip hand pump, connecting pipes, etc., which forms negative pressure inside the cup using the mechanical principles. The vacuum cup body is transparent, making it easy to observe the changes of skin in the cup. Different from the traditional tools, the suction cups do not create negative pressure by burning, and are safer and more convenient, but their drawbacks are marked by no sense of warmth and inability to move (fig. 5).

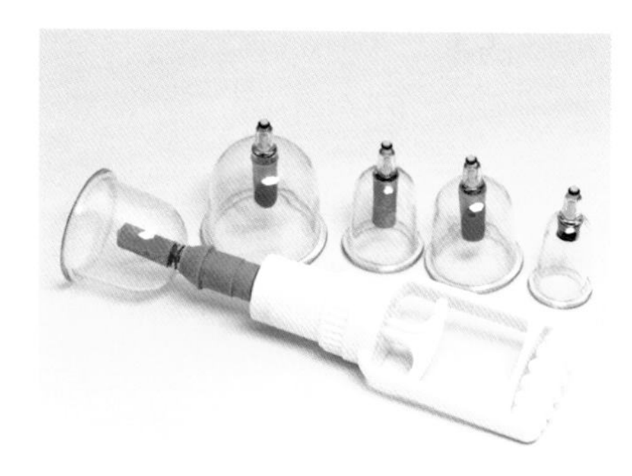

Fig. 5 The vacuum cups are more modern. Their transparency makes it convenient for the operator to observe skin changes.

In addition to those cups described above, people will also use readily available alternative cupping tools during health care at home. These tools are jointly characterized by: small mouth and large cavity, flat and smooth mouth, no hurt to skin, heat-resistant materials with no risk to burn the skin, and capability of producing certain suction force. Therefore, teacups, small bowls, glass bottles, medicine bottles, and other daily necessities which satisfy these conditions can be used to substitute special cupping tools. Of course, if the conditions permit, better results can be achieved by using special cupping tools. The demonstrations in this book use transparent glass cups to help observe the skin conditions in the cups, and make the display of gestures more visible.

Apart from the cupping tools described above, to obtain good cupping effects, auxiliary tools can be prepared based on personal needs, including materials for burning, products for disinfection and cleaning, needles, lubricants, scald ointment, etc. For example, you can prepare medical alcohol, paper, alcohol cotton balls, absorbent cotton pads, three-edged needles, plum-blossom needles, Vaseline, safflower oil (lubricants), pincers, haemostatic forceps, etc. (fig. 6).

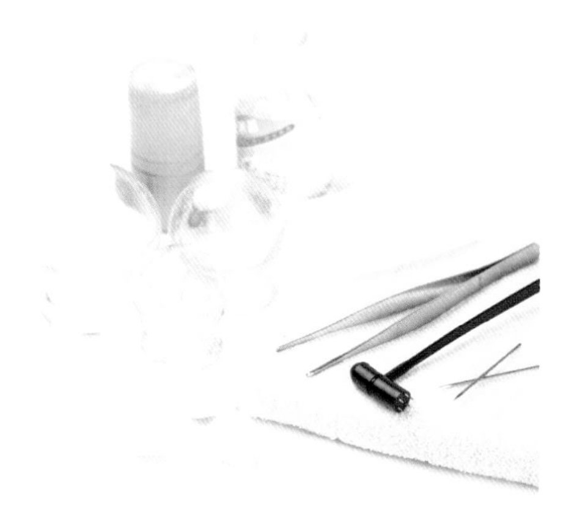

Fig. 6 Auxiliary tools.

### Selection of Cup Sizes

Cups are generally divided into large, medium, and small sizes, adaptable to different people and targeted areas. So, how do you determine an appropriate size? These are the general methods:

Depending on the characteristics of the body parts to be worked on: Large-size cups can be used on flat and muscular parts with thick subcutaneous fat, such as the chest, back, waist, abdomen, buttocks, and thighs; medium-size cups can be used on such areas as neck, shoulders, upper arms, front arms, and lower legs; and small-size cups can be used on those parts with rugged bones and weak muscles and fat, such as joints, head and face, hands and feet.

Depending on the patient's physical conditions: Use large-size cups for strong and fat patients; and use small-size ones for weak, thin patients and old people.

Depending on the patient's conditions: Use large-size cups or use several cups jointly for seriously ill patients or patients with greater extent of lesion; and use small-size cups or single cup for mildly ill patients or patients with a small extent of lesion.

## 3. Methods of Placing Cups

Placing cups is a process of evacuating the air from the cups to produce negative pressure, and sucking them onto the skin. Most of the cupping techniques evacuate the air by using a flame to heat the cup, thereby creating negative pressure within the cup before sucking the cup onto the skin. Therefore, this method of cupping is called fire cupping. Besides flame, the air can also be evacuated by using steam to generate heat, using pistol grip hand pump of the suction cup, and other methods. Below are the introductions to several most commonly used methods of placing cups. After learning these techniques of placing cups and their respective characteristics, you may choose the most suitable one or more from them.

### Flash-Fire Cupping

During operation, use a pair of haemostatic forceps to hold a 95% alcohol cotton ball, ignite and insert the cotton ball into the cup to rotate one or two seconds, and then after quickly taking out the cotton ball, place the mouth of the cup onto the appropriate body part. Be careful not to bake the cup mouth, so as not to burn the skin. Several more cups can be prepared so that quick replacement is possible if the mouth of the cup heats up. This method is applicable to various positions and cupping methods, and is the most common one (fig. 7).

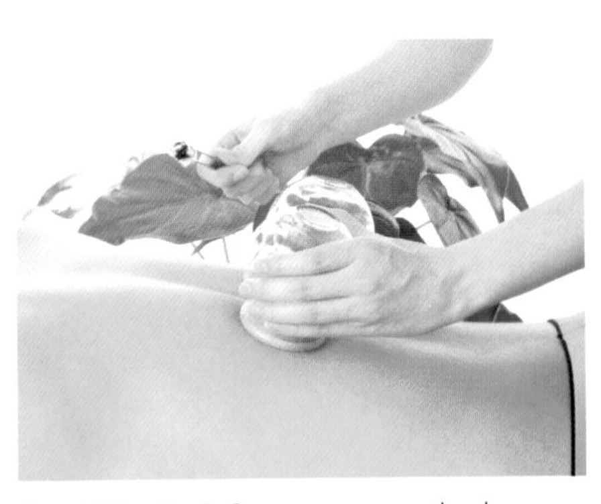

Fig. 7 The flash-fire cupping method.

### Cotton-Burning Cupping

During operation, pull the periphery of an absorbent cotton ball two centimeter in diameter thin, and slightly dip it in alcohol and paste it to the middle inner wall of the cup. After igniting, quickly apply the cup to the appropriate area. Note that the cotton ball should not be too thick to prevent it from falling while burning, and alcohol should not be too much so it will not flow down and burn the skin. This method is better applicable to horizontal cupping on lateral areas (fig. 8).

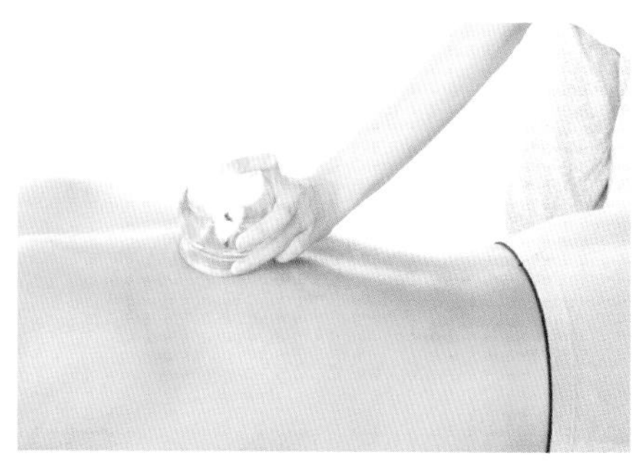
Fig. 8 The cotton-burning cupping method.

## Fire-Insertion Cupping

First fold paper into a wide strip. The operator should hold the cup bottom with one hand, ignite the paper and throw it into the cup, and then quickly apply the cup to the appropriate area before the paper burns up. This method is mainly applied to lateral parts of the body, because it prevents the paper from falling down and burning the skin (fig. 9).

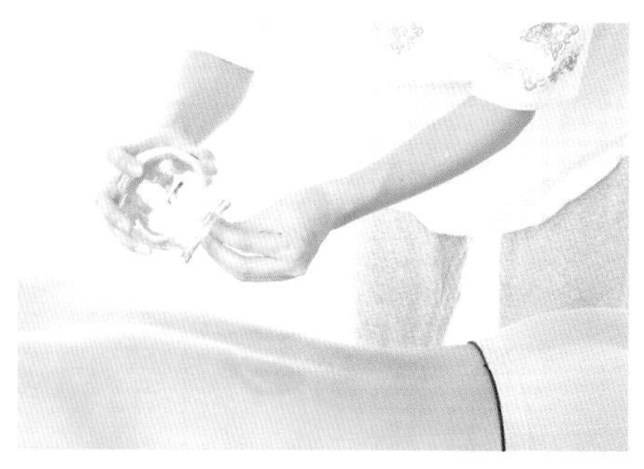
Fig. 9 The fire-insertion cupping method.

## Alcohol Fire Cupping

To operate, drip alcohol into the lower part of the cup, and then rotate the cup to make the alcohol attach to the inner wall evenly. After igniting, hold the cup bottom and quickly apply the cup to the appropriate body part. Pay attention not to drip the alcohol to the cup mouth so it will not burn the skin; do not drip too much alcohol, and 1 to 2 drips are sufficient. This method is applicable to various positions (fig. 10).

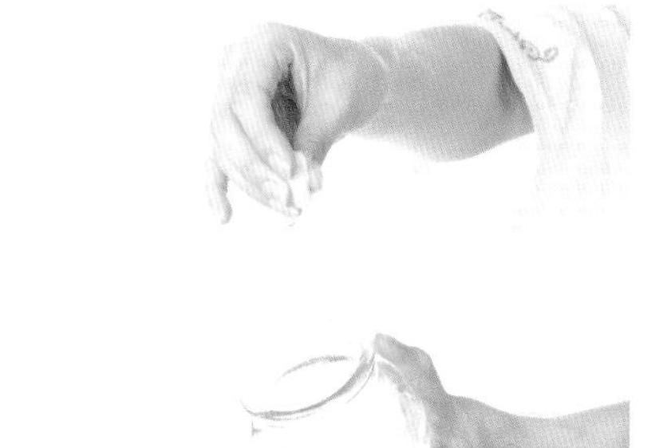
Fig. 10 The alcohol fire cupping method.

## Herbal Cupping

Herbal cupping method is an effective therapy applicable to a wide range, with dual treatment effects of cupping and medicine treatment. There are two commonly used herbal cupping methods: boiled herbal cupping and stored herbal cupping (fig. 11).

Different from the abovementioned cupping methods, boiled herbal cupping method evacuates the air from the cups through the heat generated by steam, instead of through burning. Bamboo cups are mainly used for this cupping. During operation, first boil herbs suitable for the conditions in water for a while, and then put the bamboo cup into the liquid medicine to boil for 2 to 3 minutes (not longer than 5 minutes). Take the bamboo cup out with a pair of chopsticks or a pair of pincers, hold the bamboo cup upside down to allow the liquid drain away, before immediately applying a folded disinfected wet towel over the cup mouth to absorb the liquid medicine and reduce the temperature at the mouth. Then quickly apply the cup to the appropriate area when the cup

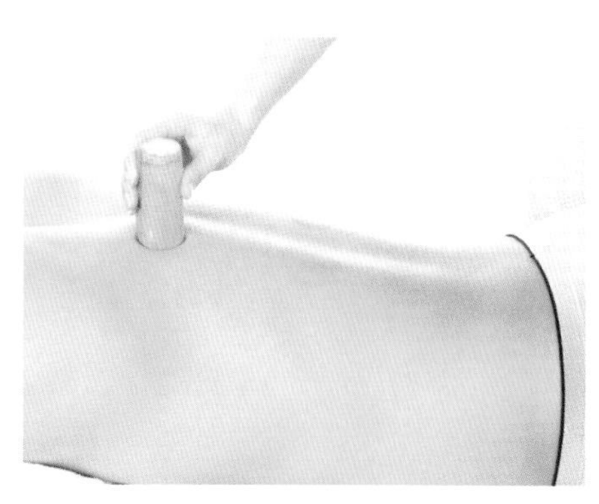
Fig. 11 The herbal cupping method.

is full of steam. After that, press the bamboo cup for about half a minute to make it suck tightly. It should be operated in a fast and accurate manner as the suction force is small.

Stored herbal cupping method is cupping with suction cups which are initially stored with an appropriate amount of liquid medicine. The cups can be sucked on the skin with flash-fire method after the glass cups are stored with appropriate liquid medicine. This method is often used for rheumatism, asthma, cough, cold, chronic gastritis, indigestion, and psoriasis.

You may choose different herbs and cups for your own needs, and also use this method combined with needle cupping, moving cupping and massage cupping methods. Despite of wide range of indications, herbal cupping method can be used only by those who have received special training as this method has high requirements for operation techniques and is prone to be burned. In general, we do not recommend the application of this method at home.

### Vacuum Cupping

Vacuum cupping method uses the suction cups and applies them over the area that needs to be worked on with suction force after negative pressure is generated by following the mechanical principles. To operate, first choose an appropriate size suction cup depending on the cupping position, and then pull upward the pressure valve at the top of the suction cup to ensure ventilation, and then slightly cover the pressure valve with pistol grip hand pump. Placing the suction cup on the chosen area, press the suction cup body with one hand, and vertically and rapidly pull the pistol grip several times, until the skin in the cup is uplifted, to the extent of feeling comfortable, but not too tight.

Vacuum cupping method is suitable for application at home. It is also portable and easy to operate by oneself. When you are cupping by yourself, you may use a connector-hose to connect the suction cup and the pistol grip hand pump to extend the operation range.

## 4. Cupping Techniques

There are different cupping methods. When cupping on the back, we may use the moving cupping method, repeatedly pushing the cups after they have been sucked to the skin. In the case of cupping on the face, immediately remove the cup after the cup is sucked, and repeat the operation several times. Each cupping method has its own characteristics and indicated diseases and areas. Depending on the conditions being treated, choose different cupping therapy methods to change the stimulation intensity and scope to the body by the cups, thereby achieving the purpose of improving health and warding off diseases. Common cupping techniques include retained cupping, moving cupping, flash cupping, etc.

### Retained Cupping

Retained cupping is the most commonly used method in which the cup is retained on the area being treated for a period of time after it is sucked, until redness, congestion or blood stasis appear on the skin. Depending on the different number of cupping tools, it is divided into the single cup method (i.e. simply use one cup) and the multi-cup method (i.e. use multiple cups). A single cup may be applied when the extent of lesion is smaller or there is one tender point; and multiple cups may be used when the extent of lesion is large and the conditions are complicated. In general, the cups are retained for 5 to 15 minutes, but they may be retained for a shorter time if the suction force is strong, or longer if the suction force is weak. Retaining time may be shortened appropriately in case of cupping for the old and weak people (fig. 12).

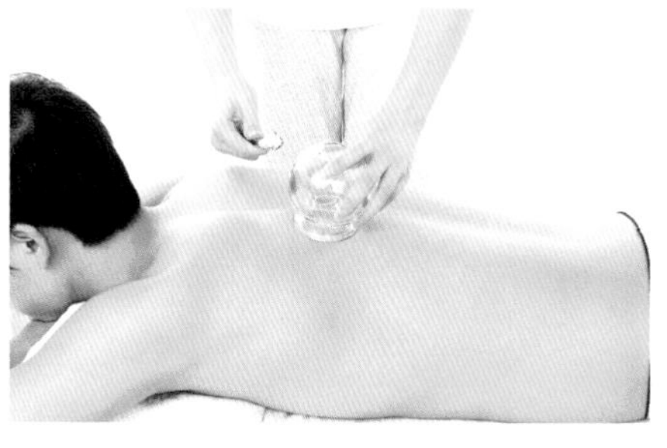

Fig. 12 The retained cupping (applied to the Geshu point).

Retained cupping can be applied to various diseases, and is often applied to cold symptoms, visceral diseases, chronic illness, as well as limited, fixed, and deep disease locations. It is also effective to other symptoms like pathogens of meridians (exogenous pathogenic factors), qi stagnation and blood stasis, exterior syndrome, skin paralysis, numbness, indigestion, neurasthenia, and hypertension.

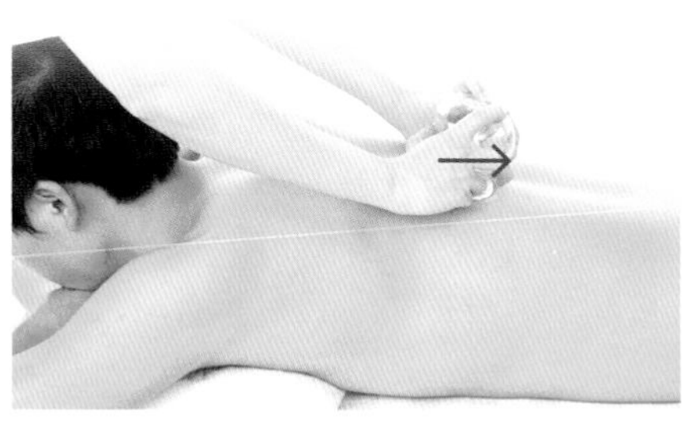

Fig. 13 After the cup is sucked, hold the cup bottom with one hand, and slowly move the up back and forth, up and down, or from left to right on the treated area with some force.

## Moving Cupping

Also known as the pushing cupping, it refers to a cupping method by which the cup is pushed repeatedly after it is sucked so as to expand the cupping area. The moving cupping is more commonly used in clinical practice as it also has the effect of massaging. Before cupping, first apply some lubricants to the cup mouth and moving areas, for example, liquid paraffin, and Vaseline, or use safflower oil, essential oil, and anti-inflammatory analgesic cream depending on the patient's condition, so as to facilitate sliding and enhance efficacy. After the cup is sucked, hold the cup bottom with one hand, and slowly move the cup back and forth, up and down or from left to right on the treated area with some force. During pushing and pulling, slightly lift half of the cup moving forward to let the other half exert force. Note that the cup should be moved immediately after it is sucked to the skin. Do not test whether it is sucked, otherwise it will be difficult to move or cause pain when pushing (fig. 13).

In general, for the waist and back, push and pull the cup back and forth along the direction of long axis of the body; for the chest rib area, push and pull along the direction of ribs; for the shoulder and abdomen, move the cup rotationally on the treated area; and for limbs, push and pull back and forth along the long axis. Push, pull, and rotation should be performed slowly, and the movement distance should not be too long each time. Stop the movement immediately when skin becomes red or crimson, appears scarlet points, or when the patient feels painful.

This method is applicable to the soreness, numbness, rheumatism, and other symptoms on large and thickly muscled areas, such as shoulders, back, waist, hips, and legs. The moving cupping is mainly applied to the Governing Vessel (GV), back-shu points (which mean the points on the bladder meridian. They are totally 12 points, i.e., Feishu, Jueyinshu, Xinshu, Ganshu, Danshu, Pishu, Weishu, Sanjiaoshu, Shenshu, Dachangshu, Xiaochangshu, and Pangguangshu points) and urinary bladder channel to stimulate the warm effect of positive qi and expel pathogenic cold. The cups employed should be very smooth at the mouth of the cup to prevent skin bruise.

## Flash Cupping

The flash cupping is a cupping method by which the cup is removed immediately after it is sucked to the treated area, and suction and removal are repeated. By using the flash cupping method, the cups should be applied in conjunction with the flash-fire method. To operate, clamp the cotton ball dipped with appropriate amount of alcohol with a pair of pincers or hemostatic forceps, ignite it and immediately place it into the cup bottom. Draw it out promptly to suck the cup onto the appropriate area, and then remove the cup immediately. Repeat this practice several times, until the skin becomes red (fig. 14).

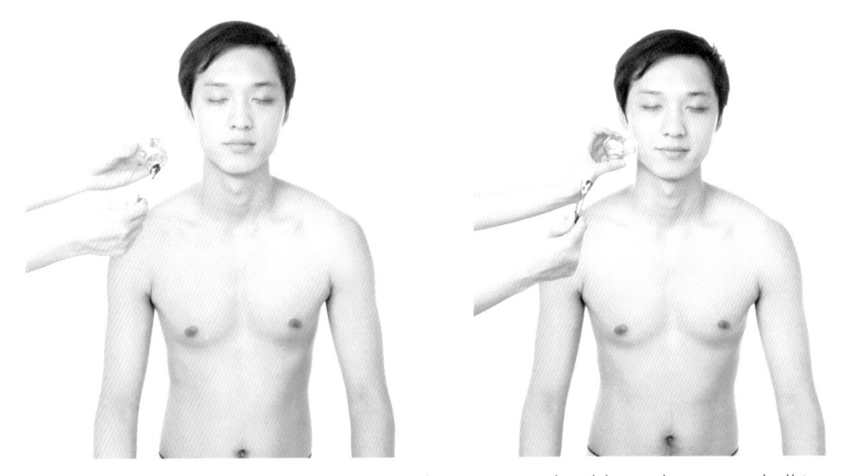

Fig. 14 During the operation of flash cupping, the operator should put the cotton ball into the cup bottom again after taking the cup off the designated part and repeat the cupping procedure.

The operator should pay attention to the cup temperature at any time, and may replace a cup to continue the operation if he/she feels the cup is too hot. Repeated cupping and removal will stimulate the nerves to some extent, and can increase the permeability of cells, thus improving local blood circulation and nutrient supply. It is mainly applicable to the diseases caused by pathogenic wind, such as skin numbness or pain, skin itching, muscle atrophy, dysfunction of internal organs, various allergic dermatitis, etc. This method is also applicable to the stroke sequelae.

The flash cupping is suitable for the face as it leaves no ecchymosis. Uneven skin and positions where cups are prone to fall are often cupped with this method.

## Cupping with Retaining of Needle

This method, also known as retained needle cupping or needle cupping, is a combination of cupping and acupuncture. First, disinfect local skin with an alcohol cotton ball. After determining the qi (the patient's acupuncture points where there are soreness, numbness, heaviness, swelling, pain, or electric shock-like reaction, or the sense of tightness when a needle is applied) following application of acupuncture needle to an appropriate acupoint, leave the needle in the original position. The needle length should be above the skin, but less than the cup height to avoid injury caused by needle hitting into the skin by the cup. Then centering on the needle, apply the cup over the needle, and the cup should be preferably transparent to facilitate observation of the conditions in the cup at any time. After 5 to 10 minutes when redness, congestion, or blood stasis is present on the skin, take off the cup gently before removing the needle. The needle tip should be applied in the vertical direction, at an even speed and with even force to reduce the patient's pain (fig. 15).

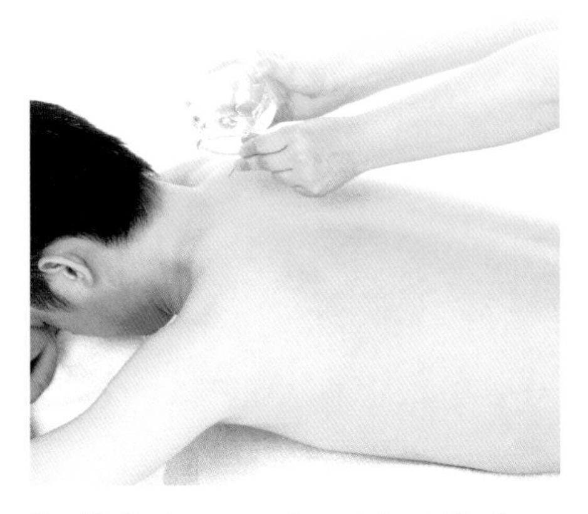

Fig. 15 During operation, qi should be first felt in the corresponding acupoint through acupuncture. The needle tip should be applied in the vertical direction; Puncture the point vertically at an even speed and with even force to reduce the pain of the patient.

This method combines the effects of needle and cupping, strengthening the acupuncture effect. In general, deep acupuncture is not suitable for the chest, back, kidney area, and limb acupoints with large blood vessels and distribution of nerves. Acupuncture for slim and weak people should not be too deep. Otherwise, the acupuncture will probably deepen adversely due to the suction force after removing the cup, which tends to cause injury.

This cupping method can only be operated by professional acupuncturists as it has high requirements for operation techniques.

## Pricking-Bloodletting Cupping

Pricking cupping is a method of pricking small blood vessels revealed on the acupoints or lesion surface with a three-edged needle or syringe needle to bleed or discharge pus, followed by immediate operation of cupping on the same area, or gently pricking the treated areas with a plum-blossom needle until the skin becomes red or bleeds followed by immediate operation of cupping.

Before cupping, first disinfect the cups and areas to be treated to avoid infection. During this practice, the cups should be removed promptly after the amount of bleeding required for treatment is reached. Regardless of the size of acupuncture area or the number of cups, the total amount of bleeding should not exceed 10 ml each time, and this amount may be increased appropriately while treating erysipelas. To facilitate observation, transparent cups are preferred. If the amount of bleeding is excessive, remove the cups immediately and press to stop bleeding. During cupping on blood stasis or abscess, if bleeding becomes slow, and the skin has wrinkled depression, it means that the blood stasis or abscess has been discharged, and the cups should be removed immediately (fig. 16 on page 24).

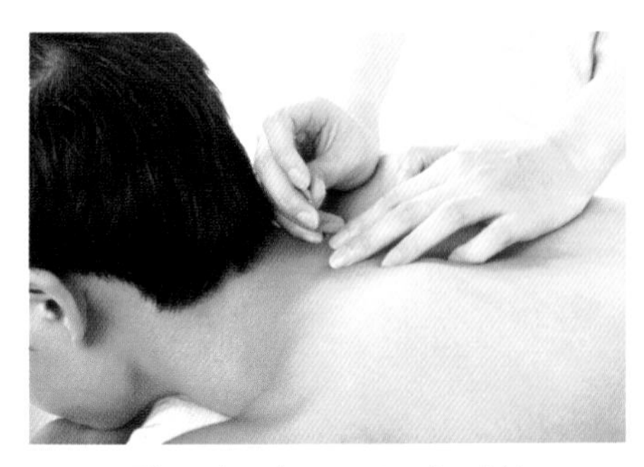

Fig. 16 The related acupoint should be pricked by a three-edged needle or a syringe needle to bring about blood or discharge pus, and then immediately operate cupping on the same area.

Pricking-bloodletting cupping is often used for those with acute and heat syndromes, excitement, and excess syrdromes characterized by being red, hot, painful, itching, or pain moving around the body (for example, fever, hypertension of liver-yang hyperactivity, skin itch, erysipelas, sore, carbuncle, acute soft tissue injury and so on).

During the pricking-bloodletting cupping, first disinfect the area to be treated with 75% alcohol. After treatment, the cups should be cleaned immediately, and disinfected and sterilized before re-use to prevent cross infection. Pricking-bloodletting cupping is contraindicated for those with serious tendency of bleeding and coagulation disorders. This cupping method should be performed by professionals, and should not be operated by patients themselves.

## 5. Methods of Removing Cups

Removing cups is the last step of the process of cupping. Depending on the employed cups and cupping methods, it is generally divided into manual, automatic, and special methods.

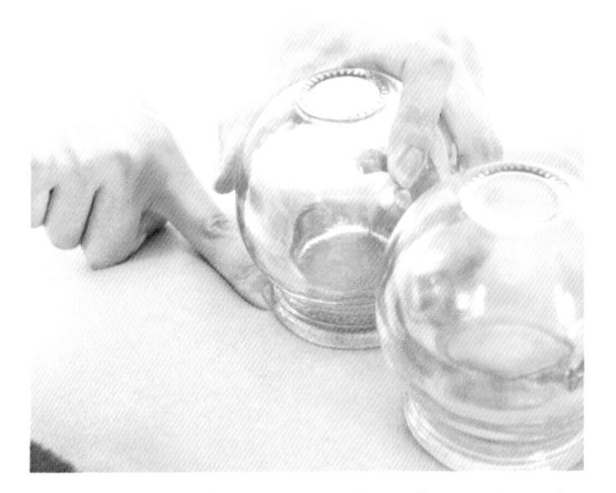

Fig. 17 Press the cup gently with one hand to make it tilt towards one side, and press the skin at the opposite side of the cup mouth with the forefinger of the other hand.

### Manual Removing

It should be performed gently and slowly. When removing the cups manually, press the cup gently with one hand to make it tilt towards one side, and press the skin at the opposite side of the cup mouth with the forefinger of the other hand to form a gap between the cup mouth and the skin. The cup will fall automatically when the suction force disappears gradually with the inflow of the air. Do not pull or rotate the cups by force when removing the cups manually to avoid injury of the skin (fig. 17).

### Automatic Removing

It is the safest and is applicable to cupping tools with automatic removing device like suction cup. When removing the cups, pull the valve core to enable the air to flow into the cup through the nozzle so that the cup will fall off.

### Special Removing

This should be performed skillfully. When stored herbal cupping is applied, particularly to horizontal treated areas (for example, cupping on the back of a patient using prone position), the cupping areas should be adjusted to a lateral position before removing the cups to prevent leakage of liquid medicine. When pricking-bloodletting cupping is used, if the amount of bleeding is large, the cups should be removed following the method of stored herbal cupping. After removing the cups, pay attention to disinfection of local skin to prevent infection.

**Post-Cupping Treatment**

Be aware of invasion of exogenous pathogenic factors.

- After removing the cups, wipe out the small drops and lubricants on the cupping marks with antiseptic gauze or a dry cotton ball. In case of local bleeding or treatment of sore and carbuncle, after removing the cups, disinfect the wound with medicinal alcohol or iodine, then cover it with sterile dressings to prevent infection. If a blister is present, prick it with a sterile needle and apply gentian violet after wiping it dry. If local skin is tight and uncomfortable, knead it gently to relax it. Purple spots on local skin appearing after removing the cups are normal reactions, so no special treatment is needed.
- With the cups removed, the patient should rest and keep warm. The patient who feels itching at the cupping area should not scratch it to avoid infection. Patients who have experienced pricking-bloodletting cupping must not take a bath within 24 hours. To prevent invasion of exogenous pathogenic factors, do not expose to fan or air-conditioner after cupping in summer.

## 6. Observation of Cupping Marks

Cupping marks will generate when local tissue is uplifted over the plane of the cup mouth due to the negative pressure in the cup, and the skin color and shape will change after the cups are retained for some time or after the flash cupping, moving cupping or other cupping methods. Patients will experience stretching, tightening, swelling, warmth, coolness, soreness, comfort, and other reactions at the cupping areas, and some patients will feel pain is alleviated gradually during cupping. For patients without obvious discomfort, cupping marks will disappear naturally in 3 to 5 days, without the need of any treatment.

After the cups are removed, the color and form of cupping marks will vary depending on the constitution and physical condition of the individual patient. In general, cupping marks include redness, red points, purple spots, and even crimson, purple black and blue spots, with patients feeling slight pain while being touched. Purple black cupping marks represent the existence of blood stasis; bright red cupping marks indicate deficiency of both qi and yin or wind-heat type of allergic constitution; steam in the cup indicates moisture at the cupping area.

Now let's learn about our own constitution and physical conditions based on the following cupping marks.

Purple black and dark marks: They indicate blood stasis in the body (for example, abnormal menstruation, dysmenorrhea, or cardiac insufficiency). Purple black and dark marks will appear if the area has been heavily affected by cold. If the marks do not disappear in several days, it represents the length of the diseases, and a longer time will be needed for cupping. If a large area of black purple marks appears following the moving cupping, it suggests a large area of wind-cold. Appropriate treatment should be employed to expel the cold and pathogens (fig. 18 on page 26).

Purple marks accompanied with plaques: They represent coagulated cold syndrome and blood stasis syndrome.

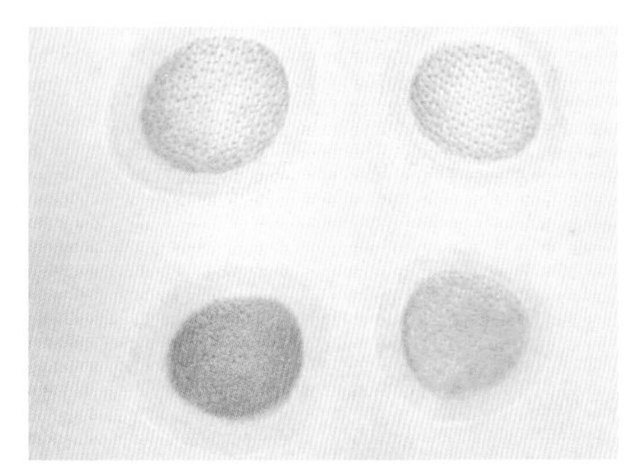

Fig. 18 The cupping marks appear dark red or purple black.

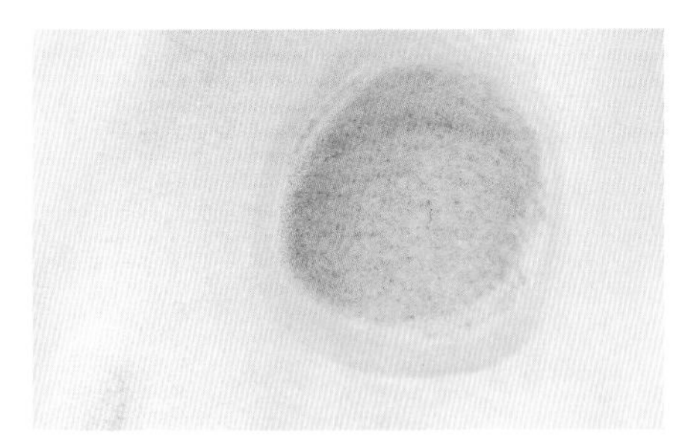

Fig. 19 The cupping marks appear scattered purple points.

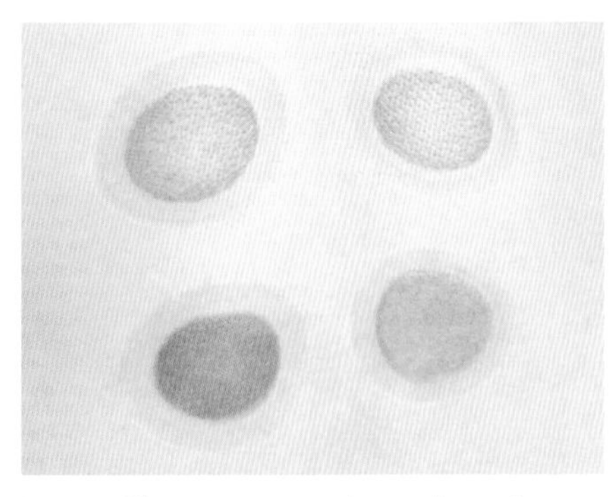

Fig. 20 The cupping marks on the waist appear crimson.

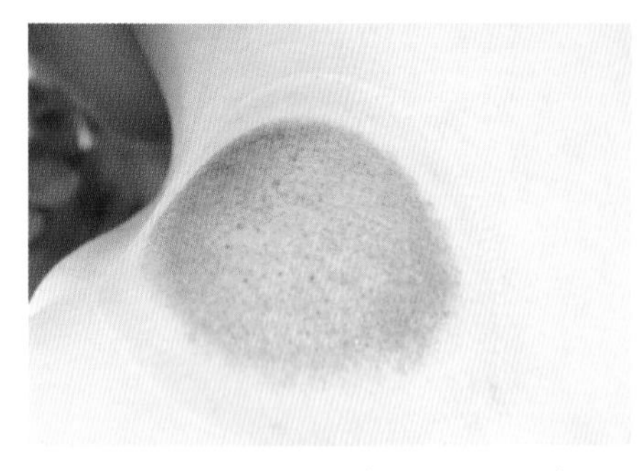

Fig. 21 The cupping marks appear scarlet points.

Cupping marks present in scattered purple points of different shades: They represent qi stagnation and blood stasis (fig. 19).

Light purple and blue marks accompanied with plaques: They represent deficiency syndrome accompanied with blood stasis. Marks at the Shenshu point represent kidney deficiency, while those at Pishu point represent qi deficiency and blood stasis. Pressing pain is often felt at the cupping areas.

Bright red marks: They suggest yin deficiency or deficiency of both qi and yin. Those suffering from wind-heat syndrome with fire excess from yin deficiency or allergic constitution can also have this mark.

Cupping marks present in scattered bright red points: They often appear after moving cupping is applied to a large area, and do not grow out of the skin. Concentration on or surrounding an acupoint represents existence of pathogens at the internal organ where the acupoint locates.

Grey marks, without feeling of warmth after touch: They represent syndromes of deficiency-cold and pathogenic damp.

Texture on cupping mark surface and slightly itchy: They indicate pathogenic wind and dampness syndrome.

Blisters on cupping marks: They represent heavy dampness in the body. Blood in the blisters reflects pathogenic heat and damp toxin.

Blisters and edema in cupping area: They indicate excessive moisture in the body, representing the syndrome of qi disease.

Appearance of crimson, purple black, or scarlet points, or slight pain if kneaded, accompanied with fever: They represent existence of heat-toxin syndrome; this circumstance without fever represents suffering from stasis syndrome (figs. 20–21).

No cupping marks after cupping, or marks disappear immediately after removing the cups: Recovery to normal color represents light pathogens. There will be no cupping marks if the acupoint is inaccurate. It is best to apply cupping several times to confirm the existence of syndrome.

No change in skin color and no feeling of warmth after touch: They suggest deficiency syndrome.

## 7. Cupping Time and Treatment Course Arrangement

Cupping time and treatment course are closely related to the efficacy of cupping. Only by grasping correct cupping and retaining time can one achieve the purpose of effectively alleviating disease or health preservation and improvement of looks to become healthier. Cupping time should be determined by taking comprehensive consideration of many factors like a patient's age, state of the illness, physique, physical condition, and cupping areas.

### Control Retaining Time

The duration of the flash cupping and moving cupping is decided by the presence of redness or scarlet points on local skin or skin under the cup, while retaining time is subject to the reaction of presence of redness or blood stasis on local skin, generally it lasts for 5 to 15 minutes, depending on different methods; in case of pricking-bloodletting cupping, cups should be removed as soon as the amount of blood required for treatment is reached or the blood stasis or pus has been completely discharged.

The time for the use of large cups should be slightly shorter, while the time for the use of small cups should be slightly longer; time may be longer for those young and strong, while shorter for those old and weak. Retaining time should be short for those with new or mild illnesses, while longer for those with old or serious diseases; retaining time should be short when cupping on the head, face, neck, shoulders, and upper limbs, while longer when cupping on the back, hips, abdomen, and lower limbs. The retaining time should be determined flexibly based on different cupping methods, combined with the tolerance degree of the patient.

### Interval between Cupping Courses

Once a day for acute illnesses (cold, fever, etc.); twice to three times a day for serious illnesses and severe pain (cupping parts should be changed); once a day for chronic diseases. However, cupping should not be applied again at the same area until ecchymosis and localized skin eruptions induced by cupping disappear, in general, once every 2 to 5 days. Apply to alternative acupoints if cupping is needed every day.

In general, 7 to 10 days is a course of treatment. Other therapies should be used if no obvious effects are achieved after 2 to 3 times of treatment of an acute disease, or after 2 to 3 courses of treatment of a chronic disease.

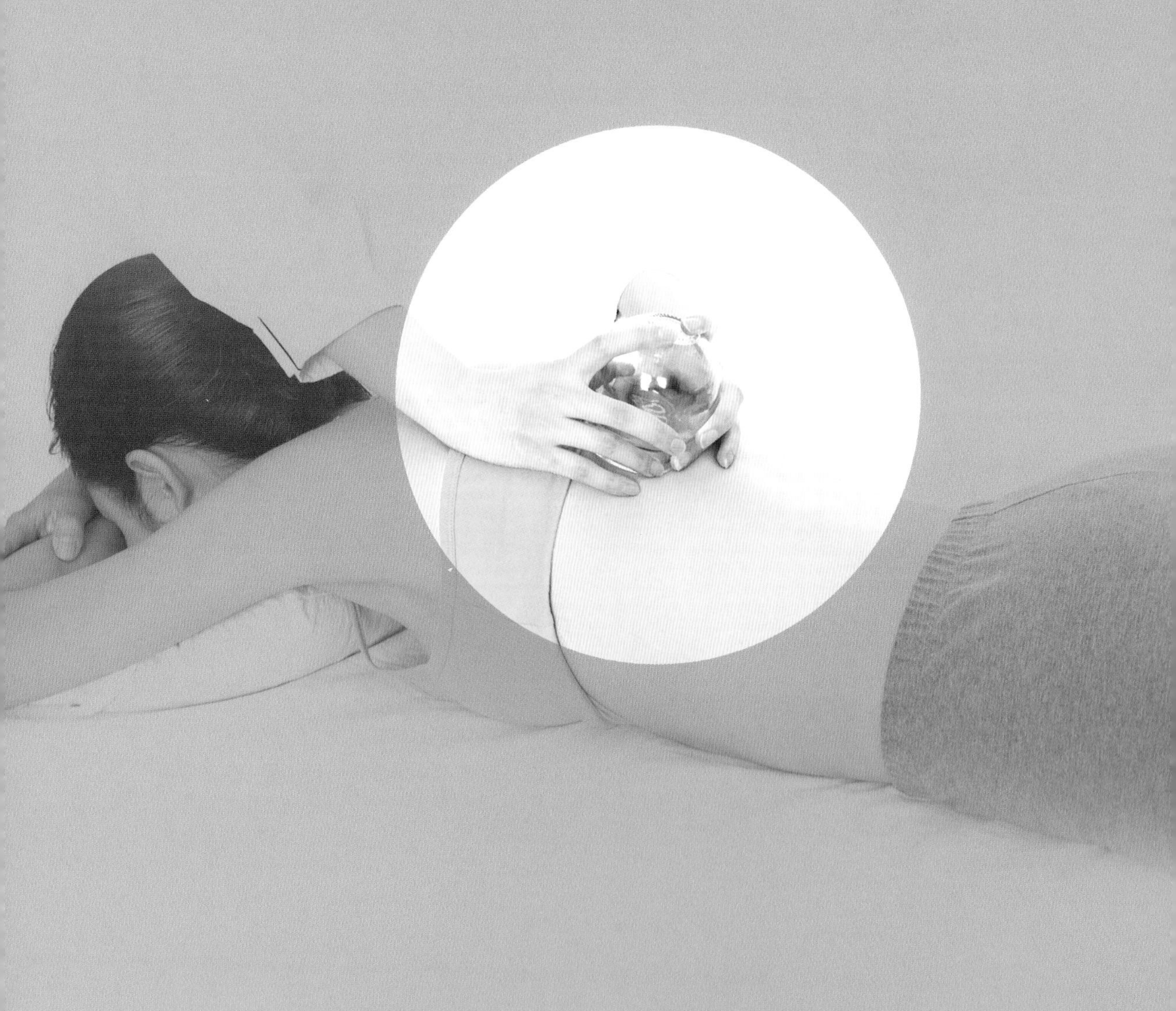

# Chapter Three
# Meridians, Collaterals, and Acupoints

As the basis of the Traditional Chinese Medicine therapy such as massage and acupuncture, meridians and points play an important role in the pathological process. In the theoretical system of Traditional Chinese Medicine, meridians and collaterals are regarded as a system that makes connections throughout the body, working their way from external points to the five internal organs (as defined by TCM) and viscera. The meridians and collaterals that run throughout the whole body serve to transport qi and blood, nourish muscles and bones. Therefore, cupping therapy, as one of the Traditional Chinese Medicine therapies, may have therapeutic effects through the meridians all over the body. Points are special parts of body surface where the qi and blood of human internal organs and meridians are infused and gathered, and reflect the changes in the internal organs through the close connection between meridians and various internal organs. The effective stimulation to meridians and points through cupping can mobilize the ability of the internal human body to resist diseases, so as to achieve the purpose of disease prevention and curing.

In the cupping therapy, other than the needle cupping method in which points should be identified accurately, for other cupping methods, the more accurately the points are identified, the better cupping effects will be achieved, although identification of points does not need to be very accurate because of the large cup mouth area. Accordingly, learning how to identify points and trying to identify them accurately are preconditions for exerting the effects of the cupping therapy. This chapter will introduce five methods to accurately identify points.

## 1. Relationship between Acupoints, Meridians, and Collaterals

Meridians are the system's major channels, and they run across the body vertically. Meridians may then branch out into finer channels called collaterals which can connect the meridians throughout the body.

In the human body there are twelve meridians, each with its own two-letter code for easy reference:

- Taiyin Lung Meridian of Hand (LU)
- Jueyin Pericardium Meridian of Hand (PC)
- Shaoyin Heart Meridian of Hand (HT)
- Yangming Large Intestine Meridian of Hand (LI)
- Shaoyang Sanjiao Meridian of Hand (TE)
- Taiyang Small Intestine Meridian of Hand (SI)
- Yangming Stomach Meridian of Foot (ST)
- Shaoyang Gallbladder Meridian of Foot (GB)
- Taiyang Bladder Meridian of Foot (BL)
- Taiyin Spleen Meridian of Foot (SP)

- Jueyin Liver Meridian of Foot (LR)
- Shaoyin Kidney Meridian of Foot (KI).

In addition there is the Conception Vessel (CV) running vertically in the front of the body and Governing Vessel (GV) at the back.

Naming conventions for meridians and collaterals:

- Those distributed in the upper limbs are called "hand meridians" while those in the lower limbs are called "foot meridians."
- According to TCM the back is associated with yang while the abdomen is concerned with yin, and the outside is concerned with yang while the inside is associated with yin. Therefore yang channels are mostly distributed in the back and the outside of the limbs, while yin channels are mostly distributed in the abdomen and inner side of the limbs. You will see "yin" in the name of the meridians running inside the limb (for example, Taiyin Meridian) while "yang" appears in the name of meridians running on the outside (for example, Taiyang Meridian).
- Meridians and collaterals are named after related internal organs. According to TCM the five main organs are the heart, liver, spleen, lungs and kidneys. The six viscera include the gallbladder, stomach, small intestine, large intestine, urinary bladder and Sanjiao, in addition to the pericardium. The heart meridian and pericardium meridian are both related to the heart, and the Sanjiao, as described in TCM, comprises three compartments in the trunk of the body.

Closely related to meridians and collaterals, acupoints are mostly distributed along the routes of meridians and collaterals. Apart from those single points on the central axis of the human body, all the other acupoints are bilaterally symmetrical. There are also extra acupoints on head and neck (EX-HN), on breast and abdomen (EX-CA), on back (EX-B) and on lower limbs (EX-LE).

In Traditional Chinese Medicine, acupoints are called "Shu points," meaning that they are points where acupuncture and moxibustion can be applied. Since these points are densely concentrated with nerve endings or quite thick nerve fibers, they will emit signals when one feels discomfort or pain.

To understand Shu points you must not picture isolated points on the surface of the body. Rather they are closely associated with tissues and inner organs deep within. Due to these connections, Shu points are reaction points for diseases and stimulation points for treatment.

The cupping steps illustrated in the cases in this book will give detailed descriptions of the specific locations of the points, which are mainly distributed in twelve meridians and on Ren Mai (Conception Vessel) and Du Mai (Governor Vessel) in the human body. The next part will introduce how to accurately identify these points. You can easily perform cupping on accurate points by referring to the meridian pictures after you have learned these methods.

## 2. How to Find Acupoints Accurately

As the combination of cupping and points can strengthen the effects of disease curing and health care, accurate identification of these points is essential to the effects of cupping. This book shows the general location of the acupoints, but it is important for you to practice finding them on your own.

Since ancient times in China, the position and measurement of acupoints have been described by the unit of the "body cun" (abbreviated as "cun" in this book).

Acupoints are of different sizes and depths. This chapter gives an introduction to several simple and quick ways for accurately finding them.

## Using Finger-Length Measurement

The finger length measurement of the body cun, a simple and convenient way to measure distance in locating acupoints, is based on the thumb width of the patient. With this highly individualized type of measurement, therefore, one cannot find the acupoints of another person according to one's own body cun, since this is not accurate.

**Two Different Concepts: Cun and Body Cun**

- "Cun" is a traditional standard unit of length in China. One cun is about 3.33 centimeters.
- "Body cun" is a measurement specific to the individual, used as the unit of length for measuring acupoints.

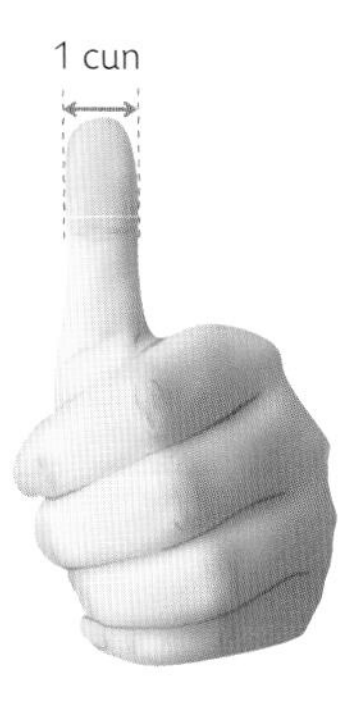


One cun: The width of the thumb joint of the patient.

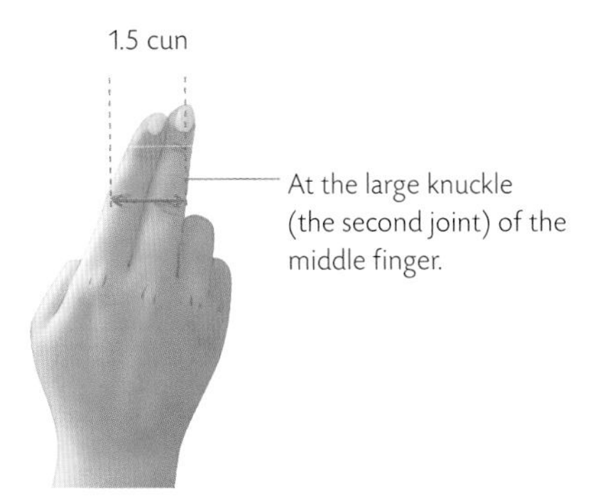


One and a half cun: Measuring at the level of the large knuckle (the second joint) of the middle finger, the width of the index and middle finger closed together is 1.5 cun.

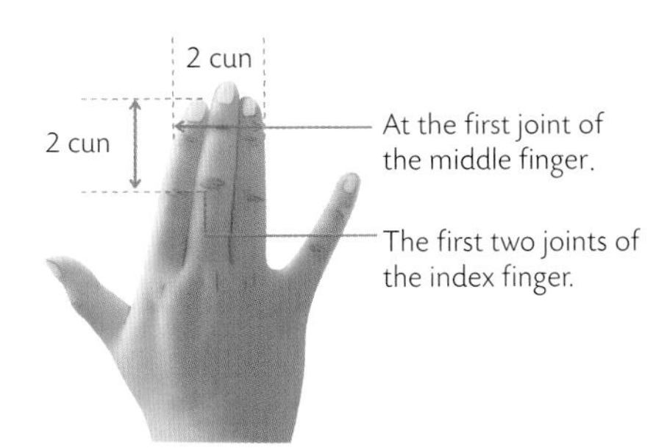


Two cun: With the index finger, middle and ring finger closed together, take the measurement at the level of the first joint of the middle finger. The length of the first two joints of the index finger is also two cun.

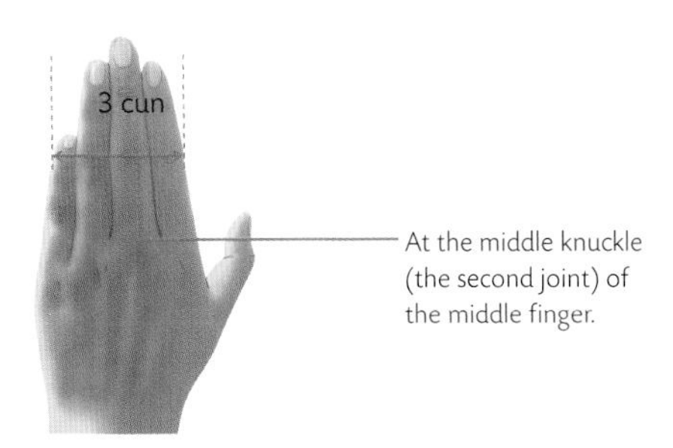


Three cun: With the four fingers closed, measure at the level of the large knuckle (the second joint) of the middle finger.

### Using Bone-Length Measurement

To ascertain the location of acupoints we can also use the measurement between bone joints. (More about the names of bones can be found in the next section.) Measurement can be made according to corresponding bone-length for people of different sexes, ages, height and weight. For any individual, the vertical cun and horizontal cun are the same length; the difference in name relates solely to direction (fig. 22).

- Horizontal cun: Mostly applied to measuring the front and rear of the body, one measures acupoints on each side in relation to their distance from the front central line.
- Vertical cun: Mostly applied to measuring acupoints upward and downward, with joints used as the basis for measurement.

### Using Physical Marks of the Body

Physical marks on human body, such as eyebrows, nipples and ankles can also serve as locators of acupoints.

- The eyes, nose, mouth, ears, eyebrows and hairline serve as marks on the head. For instance the Yintang point lies between the eyebrows.
- On the abdomen, the nipples, xiphoid process and navel serve as marks. For instance the Zhongwan point lies between the xiphoid process and navel, while the Danzhong point lies between the nipples.
- Joints and ankles serve as marks on four limbs. For instance, Yanglingquan point lies in the anterior inferior part of the fibular head.

| Location | Starting and Ending Points | Cun | Measurement |
|---|---|---|---|
| Head and face | A: From middle of frontal hairline to middle of rear hairline. | 12 cun | vertical cun |
| | B: From Yintang point to middle of frontal hairline. | 3 cun | vertical cun |
| | C: From Dazhui point to middle of rear hairline. | 3 cun | vertical cun |
| | D: From Yintang point to Dazhui point. | 18 cun | vertical cun |
| | E: Between two Touwei points on forehead. | 9 cun | horizontal cun |
| | F: Between two mastoids (Wangu points) behind ears. | 9 cun | horizontal cun |
| Chest and abdomen | G: From Tiantu point to bottom of sternum. | 9 cun | vertical cun |
| | H: From bottom of sternum to Qizhong point. | 8 cun | vertical cun |
| | I: From Qizhong point to Qugu point. | 5 cun | vertical cun |
| | J: Between two nipples. | 8 cun | horizontal cun |
| | K: From top of armpit to Zhangmen point. | 12 cun | vertical cun |
| Back | L: From margo medialis of scapula to posterior midline. | 3 cun | horizontal cun |
| Arms | M: From frontal crease and rear crease of armpit to cubital crease (inside of elbow). | 9 cun | vertical cun |
| | N: From inside of elbow to side bend of wrist. | 12 cun | vertical cun |
| Legs | O: From upper margin of pubic bone to upper margin of epicondyle of femur. | 18 cun | vertical cun |
| | P: From lower margin of condylus medialis tibiae to inner ankle tip. | 13 cun | vertical cun |
| | Q: From greater trochanter of femur to bend at back of knee. | 19 cun | vertical cun |
| | R: From bend at back of knee to outer ankle tip. | 16 cun | vertical cun |

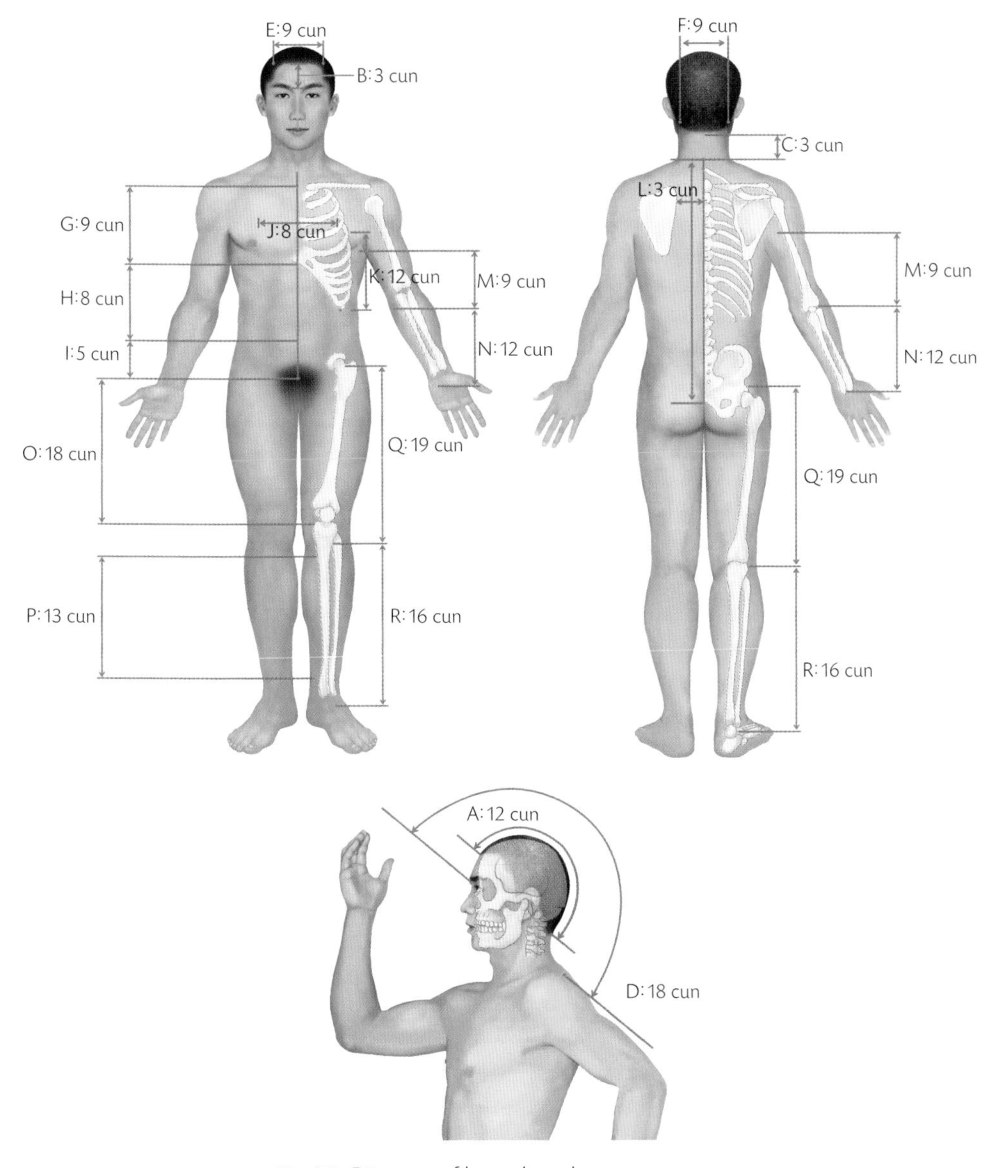


Fig. 22 Diagram of bone-length measurement.

## Using Pressing

Most of the acupoints are in a cavity, which is the key to the positioning. The patient will feel a sense of tingling, numbness, swelling and pain when the correct location of the acupoint is pressed.

## Using Special Postures

You can also make use of some special postures to find acupoints. For instance the Quchi point lies at the end of a bent elbow. The Jiexi point can be found on the back of the foot when it is bent, between the two tendons bordering the heel and the lower leg. The Ququan point lies at the end of the bend of the knee.

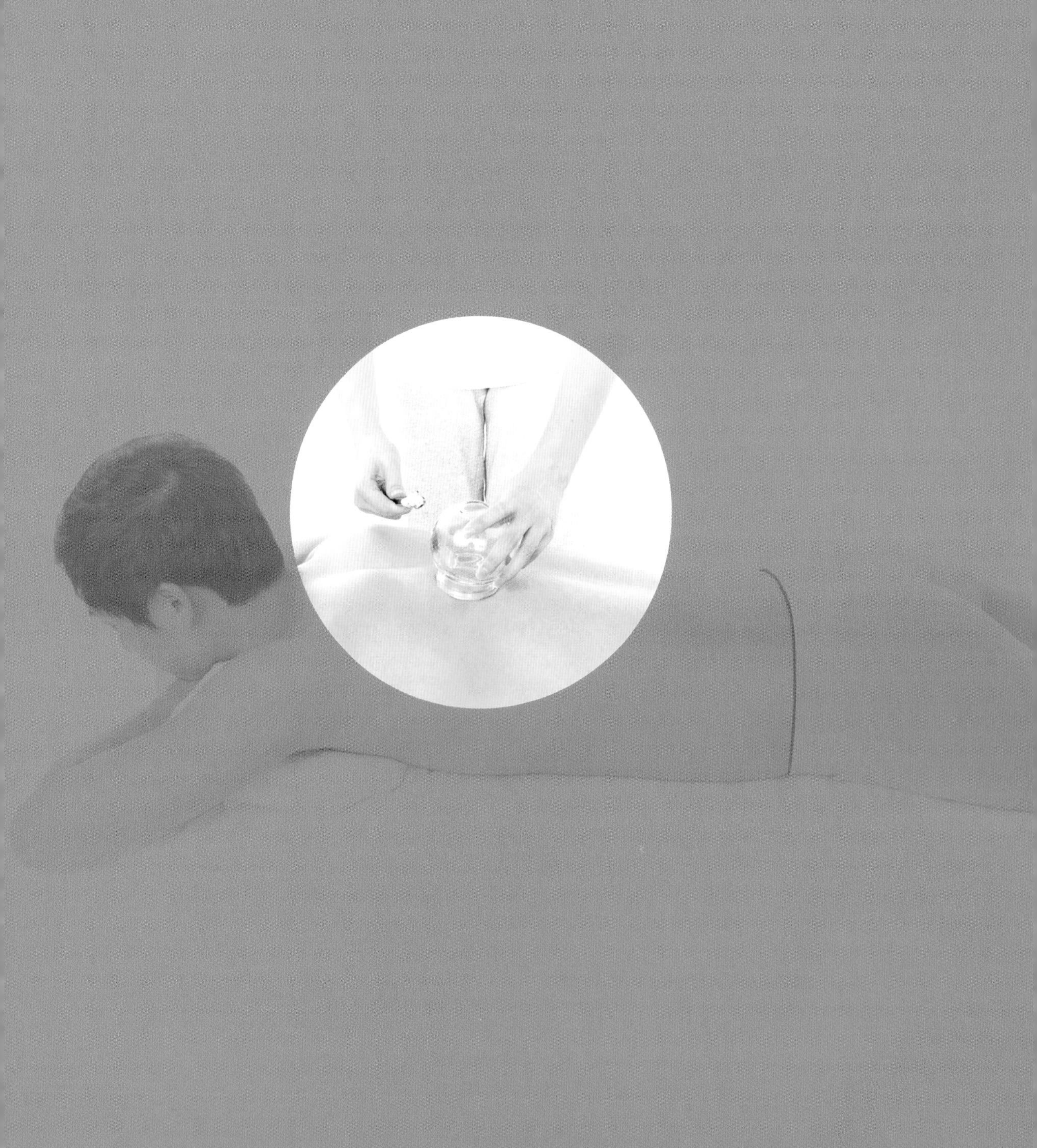

# Chapter Four
## Sub-Health

Do you always feel depressed and sleepy in the day, but often cannot fall asleep at night? It means that you are suffering from sub-health problems. Many people nowadays are troubled by these problems. Insomnia, physical weakness, neurasthenia, and other sub-health symptoms seriously affect people's life and work. In fact, these sub-health conditions can be eliminated simply by cupping on appropriate acupoints.

## 1 Insomnia

Insomnia patients often have difficulty in falling asleep, sleep lightly, or cannot fall asleep after waking up. In a serious case, they cannot fall asleep all night, often accompanied with such syndromes as the lack of energy, headache, dizziness, palpitations, and amnesia.

Good diet and rest habits should be developed in daily life. In terms of diet, one is advised to often eat porridge made with coix seeds, red dates, corns, black sesame seeds, and other food materials to tonify qi and blood. Second, one should develop a good sleep habit by drinking some milk, millet porridge, etc., before going to bed; avoid drinking coffee or strong tea, or smoking, as these habits have certain negative impacts on sleep. Besides, before going to sleep, one may soak his feet in mildly hot water, until small amount of sweat oozes on the forehead, or rub one's feet on a pumice stone, which can promote blood circulation, thereby improving sleep quality.

This type of patients may be cupped mainly on Shenmen point. The patients who also suffer from poor appetite, loose stool, or sticky stool, may also be cupped on Pishu point or Weishu point. The patients who suffer from insomnia due to frequent urination may also be cupped on Shenshu point.

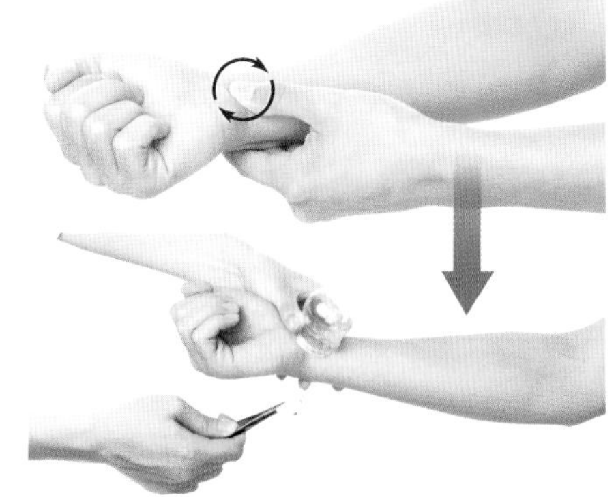

### Cupping Methods

**1. Shenmen Point**

**Location:** On the inner wrist near the small finger when the palm is turned upward.

**Method:** First knead Shenmen point with the thumb pulp for 2–3 minutes, and then select and apply a small cup to the point, retaining for 5–10 minutes.

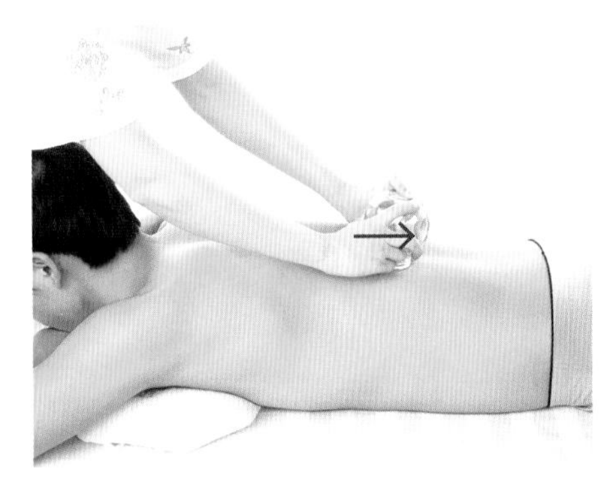

### 2. Pishu Point

**Location:** At the point 1.5 cun away horizontally from the eleventh thoracic vertebra.

**Method:** Use the moving cupping method. Move the cup on the bladder meridian on the back by segment along the meridian, and move it several times mainly on the Pishu point. Repeatedly push and pull on the point back and forth, until the skin becomes red. The cup may be retained on the above mentioned point for 5 minutes after the moving cupping.

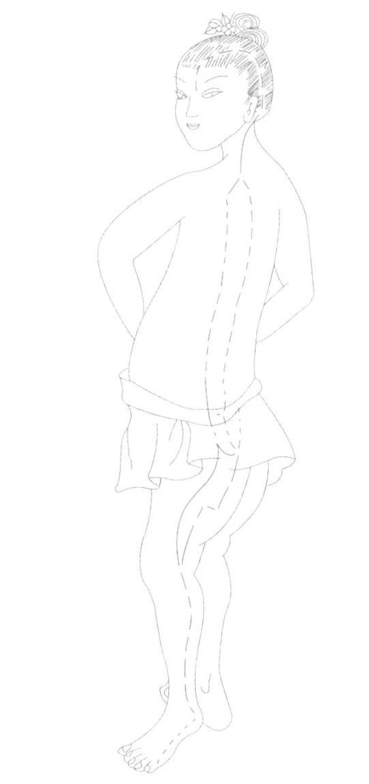

Fig. 23 Taiyang Bladder Meridian of Foot (BL).

### 3. Weishu Point

**Location:** About 1.5 cun below the spinous process of the twelfth thoracic vertebra.

**Method:** Use the moving cupping method. Move the cup on the bladder meridian on the back by segment along the meridian, and move it several times mainly on the Weishu point. Repeatedly push and pull on the point back and forth, until the skin becomes red. The cup may be retained on the abovementioned point for 5 minutes after the moving cupping.

### 4. Shenshu Point

**Location:** 1.5 cun horizontally from the second lumbar spinal process.

**Method:** Use the moving cupping method. Move the cup on the bladder meridian (fig. 23) on the back by segment along the meridian, and move it several times mainly on the Shenshu point. Repeatedly push and pull on the point back and forth, until the skin becomes red. The cup may be retained on the above mentioned point for 5 minutes after the moving cupping.

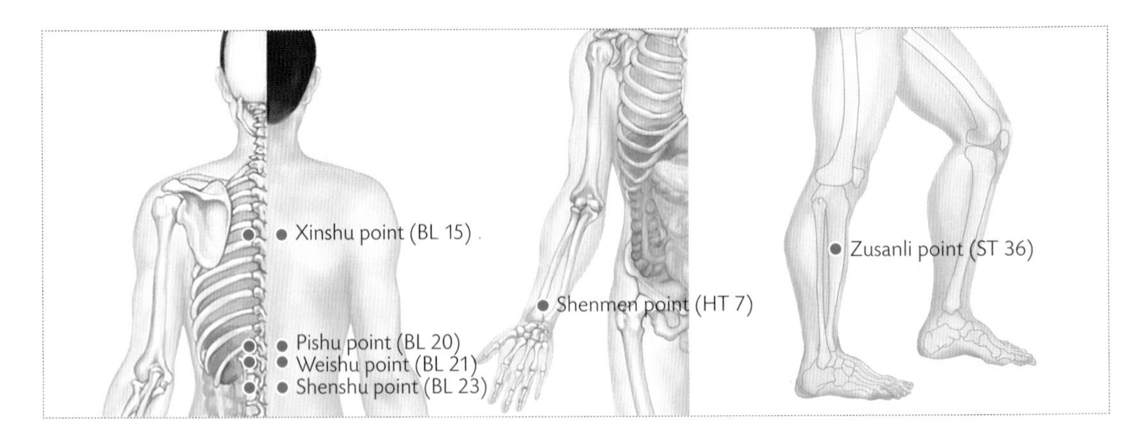

# 2 Amnesia

Amnesia means poor memory and being apt to forget things. It often occurs among people who are over forty years old. With the increase of age, more and more people suffer from this disease.

In daily life, one may read more books and newspapers, play chess and cards, and participate in other brain-consuming activities to enhance memory and improve thinking ability. From the perspective of the diet, amnesiacs may often eat walnuts, carrots, kelp, fish and other food that are conducive to improving memory. In addition, chewing frequently is not only good for teeth and better enjoying the food, but also enhances learning and memorizing abilities.

Amnesia patients should be cupped mainly on Shenmen, Zusanli, Xinshu, Pishu, and Shenshu points.

## Cupping Methods

### 1. Shenmen Point

**Location:** On the inner wrist near the small finger when the palm is turned upward.

**Method:** First knead Shenmen point with the thumb pulp for 2–3 minutes, and then select a cup of appropriate size and apply it to the point, retaining for 10–15 minutes. With the cup removed, perform moxibustion with a moxa stick for 3–5 minutes until warmth is felt.

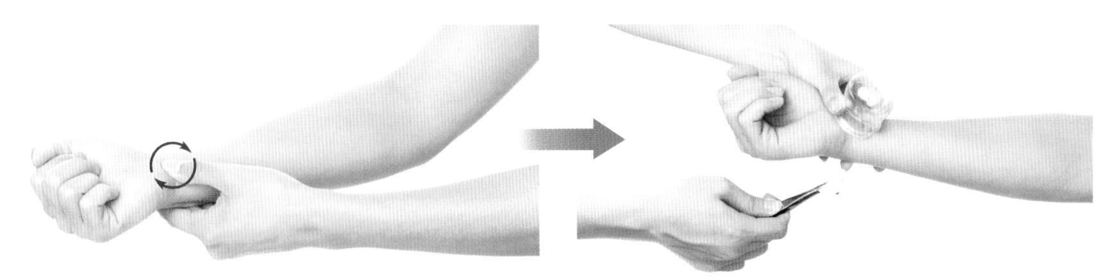

### 2. Zusanli Point

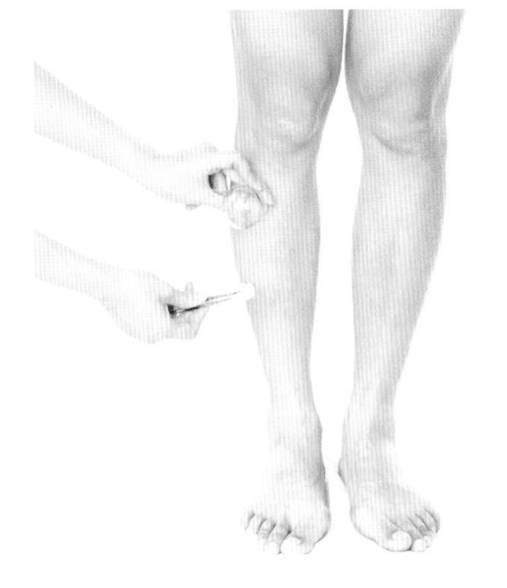

**Location:** About 3 cun below the knee on the outer side of the tibia.

**Method:** First knead Zusanli point with the thumb pulp for 2–3 minutes, and then select a cup of appropriate size and apply it to the point, retaining for 10–15 minutes. With the cup removed, perform moxibustion with a moxa stick for 3–5 minutes until warmth is felt.

### 3. Xinshu Point

**Location:** Under the fifth thoracic vertebra on the inner side of the scapula, 1.5 cun horizontally away.

**Method:** Use the moving cupping method.

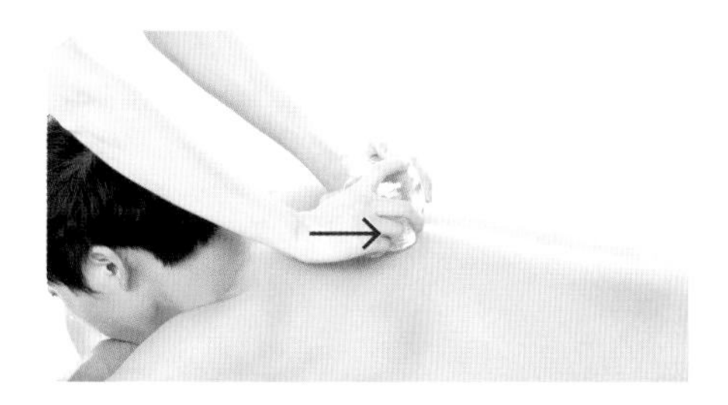

Move the cup on the bladder meridian on the back by segment along the meridian, and move the cup several times mainly on the Xinshu point. Repeatedly push and pull on the point back and forth, until the skin becomes red. The cup may be retained on the abovementioned point for 5 minutes after the moving cupping.

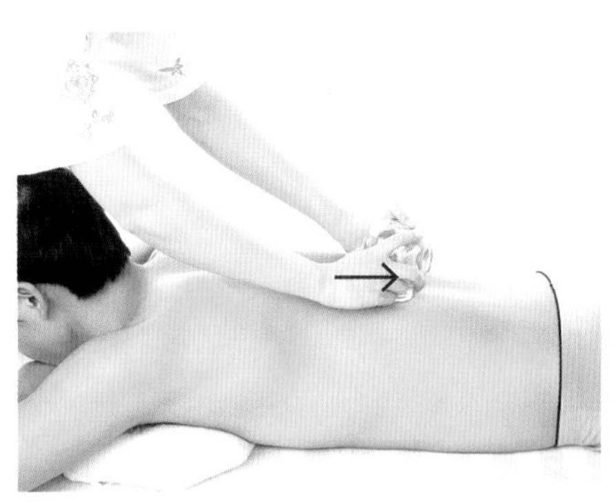

### 4. Pishu Point

**Location:** 1.5 cun away horizontally from the eleventh thoracic vertebra.

**Method:** Use the moving cupping method. Move the cup on the bladder meridian on the back by segment along the meridian, and move it several times mainly on the Pishu point. Repeatedly push and pull on the point back and forth, until the skin becomes red. The cup may be retained on the abovementioned point for 5 minutes after the moving cupping.

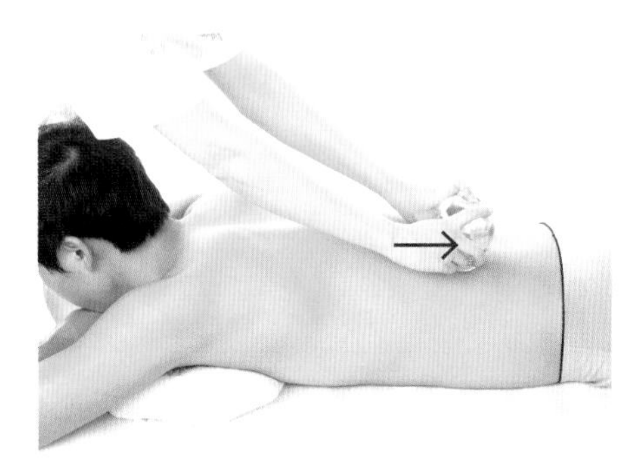

### 5. Shenshu Point

**Location:** 1.5 cun horizontally from the second lumbar spinal process.

**Method:** Use the moving cupping method. Move the cup on the bladder meridian on the back by segment along the meridian, and move it several times mainly on the Shenshu point. Repeatedly push and pull on the point back and forth, until the skin becomes red. The cup may be retained on the abovementioned point for 5 minutes after the moving cupping.

#### Moxibustion

Moxibustion is one of the most ancient therapies in China, by which a moxa stick or shorter moxa cone made of moxa floss is burned above an acupoint or a specific area on body surface to produce heat stimulation, thereby stimulating the meridian qi activities and adjusting the body's physical disorders. It has the effects of warming and activating the meridians, eliminating blood stasis and dispersing accumulation of pathogens, tonifying the middle warmer and replenishing qi, and so on. Applied in combination with cupping, it can strengthen the stimulation to acupoints, and offer better curative effects (fig. 24). During moxibution, pay attention not to touch the skin with the moxa sticks or moxa cones to avoid burning. They can be used together with a moxa box when necessary, so that the operation will be safer and more reliable (fig. 25).

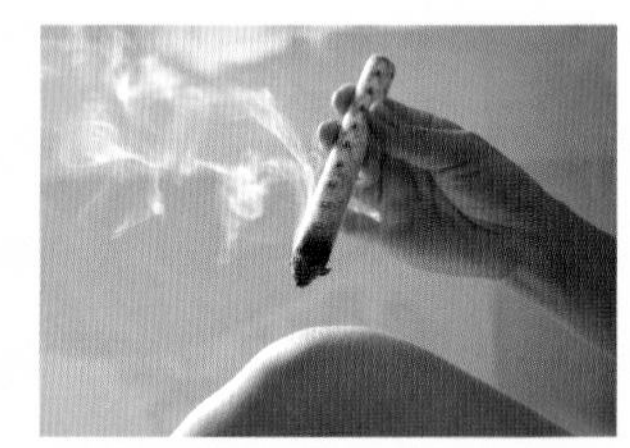

Fig. 24 Moxibustion.

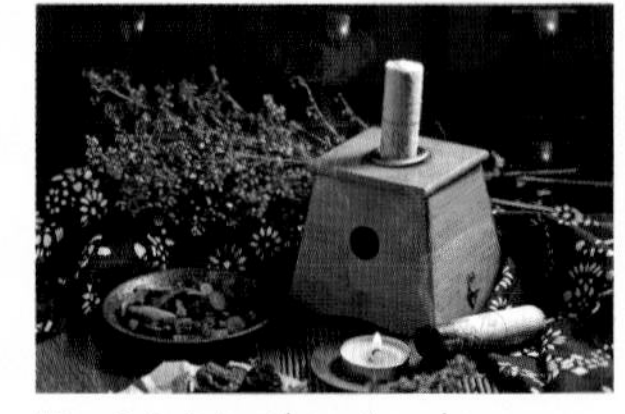

Fig. 25 Moxibustion box.

# 3 Fatigue

Fatigue is a feeling by a patient of weakness all over the body, drowsiness, limpness of legs and laziness.

There are many causes for fatigue, and one should find out the causes in time. It can appear after lack of sleep, in hot weather, after heavy labor, or with physical problems. To restore health as soon as possible, get more sleep to avoid chronic fatigue. If fatigue is induced by other diseases, the primary illness should be treated in time without delay. For diet, one should eat more high protein food, and the food should not taste too light. Necessary daily intake of salt should be ensured.

Those who feel fatigue should be cupped mainly on the Mingmen, Guanyuan, Ganshu, Pishu, and Shenshu points, plus the Shousanli point for those who mainly feel weakness in their upper limbs, or the Chengshan point for those who mainly lack strength in their lower limbs.

## Cupping Methods

### 1. Mingmen Point

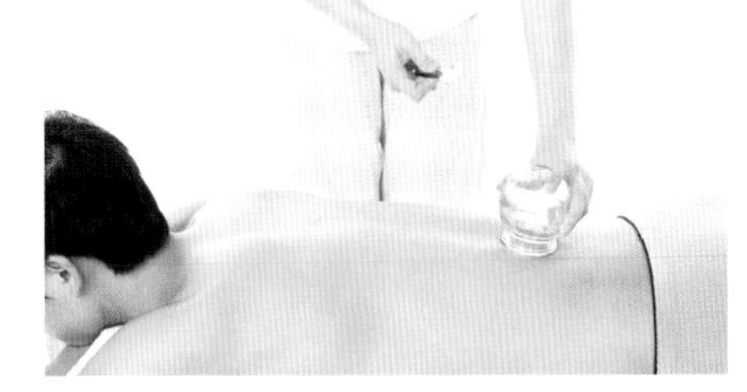

**Location:** In a cavity below the spinous process of the second cervical vertebra.

**Method:** First knead Mingmen point with the thumb pulp for 2–3 minutes, and then select and apply a cup of appropriate size to the point, retaining the cup for 5–10 minutes.

### 2. Guanyuan Point

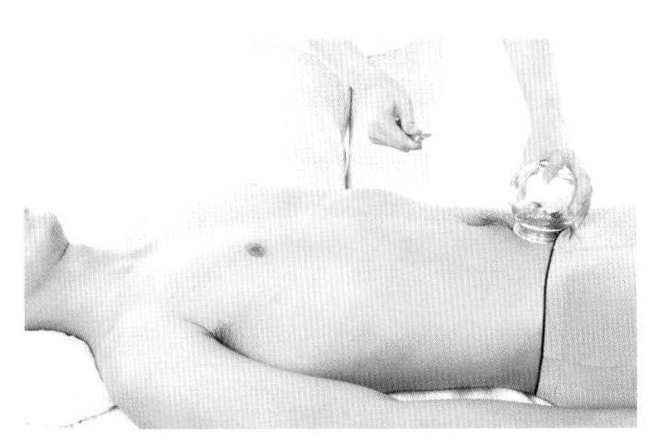

**Location:** About 3 cun below the navel.

**Method:** First knead Guanyuan point with the thumb pulp for 2–3 minutes, and then select and apply a cup of appropriate size to the point, retaining the cup for 10–15 minutes. With the cup removed, perform moxibustion with a moxa box or moxa cone for 3–5 minutes until warmth is felt.

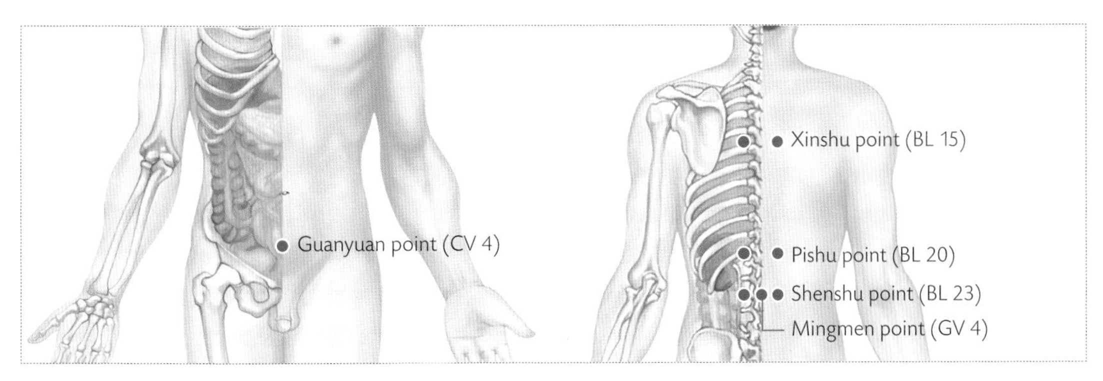

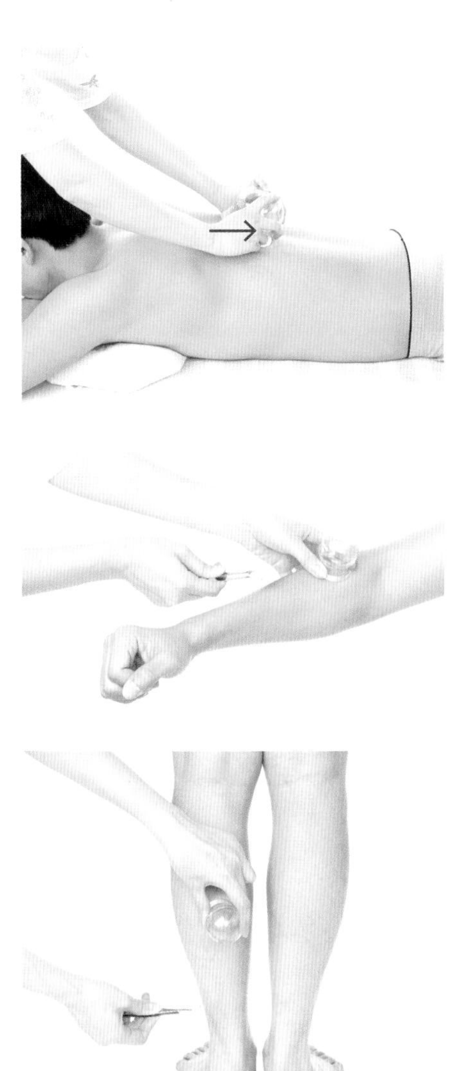

### 3. Ganshu, Pishu and Shenshu Points

**Location:** Ganshu point is 1.5 cun away from the ninth thoracic spinal process on the inner side of the scapula; Pishu point is at the point 1.5 cun away horizontally from the eleventh thoracic vertebra; Shenshu point is 1.5 cun horizontally from the second lumbar spinal process.

**Method:** Use the moving cupping method by moving the cup on the bladder meridian on the back by segment along the meridian. Move the cup several times mainly on Ganshu, Pishu and Shenshu points, and repeatedly push and pull on the points back and forth, until the skin becomes red. The cup may be retained on the abovementioned points for 5 minutes after the moving cupping.

### 4. Shousanli Point

**Location:** 2 cun below the Quchi point.

**Method:** First knead Shousanli point with the thumb pulp for 2–3 minutes, and then select and apply a small cup to the point, retaining the cup for 5–10 minutes.

### 5. Chengshan Point

**Location:** In a cavity in the middle of the rear of the lower leg, at the top of the depression between the two muscles of the calf.

**Method:** First knead Chengshan point with the thumb tip for 2–3 minutes, preferably with a heavy force, until one feels sore and swelling at the point. Then apply a cup of appropriate size to the point, and retain the cup for 5–10 minutes.

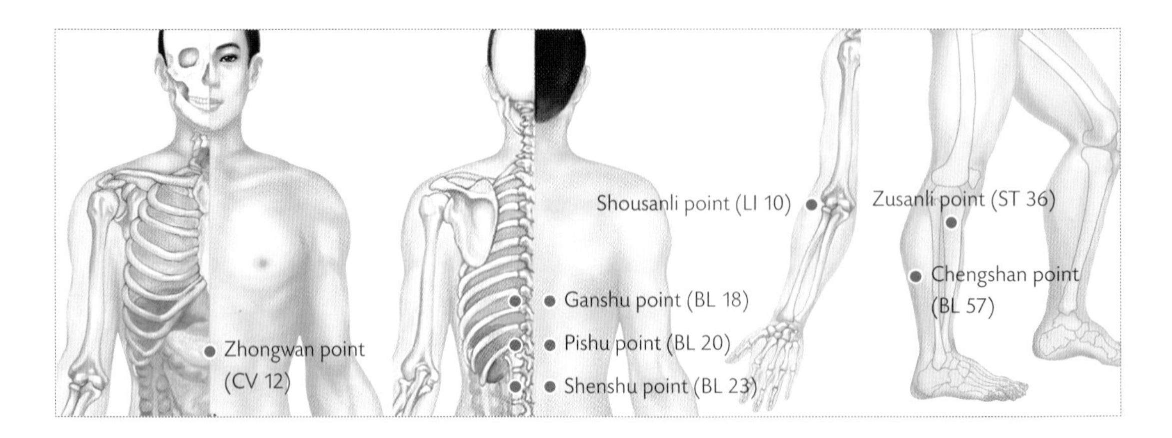

# 4 Loss of Appetite

Loss of appetite means no appetite or no desire to eat. Occasional loss of appetite is mainly caused by disorder in emotion, or improper diet, which can be relieved after the cause is removed.

To avoid loss of appetite, one should have a healthy and regular diet, reduce the intake of fried food, and insist on eating regularly and properly, instead of being very hungry or eating too much. In this way, one will have an appetite to eat and excrete a variety of digestive juices at meal time, thereby being conducive to the absorption of various nutrients in the food. One can also try to improve cooking food with good color, aroma, and taste, which will help the human body secrete a lot of digestive juices, thus working up a strong appetite and being conducive to the digestion and absorption of food. One should also do appropriate exercise to help digestion and absorption of food. For example, walking, jogging, and *taijiquan* are good choices for gastrointestinal patients. But do not engage in strenuous exercise after a meal.

In addition, the Traditional Chinese Medicine for recuperating intestines and stomach can be taken for curing loss of appetite caused by long-term use of drugs. A child experiencing loss of appetite should supplement with an appropriate amount of zinc.

Patients with this symptom may be cupped mainly on Zhongwan, Neiguan, and Zusanli points.

## Cupping Methods

### 1. Zhongwan Point

**Location:** On the upper abdomen, 4 cun above the center of the umbilicus, on the anterior midline.

**Method:** First, massage the upper abdomen above the belly button for about ten circles with the palm or with the index finger, the middle finger, and the ring finger together. This should be performed gently. Then select a cup of appropriate size, and apply it to Zhongwan point, retaining the cup for 10–15 minutes.

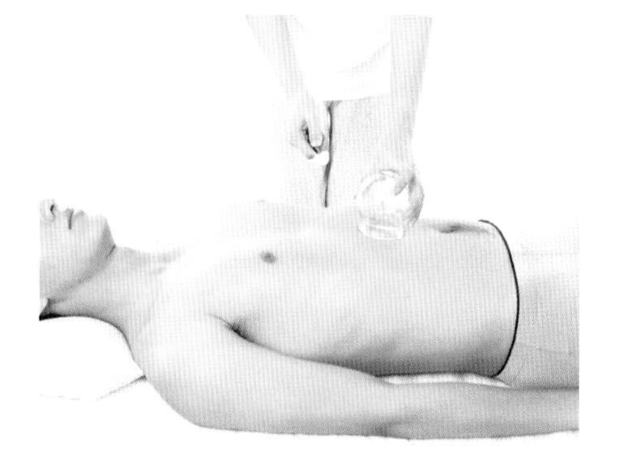

### 2. Zusanli Point

**Location:** About 3 cun below the knee on the outer side of the tibia.

**Method:** First knead Zusanli point with the thumb pulp for 2–3 minutes, and then select a cup of appropriate size and apply it to the point, retaining for 10–15 minutes. With the cup removed, perform moxibustion with a moxa stick for 3–5 minutes until warmth is felt.

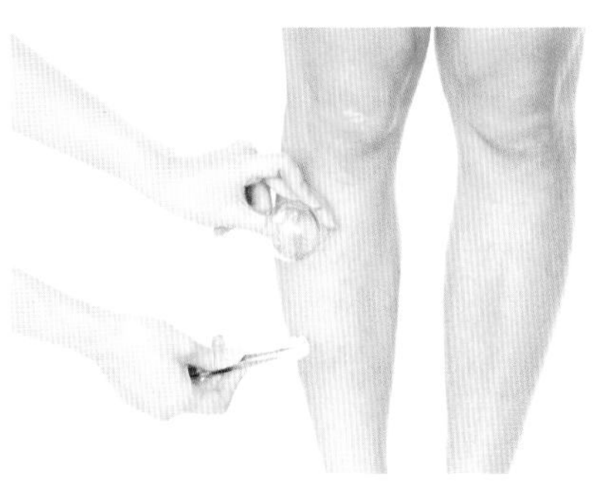

### 3. Neiguan Point

**Location:** Between the two tendons about 2 cun above the wrist joint bend on the inside of the arm.

**Method:** First knead Neiguan point with the thumb pulp, and then select and apply a cup of appropriate size to the point, retaining the cup for 10–15 minutes.

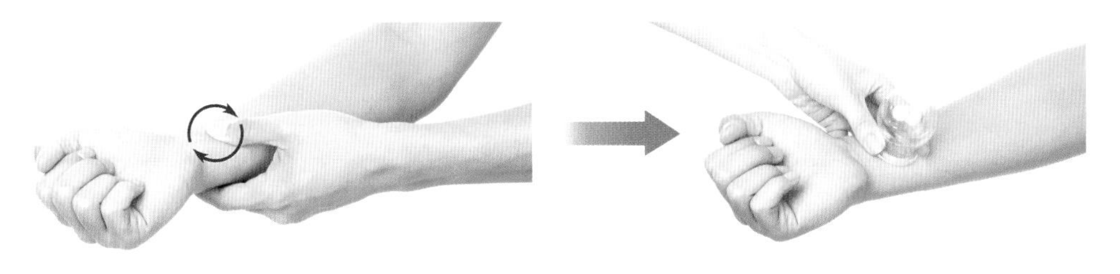

# 5 Leg Cramps

Leg cramps are often a result of strenuous exercise, work fatigue, a severe twist of the tibia, or the calcium deficiency, coldness, and pressure of local nerve vessels. It usually happens when one is lying or sleeping.

One who is prone to leg cramps should often do exercise to prevent excessive fatigue of muscles during exercise. Make full preparations before exercise, and do not be too hasty, so as to avoid being hurt. Pay attention to balanced diets, supplementation of calcium, and drinking of more milk, soybean milk, etc. In addition, eating vegetables and fruits can help supplement various trace elements. Drink water often; do not drink only when you feel thirsty. Supplement with nutrition fortifying sports drinks after profuse sweating. One who often suffers from leg cramps at night should, in particular, pay attention to keeping warm, and may stretch the muscles prone to cramps before sleeping.

The patient can be cupped mainly on Weizhong, Chengshan, and Yanglingquan points.

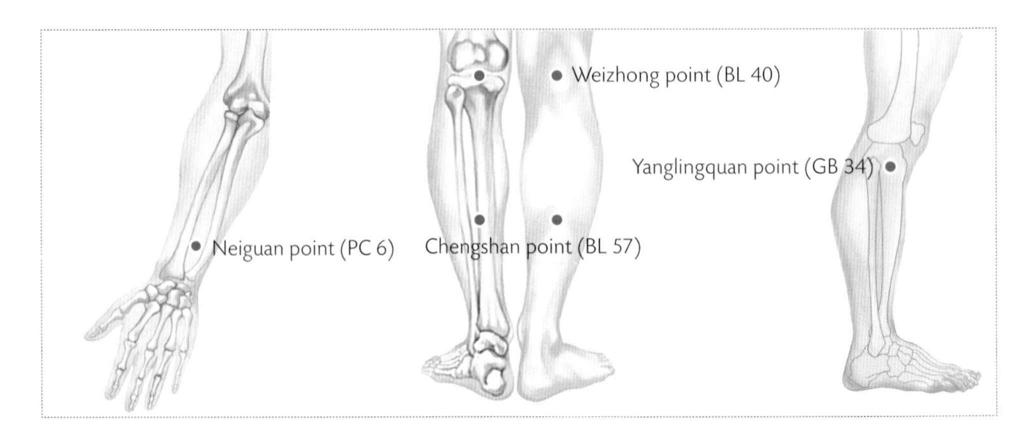

## Cupping Methods

### 1. Weizhong Point

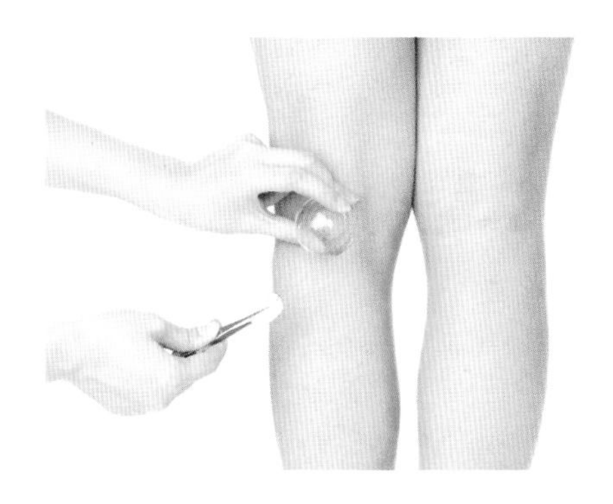

**Location:** Right in the middle of popliteal crease (at the back of the knee).

**Method:** First knead Weizhong point with the thumb tip for 2–3 minutes, preferably with a heavy force, until one feels sore and swelling at the point. Then apply a cup of appropriate size to the point, and retain the cup for 5–10 minutes.

### 2. Chengshan Point

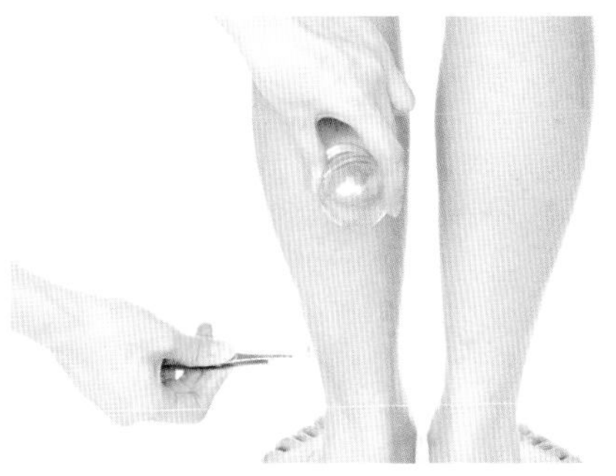

**Location:** In a cavity in the middle of the rear of the lower leg, at the top of the depression between the two muscles of the calf.

**Method:** First knead Chengshan point with the thumb tip for 2–3 minutes, preferably with a heavy force, until one feels sore and swelling at the point. Then apply a cup of appropriate size to the point, and retain the cup for 5–10 minutes.

### 3. Yanglingquan Point

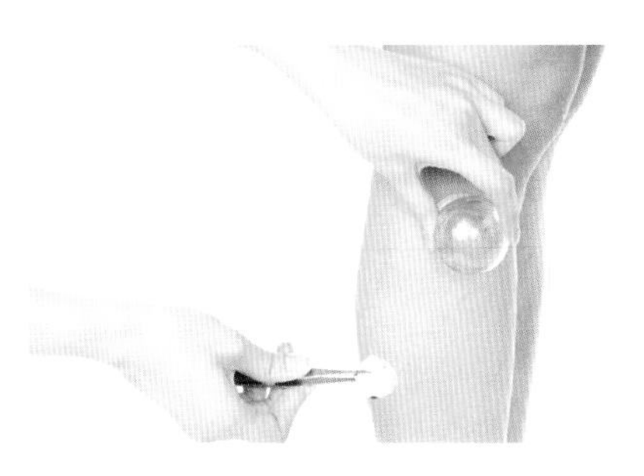

**Location:** On the outer side of the shin in a notch at the front lower part of the fibula.

**Method:** First knead Yanglingquan point with the thumb tip for 2–3 minutes, preferably with a heavy force, until one feels sore and swelling at the point. Then apply a cup of appropriate size to the point, and retain the cup for 5–10 minutes.

# 6 Muscle Soreness

Muscle soreness is a local or a large range of muscular pain mainly due to abruptly strenuous exercise, or long-term muscle strain. The pain increases when the affected muscle is pressed.

In order to avoid muscle soreness, during exercise, one should make a scientific arrangement of the exercise load depending on his/her own physique and health conditions. Try to avoid focusing on exercising a certain part for a long time, so as to avoid overload of local muscles. Make full preparation before exercise. One who suffers from muscle soreness for a long time should avoid high-intensity manual labor, and pay attention to resting and keeping warm.

For those who suffer from muscle soreness, cupping locations should be chosen according to different parts, mostly on the parts with muscle soreness.

## Cupping Methods

### 1. Jianjing Point (Soreness in Shouler and Neck)

**Location:** At the midpoint of the top on the shoulder.

**Method:** First knead Jianjing point with the thumb tip for 2–3 minutes, preferably with a heavy force, until one feels sore and swelling at the point. Then apply a cup of appropriate size to the point, and retain the cup for 5–10 minutes.

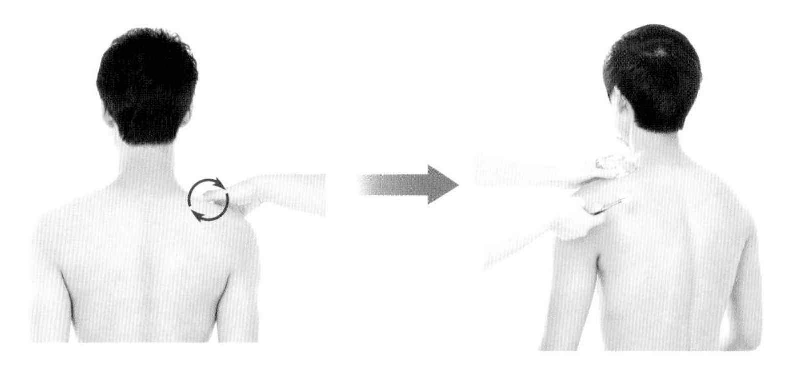

### 2. Weizhong Point (Soreness in Leg and Ankle)

**Location:** Right in the middle of popliteal crease (at the back of the knee).

**Method:** First knead Weizhong point with the thumb tip for 2–3 minutes, preferably with a heavy force, until one feels sore and swelling at the point. Then apply a cup of appropriate size to the point, and retain the cup for 5–10 minutes.

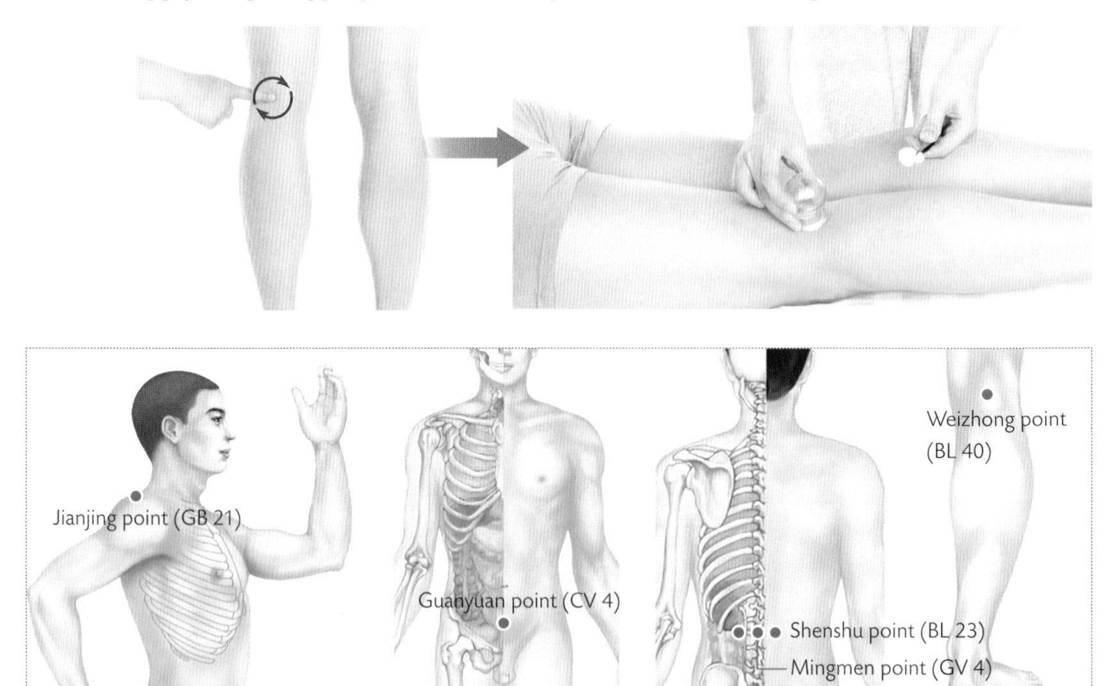

# 7 Fear of Cold

Fear of cold is feeling cold, a symptom which will be aggravated by exposure to cold, but alleviated by exposure to heat. According to Traditional Chinese Medicine, it is caused by deficiency of yang.

People who have fear of cold should do exercise actively to enhance their physique, and prevent cold to keep warm. According to the principles of "nourishing yang in spring and summer," they should bask more in the sun in spring and summer, so as to nourish and supplement yang by virtue of the yang in the nature. They may also eat more food with warming yang, such as lamb, pork stomach, chicken and leeks, or add gingers, cinnamon, and other pungent and fragrant condiments in food. They should not eat raw and cold food.

The cupping should be performed mainly on Shenshu, Guanyuan, and Mingmen points.

## Cupping Methods

### 1. Shenshu Point

**Location:** 1.5 cun horizontally from the second lumbar spinal process.

**Method:** Select and apply a cup of appropriate size to Shenshu point, retaining the cup for 10–15 minutes. With the cup removed, perform moxibustion with a moxa box or a moxa cone for 3–5 minutes until warmth is felt.

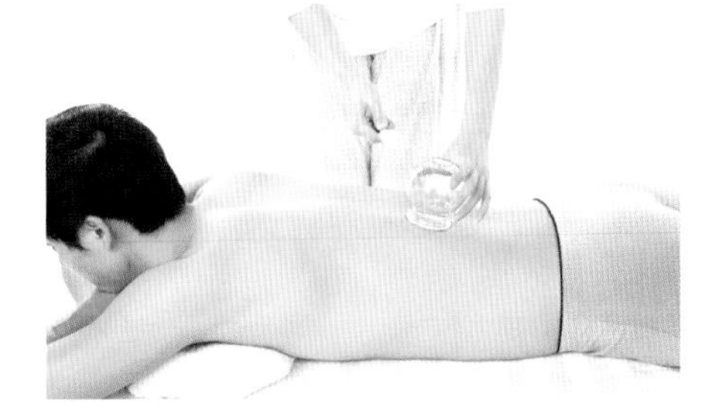

### 2. Guanyuan Point

**Location:** About 3 cun below the navel.

**Method:** Select and apply a cup of appropriate size to Guanyuan point, retaining the cup for 10–15 minutes. With the cup removed, perform moxibustion with a moxa box or a moxa cone for 3–5 minutes until warmth is felt.

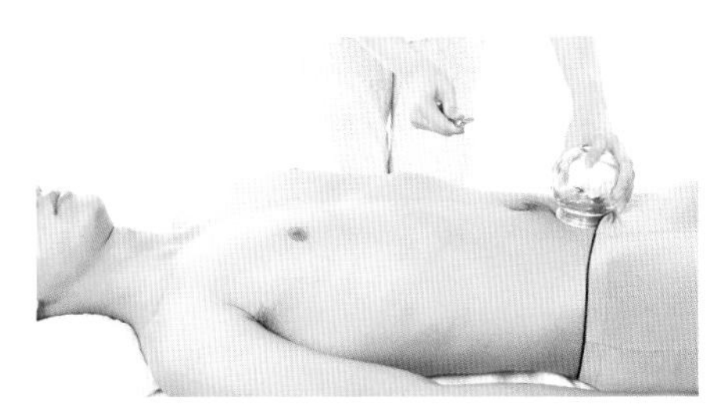

### 3. Mingmen Point

**Location:** In a cavity below the spinous process of the second cervical vertebra.

**Method:** First knead Mingmen point with the thumb pulp for 2–3 minutes, and then select and apply a cup of appropriate size to the point, retaining the cup for 10–15 minutes. With the cup removed, perform moxibustion with a moxa box or a moxa cone for 3–5 minutes until warmth is felt.

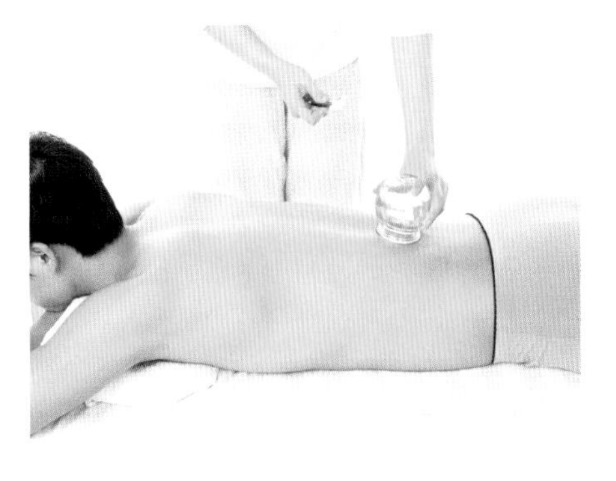

# 8 Excessive Internal Heat

The symptoms of excessive internal heat include repeated oral ulcers, swelling in the gum, dry mouth, bitter taste in the mouth, dry cough with little sputum, angina and hoarse voice, oliguria with reddish urine, upset and irritability, skin sores, etc.

Once having excessive internal heat, one may eat more heat-clearing, fire-purging, and detoxifying food like chrysanthemum, lotus seeds, tomatoes, green beans, red beans, bitter gourd, bitter herbs, bracken, escargots, eggplants, millet, and buckwheat, and eat less warm, pungent, and stimulating food. In addition, one should have enough sleep and regulate his/her emotions. One who often has mouth sores should pay attention to cleaning and hygiene of oral cavity, and consult a surgeon dentist when necessary.

One who has excessive internal heat shall be cupped mainly on Dazhui, Quchi, Taichong, and Hegu points.

## Cupping Methods

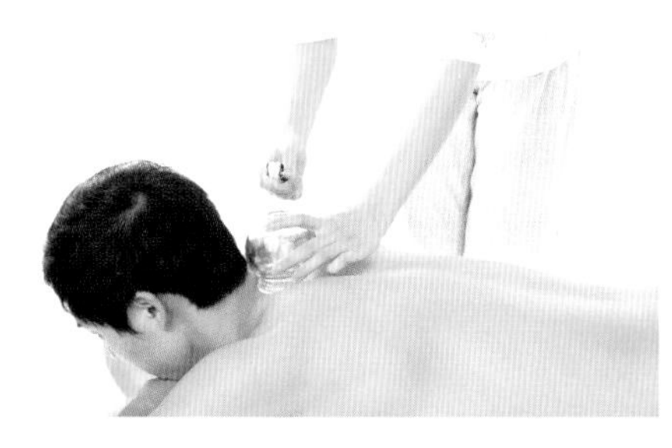

### 1. Dazhui Point

**Location:** Under the spinous process of the seventh cervical vertebrae.

**Method:** Select a cup of appropriate size and apply it to Dazhui point. Retain the cup for 10–15 minutes.

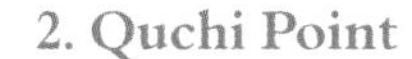

### 2. Quchi Point

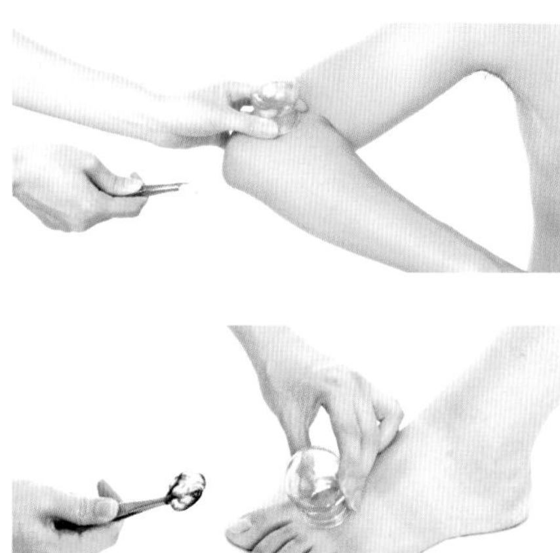

**Location:** With the elbow bent halfway, on the outer side of the cubital transverse crease.

**Method:** Select a cup of appropriate size and apply it to Quchi point. Retain the cup for 10–15 minutes.

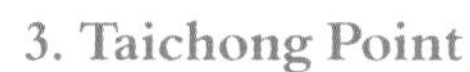

### 3. Taichong Point

**Location:** On the foot in a notch between the first and second metatarsal bones.

**Method:** First knead Taichong point with the thumb pulp for 2–3 minutes, and then select and apply a cup of appropriate size to the point, retaining the cup for 10–15 minutes.

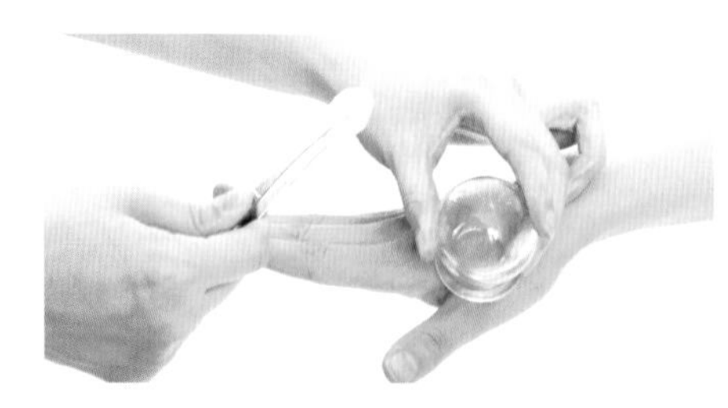

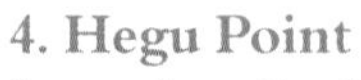

### 4. Hegu Point

**Location:** In the highest point on the back of the hand between the thumb base and the base of the index finger (in the webbing between these two fingers).

**Method:** First knead Hegu point with the thumb pulp for 2–3 minutes, and then select and apply a cup of appropriate size to the point, retaining the cup for 10–15 minutes.

# 9 Anxiety

People with anxiety often worry too much, and are nervous and afraid, but often without specific reasons. Some patients may have headache, insomnia, and other symptoms.

Anxiety should be treated mainly by self-regulation, and regulating emotions, relaxing, and developing interests and hobbies to transfer the attention to other aspects. They can listen to music, practice mediation, receive massage, ensure enough sleep, try to actively practice self-relief and self-relaxation, and maintain an optimistic attitude.

The cupping can be applied mainly on Shenmen, Taichong, Dazhui, and Xinshu points.

## Cupping Methods

### 1. Shenmen Point

**Location:** On the inner wrist near the small finger when the palm is turned upward.

**Method:** First knead Shenmen point with the thumb pulp for 2–3 minutes, and then select and apply a small cup to the point, retaining for 5–10 minutes.

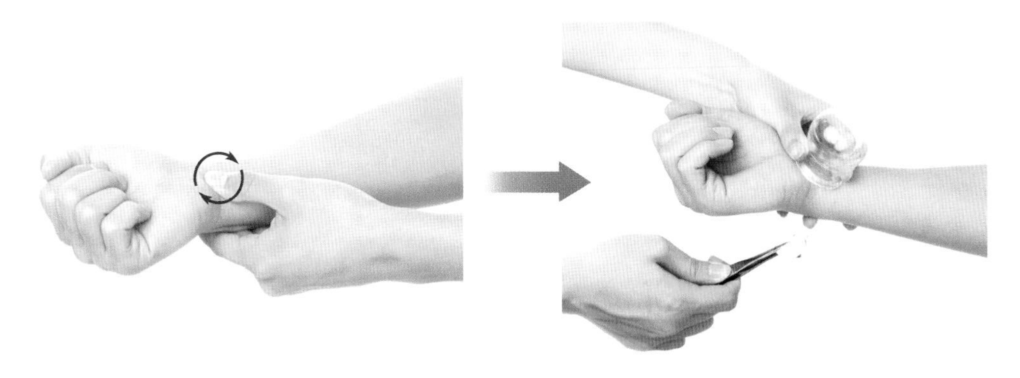

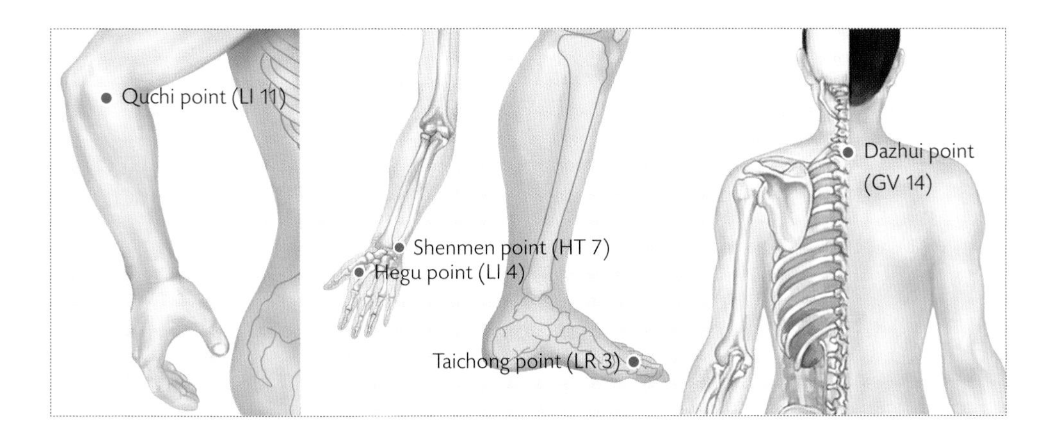

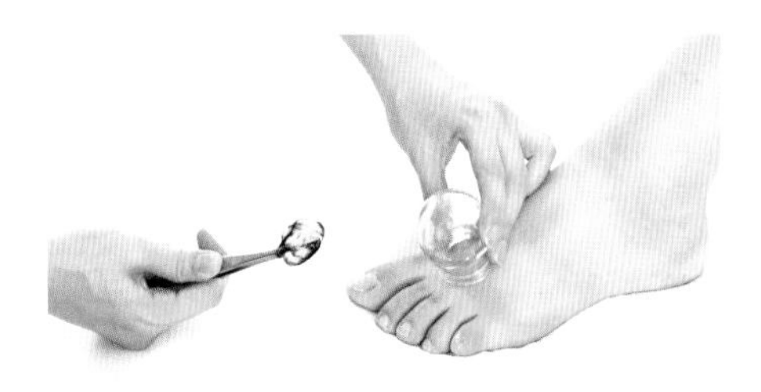

### 2. Taichong Point

**Location:** On the foot in a notch between the first and second metatarsal bones.

**Method:** First knead Taichong point with the thumb pulp for 2–3 minutes, and then select and apply a cup of appropriate size to the point, retaining the cup for 10–15 minutes.

### 3. Dazhui Point

**Location:** Under the spinous process of the seventh cervical vertebrae.

**Method:** Select a cup of appropriate size and apply it to Dazhui point. Retain the cup for 10–15 minutes.

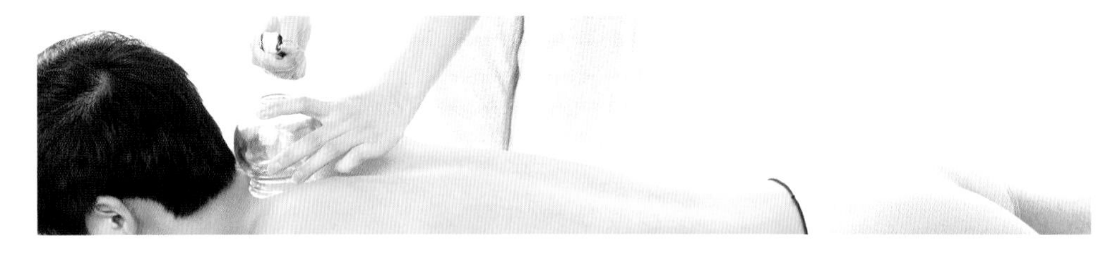

### 4. Xinshu Point

**Location:** Under the fifth thoracic vertebra on the inner side of the scapula, 1.5 cun horizontally away.

**Method:** Select a cup of appropriate size and apply it to Xinshu point. Retain the cup for 10–15 minutes.

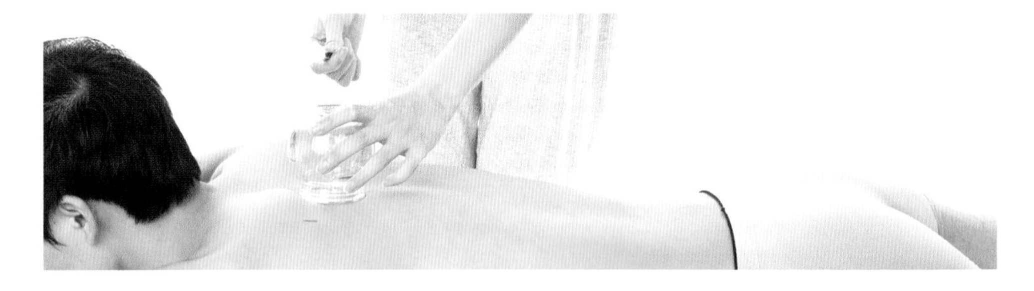

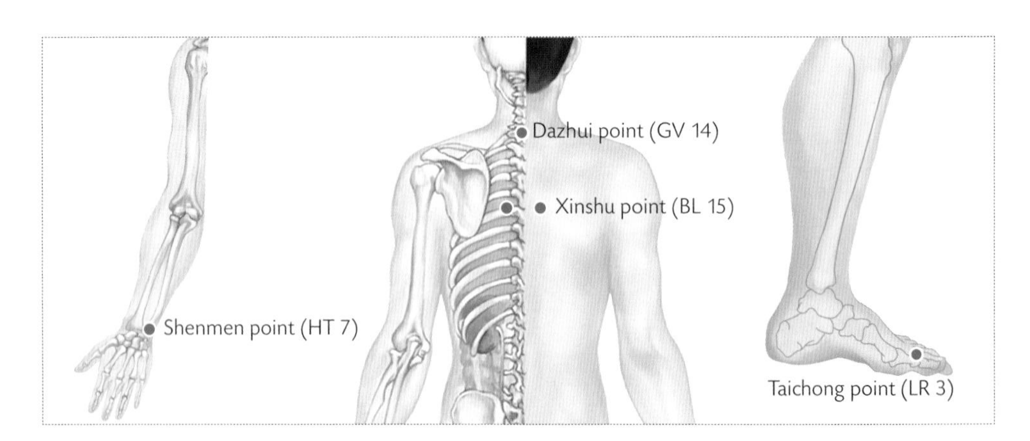

# 10 Neurasthenia

Neurasthenia is neurological dysfunction characterized by such symptoms as proneness to mental excitation, mental fatigue and emotional instability, often accompanied by serious sleep disorders and hypomnesia.

Those suffering from neurasthenia should learn self-regulation, strengthen self-cultivation, and develop interests and hobbies, in order to vent their intrapsychic dissatisfaction and depression in an appropriate way, and to relieve their psychological depression and mental stress. They should participate in physical exercise, such as *taijiquan*, fitness walking, jogging and playing table tennis which help alleviate neurasthenia. In terms of diet, they should eat more food rich in vitamin C, and may add medlar, lilies, pearl barley, red dates, corn, lotus seeds, and other ingredients to regulate qi and blood. They should also pay attention to reducing smoking, drinking less coffee, and so on.

The cupping should be mainly applied to Shenmen, Taichong, Xinshu, Ganshu, and Yongquan points.

## Cupping Methods

### 1. Shenmen Point

**Location:** On the inner wrist near the small finger when the palm is turned upward.

**Method:** First knead Shenmen point with the thumb pulp for 2–3 minutes, and then select and apply a small cup to the point, retaining for 5–10 minutes.

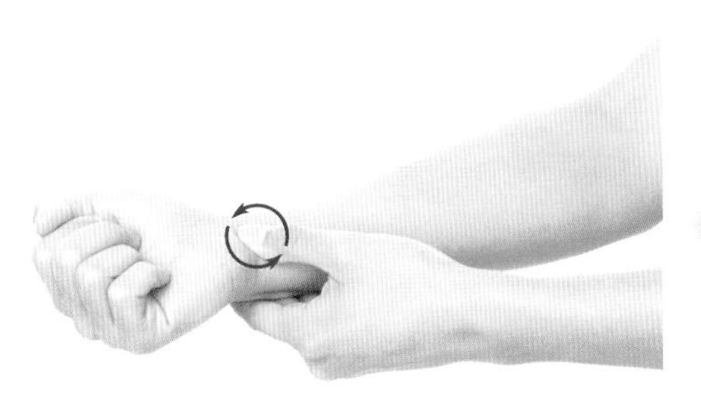

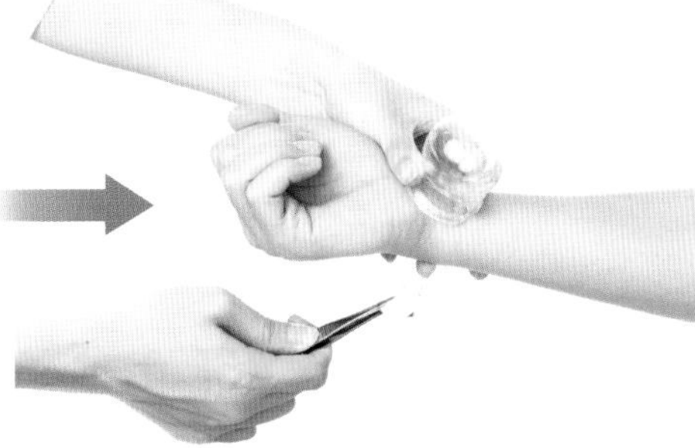

### 2. Taichong Point

**Location:** On the foot in a notch between the first and second metatarsal bones.

**Method:** First knead Taichong point with the thumb pulp for 2–3 minutes, and then select and apply a cup of appropriate size to the point, retaining the cup for 10–15 minutes.

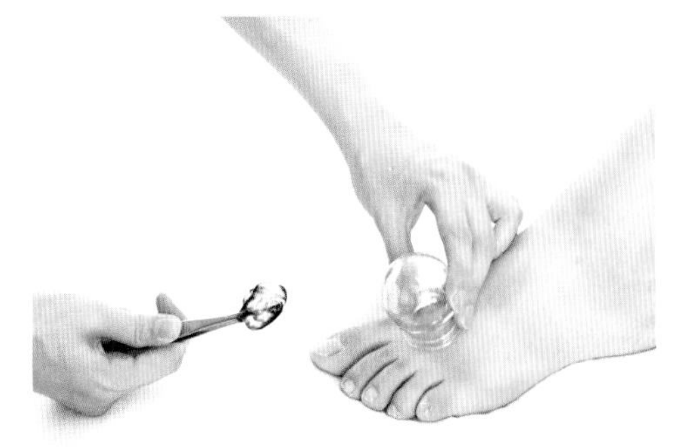

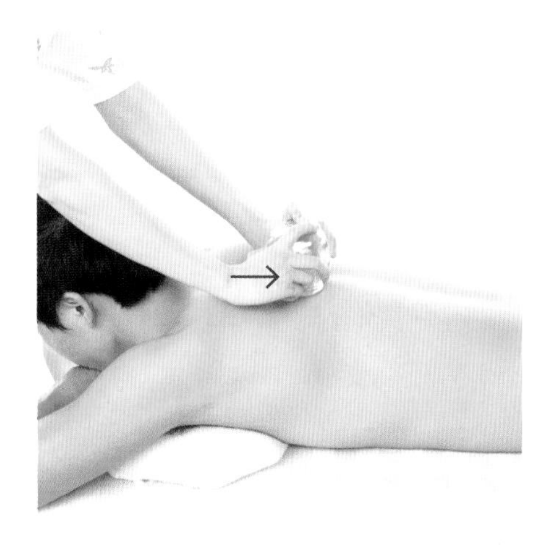

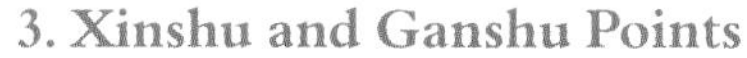

### 3. Xinshu and Ganshu Points

**Location:** Xinshu point is under the fifth thoracic vertebra on the inner side of the scapula, 1.5 cun horizontally away; Ganshu point is 1.5 cun away from the ninth thoracic spinal process on the inner side of the scapula.

**Method:** Use the moving cupping method. Move the cup on the bladder meridian on the back by segment along the meridian, and move the cup several times mainly on Xinshu and Ganshu points. Repeatedly push and pull on the points back and forth, until the skin becomes red. The cup may be retained on the abovementioned points for 5 minutes after the moving cupping.

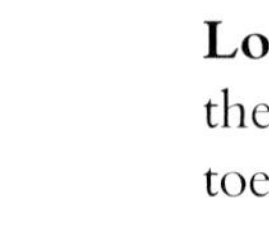

### 4. Yongquan Point

**Location:** In a depression in the front of the sole of the foot, about one-third of the way down from the toes.

**Method:** First knead Yongquan point with the palm for 2–3 minutes, until a feeling of heat is present. Then select a cup of appropriate size and apply it to the point, retaining the cup for 10–15 minutes. With the cup removed, perform moxibustion with a moxa stick for 3–5 minutes until warmth is felt.

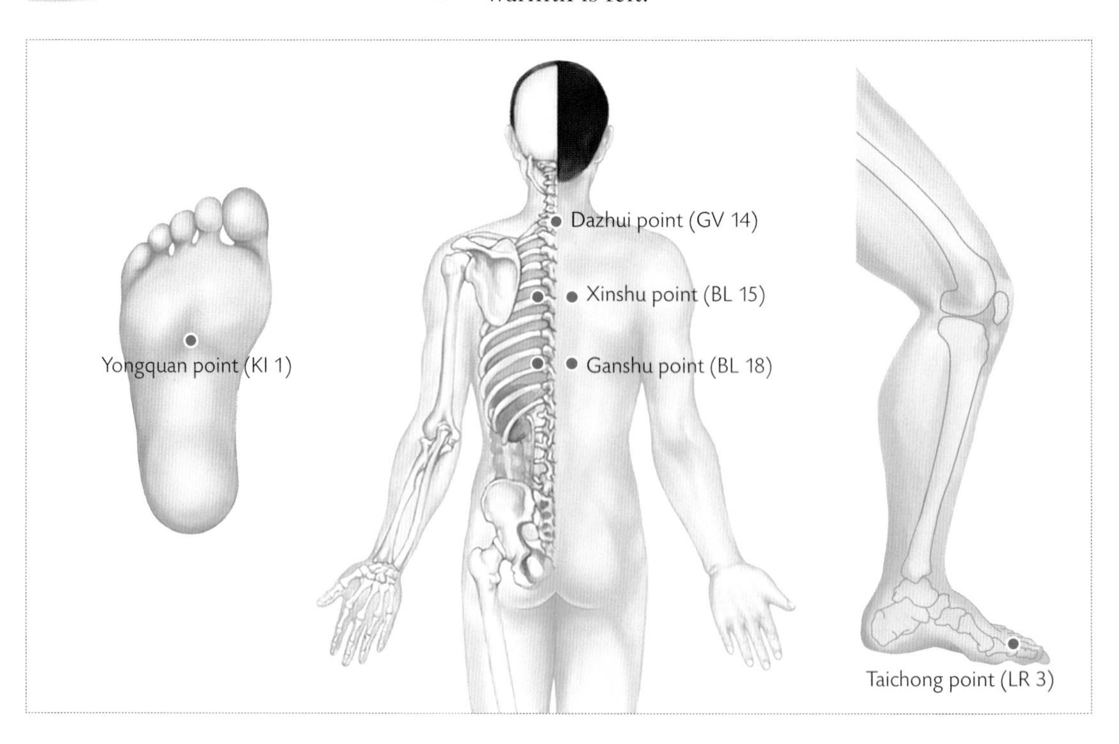

# 11 Rashness and Irritation

This type of patients has symptoms such as rashness, proneness to irritation, and emotional instability, which are caused by hyperactivity of liver fire according to Traditional Chinese Medicine.

Rash and irritable people should strive to maintain a good mood, behave peacefully in social life, learn to tolerate, and develop interests and hobbies like calligraphy, gardening, *taijiquan*, and so on to cultivate their minds. In terms of diet, they should eat less spicy, stimulating, or fried food, but drink more such drinks as chrysanthemum tea and lotus seed tea.

The cupping should be mainly applied to Dazhui, Taichong, Xinshu, and Ganshu points.

## Cupping Methods

### 1. Dazhui Point

**Location:** Under the spinous process of the seventh cervical vertebrae.

**Method:** Select a cup of appropriate size and apply it to Dazhui point. Retain the cup for 10–15 minutes.

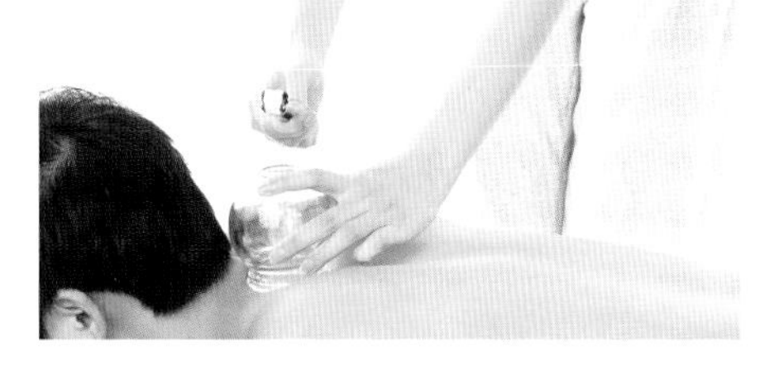

### 2. Taichong Point

**Location:** On the foot in a notch between the first and second metatarsal bones.

**Method:** First knead Taichong point with the thumb pulp for 2–3 minutes, and then select and apply a cup of appropriate size to the point, retaining the cup for 10–15 minutes.

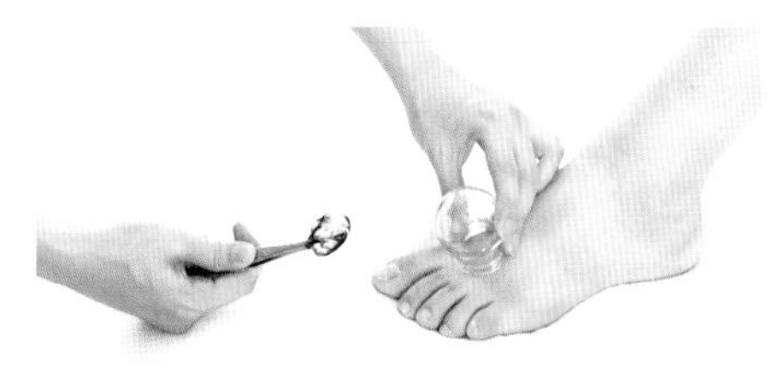

### 3. Xinshu and Ganshu Points

**Location:** Xinshu point is under the fifth thoracic vertebra on the inner side of the scapula, 1.5 cun horizontally away; Ganshu point is 1.5 cun away from the ninth thoracic spinal process on the inner side of the scapula.

**Method:** Use the moving cupping method. Move the cup on the bladder meridian on the back by segment along the meridian, and move the cup several

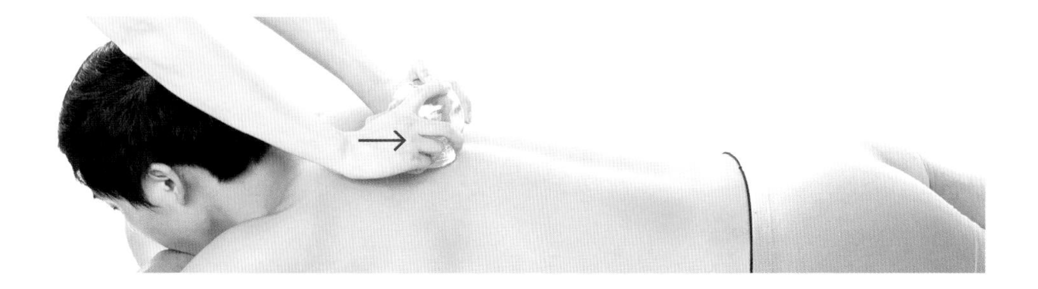

times mainly on Xinshu and Ganshu points. Repeatedly push and pull on the points back and forth, until the skin becomes red. The cup may be retained on the abovementioned points for 5 minutes after the moving cupping.

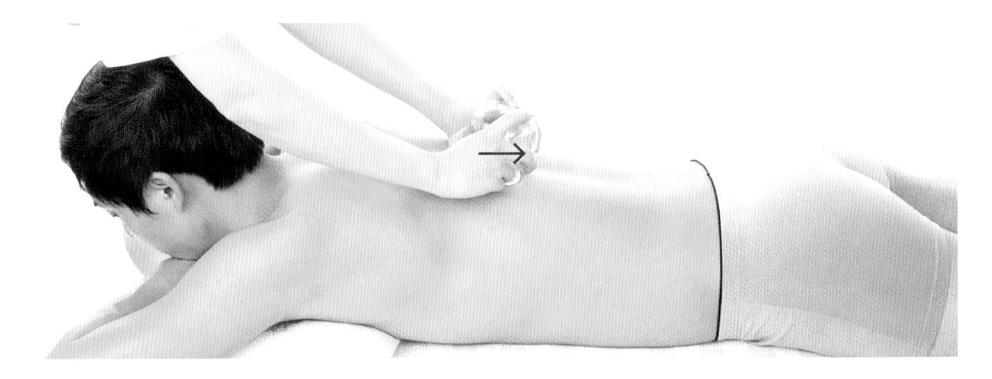

# 12 Depression

Depressed persons are mainly characterized by low spirit, manifested by being depressed or distraught, and may have such symptoms as loss of appetite and poor sleep.

Patients should try to build confidence, establish a good lifestyle, participate in physical exercise, hang out with funny and humorous intimate friends to whom they can open their heart, keep in touch with friends, and let them know when they're unhappy. In addition, they may eat more food containing vitamin B and amino acids to supplement elements required by their bodies.

The cupping should be applied mainly on Shenmen, Jueyinshu, Xinshu, and Shenshu points.

## Cupping Methods

### 1. Shenmen Point

**Location:** On the inner wrist near the small finger when the palm is turned upward.

**Method:** First knead Shenmen point with the thumb pulp for 2–3 minutes, and then select and apply a small cup to the point, retaining for 5–10 minutes.

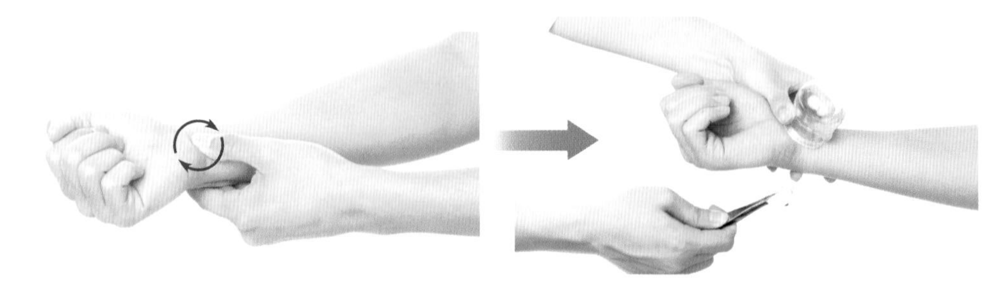

## 2. Jueyinshu Point

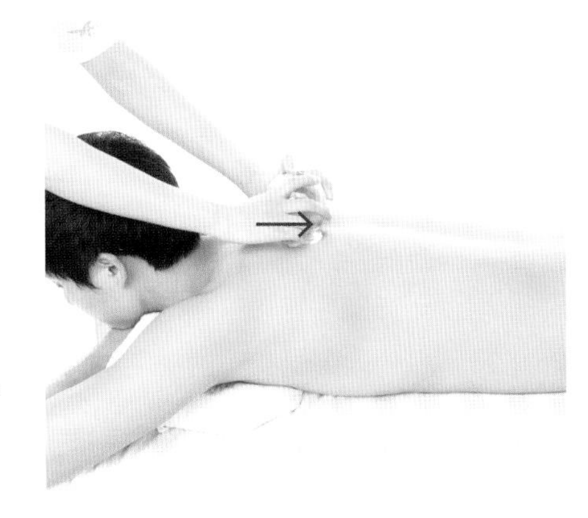

**Location:** In the spine area, 1.5 cun lateral to the posterior midline of the lower border of the spinous process of the fourth thoracic vertebra.

**Method:** Use the moving cupping method. Move the cup on the bladder meridian on the back by segment along the meridian, and move the cup several times mainly on the Jueyinshu point. Repeatedly push and pull on the point back and forth, until the skin becomes red. The cup may be retained on the abovementioned point for 5 minutes after the moving cupping.

## 3. Xinshu Point

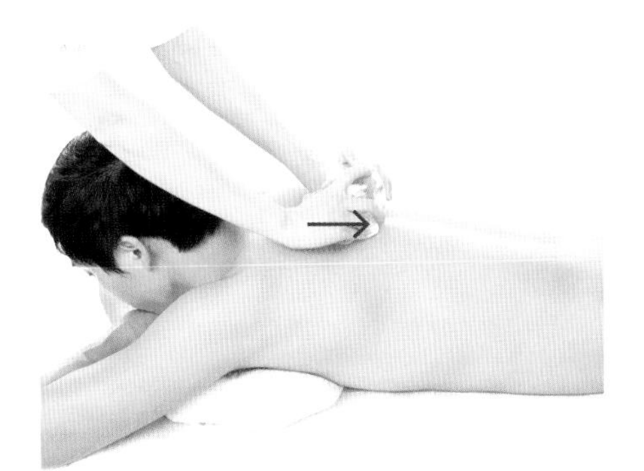

**Location:** Under the fifth thoracic vertebra on the inner side of the scapula, 1.5 cun horizontally away.

**Method:** Use the moving cupping method. Move the cup on the bladder meridian on the back by segment along the meridian, and move the cup several times mainly on the Xinshu point. Repeatedly push and pull on the point back and forth, until the skin becomes red. The cup may be retained on the abovementioned point for 5 minutes after the moving cupping.

## 4. Shenshu Point

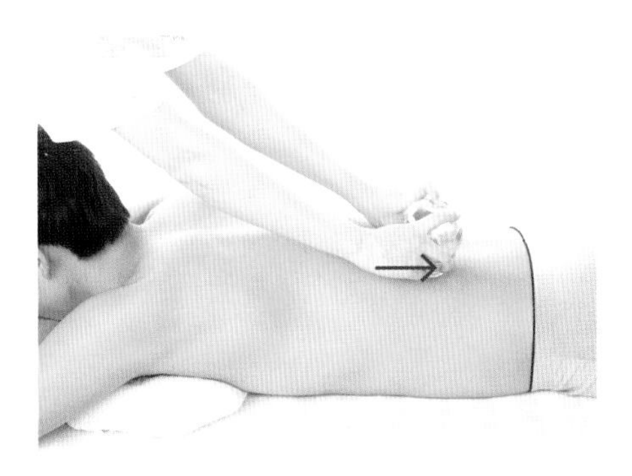

**Location:** 1.5 cun horizontally from the second lumbar spinal process.

**Method:** Use the moving cupping method. Move the cup on the bladder meridian on the back by segment along the meridian, and move it several times mainly on the Shenshu point. Repeatedly push and pull on the point back and forth, until the skin becomes red. The cup may be retained on the abovementioned point for 5 minutes after the moving cupping.

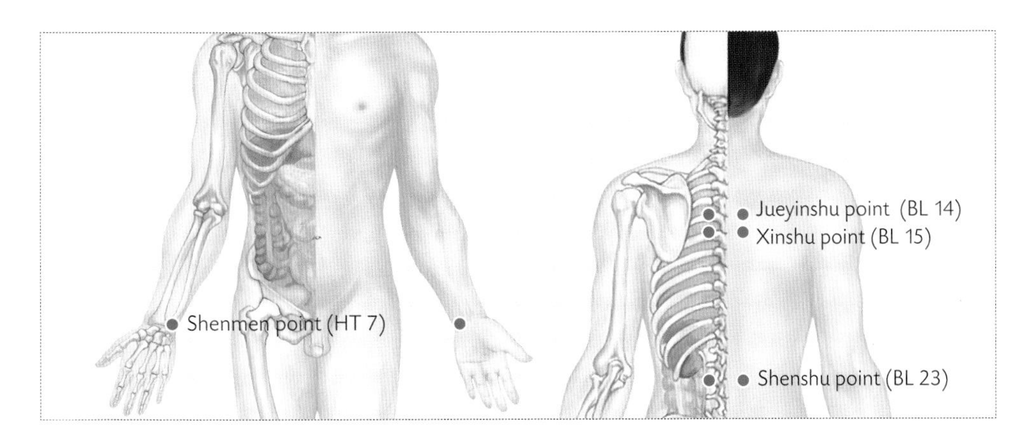

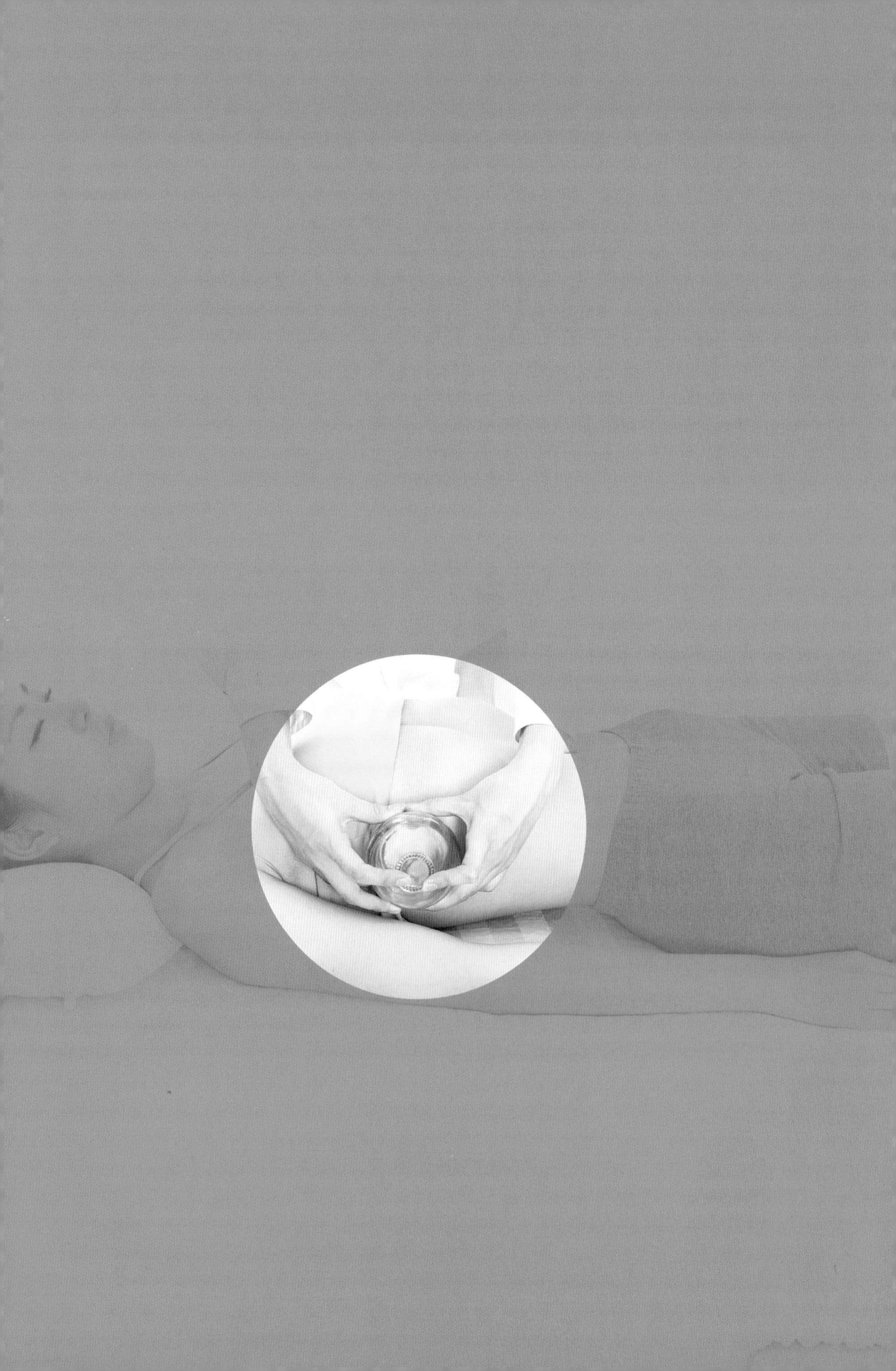

# Chapter Five
# Internal Diseases

Internal diseases include not only coronary heart disease, high blood pressure, diabetes, and other diseases often associated with the old people, but also cold, cough, headache, constipation and other common diseases. Though some diseases are not serious, they will cause a variety of discomforts to our body. Cupping therapy can eliminate various internal diseases and allow a refreshed and healthy body.

## 1 Coronary Heart Disease

Some patients have a symptom of paroxysmal crushing tight pain in the chest, or have a symptom of persistent severe retrosternal pain, palpitations, and shock. Those with mild symptoms suffer from chest distress and suppression of breath, while those with severe symptoms suffer from chest pain spreading all the way to the back with pale complexion.

In the case of the outbreak of myocardial infarction or heart failure in a severe condition, the patient should stay in bed, and receive combined treatment of Traditional Chinese Medicine and the Western medicine, supported by the cupping therapy under the close observation. Though the cupping therapy may alleviate the onset and frequency of symptom, it cannot completely replace other therapies. At ordinary times, one should avoid fatigue and emotional fluctuation, and eat light food, while abstaining themselves from smoking and drinking alcohol.

For this disease, cupping may be applied to three groups of points, one group a day and three groups in turn, until the symptoms are alleviated or disappear. The first group includes Danzhong, Xinshu, and Geshu points. The second group includes Zhiyang, Juque and Neiguan points. The third group includes Shenmen, Sanyinjiao, and Quze points.

### Cupping Methods

**The First Group of Points**

#### 1. Danzhong Point

**Location:** Directly in the middle of the chest between the nipples.

**Method:** First knead Danzhong point with the thumb pulp for 2–3

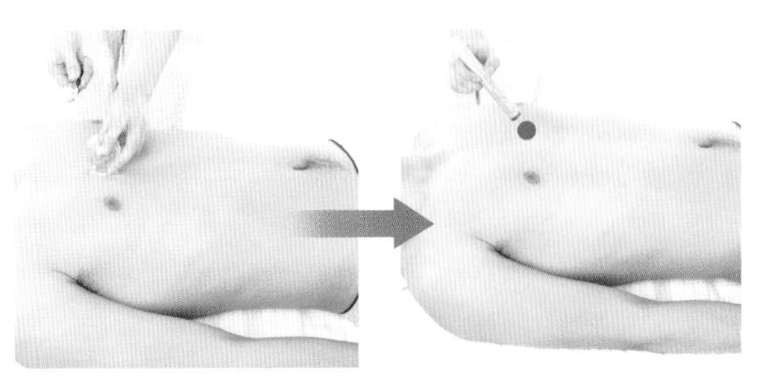

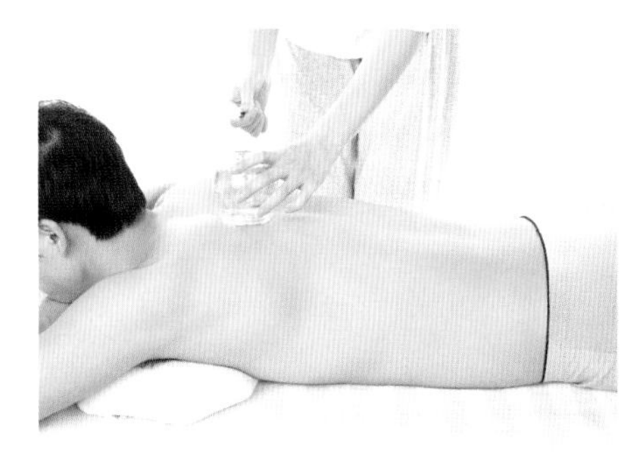

minutes, and then select and apply a cup of appropriate size to the point, retaining the cup for 10–15 minutes. After the cup is removed, perform moxibustion with a moxa stick for 3–5 minutes until warmth is felt.

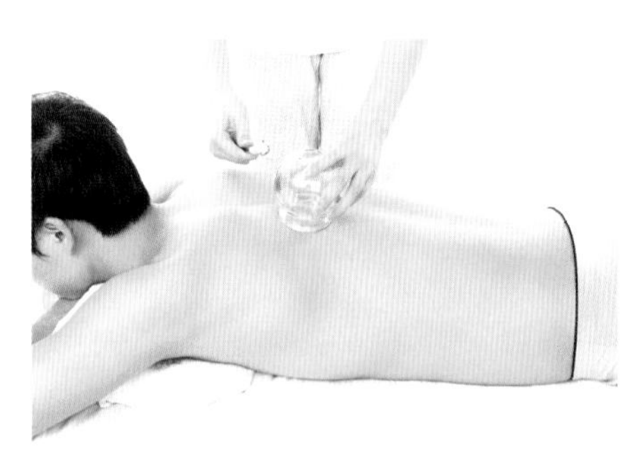

### 2. Xinshu Point

**Location:** Under the fifth thoracic vertebra on the inner side of the scapula, 1.5 cun horizontally away.

**Method:** Select a cup of appropriate size and apply it to Xinshu point. Retain the cup for 10–15 minutes. With the cup removed, perform moxibustion with a moxa box for 3–5 minutes.

### 3. Geshu Point

**Location:** At the point 1.5 cun away from the spinous process of the seventh thoracic vertebra.

**Method:** Select a cup of appropriate size and apply it to Geshu point. Retain the cup for 10–15 minutes.

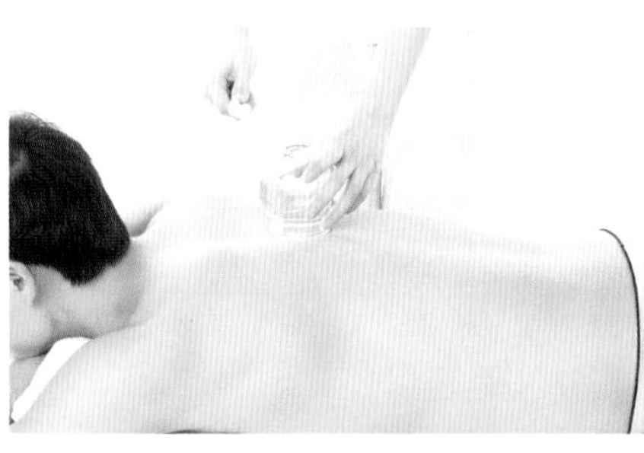

## The Second Group of Points

### 1. Zhiyang Point

**Location:** In a cavity below the spinous process of the seventh thoracic vertebra on the midline of the back.

**Method:** Select a cup of appropriate size and apply it to Zhiyang point. Retain the cup for 10–15 minutes. With the cup removed, perform moxibustion with a moxa box for 3–5 minutes.

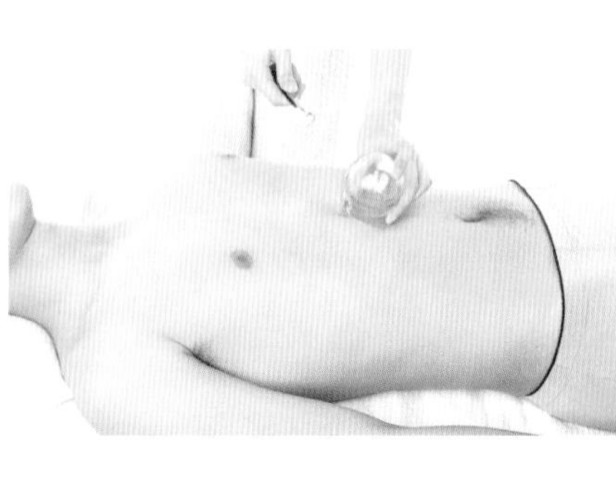

### 2. Juque Point

**Location:** On the upper abdomen, 6 cun above the center of the umbilicus, on the anterior midline.

**Method:** Knead Juque point with the thumb pulp for 2–3 minutes, and then cup the point, retaining the cup for 10–15 minutes. After the cup is removed, perform moxibustion with a moxa stick for 3–5 minutes until warmth is felt.

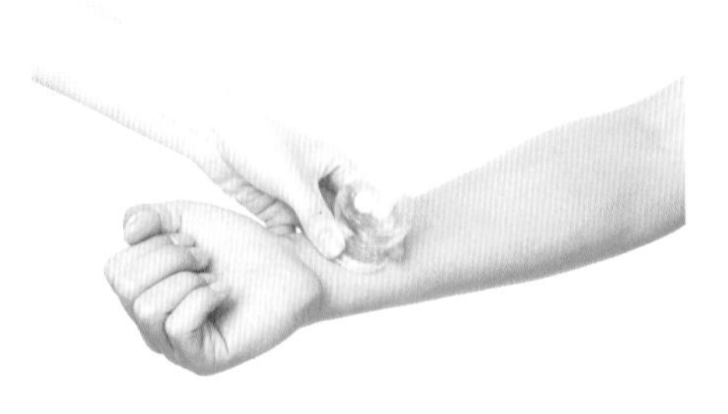

### 3. Neiguan Point

**Location:** Between the two tendons about 2 cun above the wrist joint bend.

**Method:** First knead Guanyuan point with the thumb pulp for 2–3 minutes, and then select and apply a cup of appropriate size to the point, retaining the cup for 10–15 minutes.

## The Third Group of Points

### 1. Shenmen Point

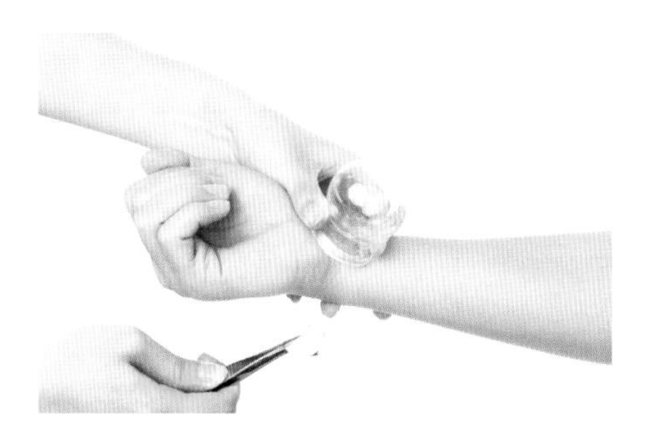

**Location:** On the inner wrist near the small finger when the palm is turned upward.

**Method:** First knead Shenmen point with the thumb pulp for 2–3 minutes until one feels sore and swelling at the point, and then apply a cup to the point, retaining the cup for 5–10 minutes.

### 2. Sanyinjiao Point

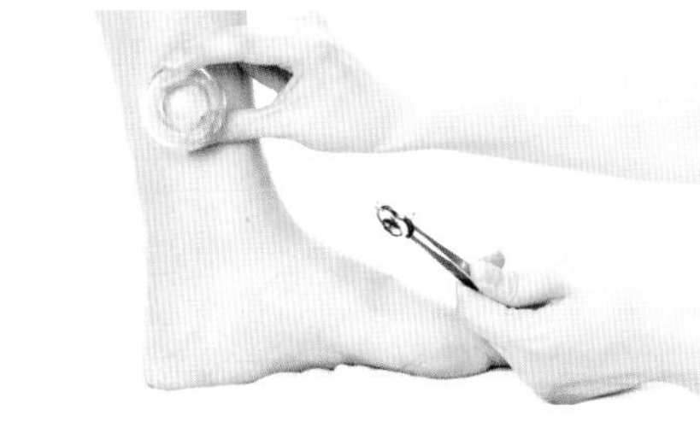

**Location:** At the rear edge of the shinbone, 3 cun above the ankle.

**Method:** First knead Sanyinjiao point with the thumb pulp for 2–3 minutes, and then select and apply a cup of appropriate size to the point, retaining the cup for 10–15 minutes.

### 3. Quze Point

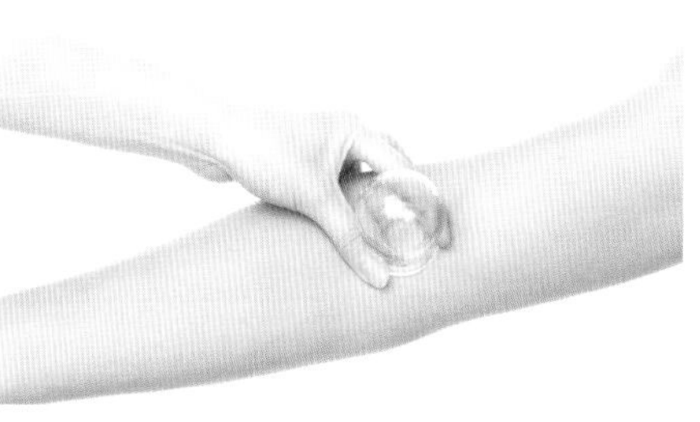

**Location:** With the elbow bent slightly, within the inner lateral margin of the biceps brachii on the cubital crease.

**Method:** Select and apply a cup of appropriate size to Quze point, retaining the cup for 10–15 minutes.

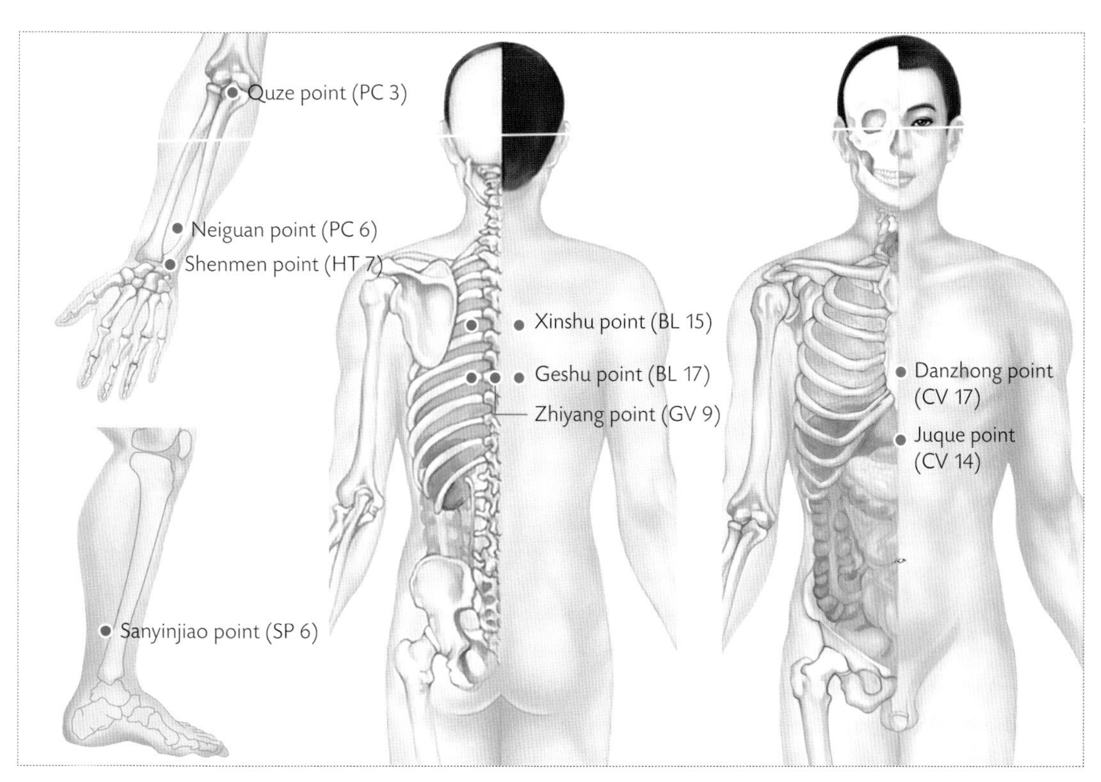

# 2 Diabetes

Diabetic patients often experience polyuria, polydipsia, polyphagia, and are lean with little flesh. The disease is often accompanied by hypodynamia, weakness, skin itch, soreness of limbs, loss of libido, impotence infertility, menstrual disorders, constipation, visual impairment, and so on.

At ordinary times, the patients should pay attention to the diet, enhance physical exercise, and test blood sugar by themselves. The cupping therapy is effective on light and medium stages of diabetes, and can alleviate the abovementioned symptoms and other accompanied symptoms. But the course of treatment is generally long. During the course of treatment, drugs should be taken to control blood sugar to delay harm to other internal organs.

The cupping is mainly applied to Feishu, Pishu, Shenshu, Yishu (i.e. Weiwanxiashu) and other back-shu points. In case of polydipsia, the cupping is mainly applied to Feishu point. In case of polyphagia, the cupping is mainly applied to Pishu point. And in case of polyuria, the cupping is mainly applied to Shenshu point. It may also be applied to Sanyinjiao, Guanyuan, Taixi, Zusanli, Neiguan, and Yinlingquan points.

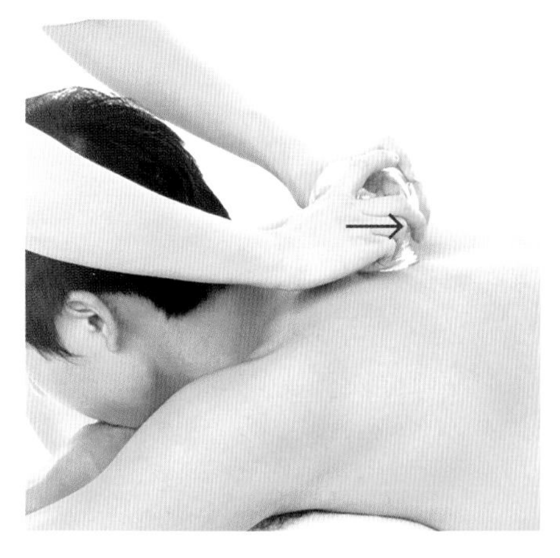

## Cupping Methods

### 1. Feishu Point

**Location:** At the point 1.5 cun beside the third thoracic vertebra on the inner side of the scapula.

**Method:** Use the moving cupping method by moving the cup on the bladder meridian on the back by segment along the meridian. Move the cup several times mainly on Feishu point, and repeatedly push and pull on the point back and forth, until the skin becomes red. The cup may be retained on the abovementioned point for 10–15 minutes after the moving cupping.

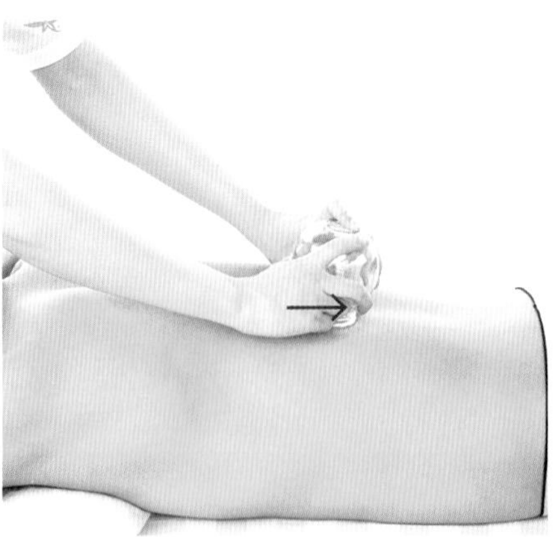

### 2. Pishu Point

**Location:** At the point 1.5 cun away horizontally from the eleventh thoracic vertebra.

**Method:** Use the moving cupping method by moving the cup on the bladder meridian on the back by segment along the meridian. Move the cup several times mainly on Pishu point, and repeatedly push and pull on the point back and forth, until the skin becomes red. The cup may be retained on the abovementioned point for 10–15 minutes after the moving cupping.

### 3. Shenshu Point

**Location:** 1.5 cun horizontally from the second lumbar spinal process.

**Method:** Use the moving cupping method by moving the cup on the bladder meridian on the back by segment along the meridian. Move the cup several times mainly on Shenshu point, and repeatedly push and pull on the point back and forth, until the skin becomes red. The cup may be retained on the abovementioned point for 10–15 minutes after the moving cupping.

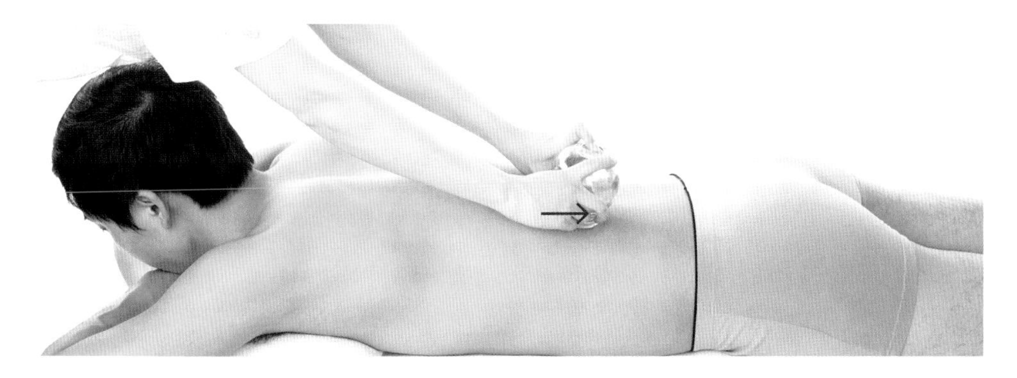

### 4. Guanyuan Point

**Location:** About 3 cun below the navel.

**Method:** Select a cup of appropriate size and apply it to Guanyuan point, retaining the cup for 10–15 minutes. With the cup removed, perform moxibustion with a moxa box for 3–5 minutes.

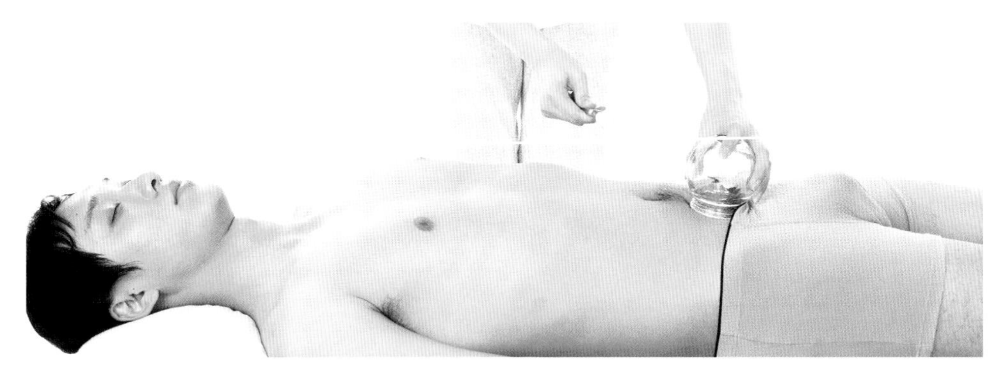

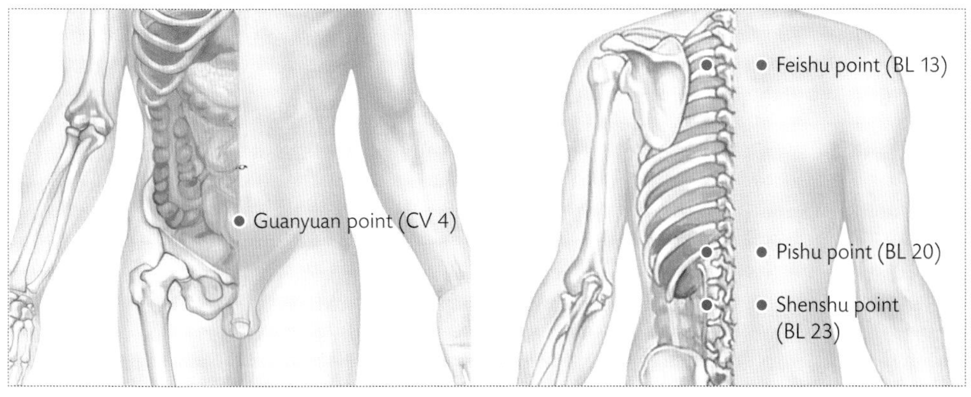

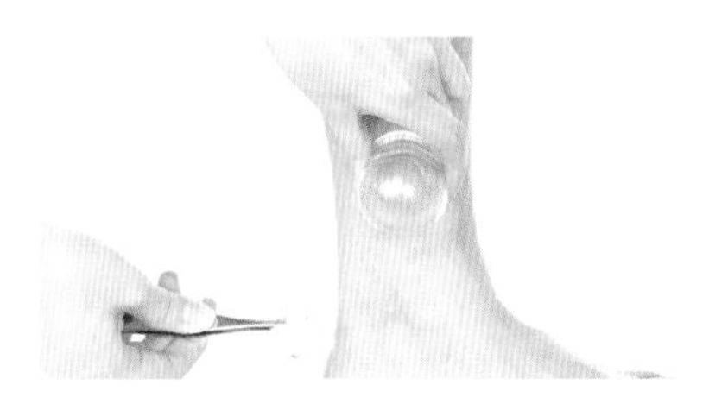

### 5. Sanyinjiao Point

**Location:** At the rear edge of the shinbone, 3 cun above the ankle.

**Method:** Knead Sanyinjiao point with the thumb pulp for 2–3 minutes, and then cup this point, retaining the cup for 10–15 minutes.

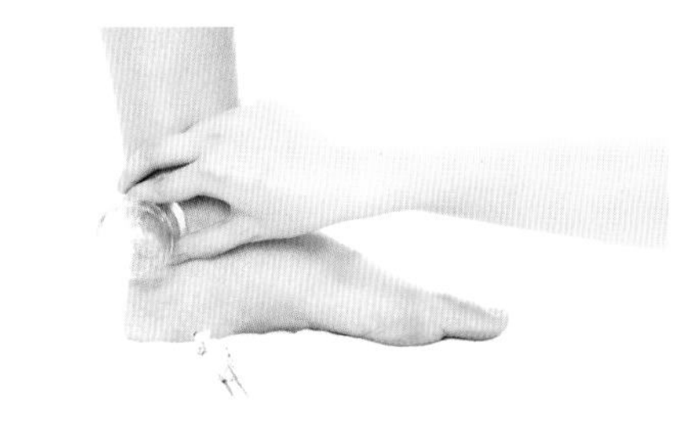

### 6. Taixi Point

**Location:** In a cavity between the medial malleolus and Achilles tendon.

**Method:** First knead Taixi point with the thumb pulp for 2–3 minutes, and then select a cup of appropriate size and apply it to the point, retaining the cup for 10–15 minutes.

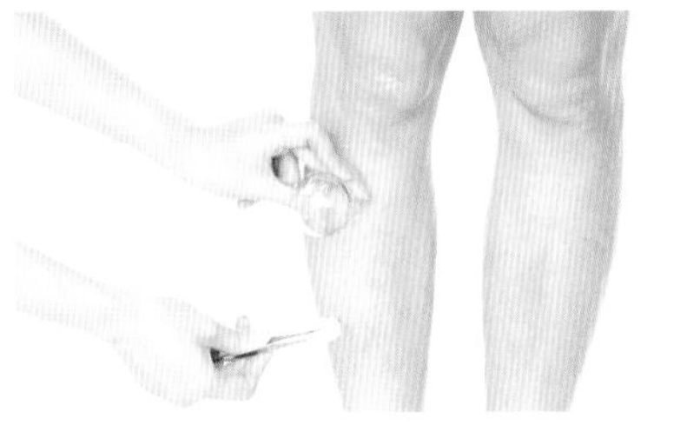

### 7. Zusanli Point

**Location:** About 3 cun below the knee on the outer side of the tibia.

**Method:** First knead Zusanli point with the thumb pulp for 2–3 minutes, and then select a cup of appropriate size and apply it to the point, retaining the cup for 10–15 minutes.

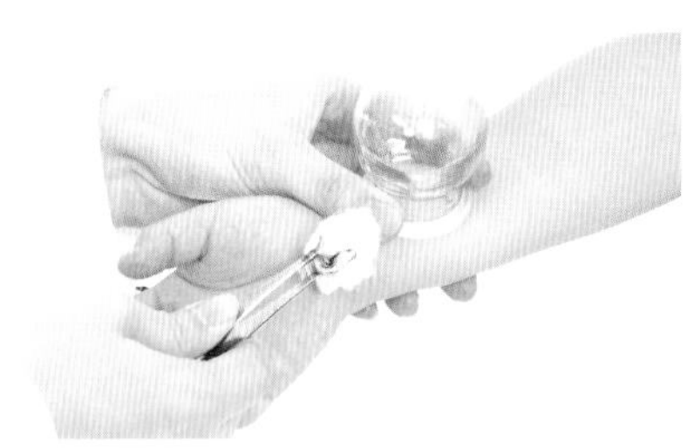

### 8. Neiguan Point

**Location:** Between the two tendons about 2 cun above the wrist joint bend.

**Method:** First knead Guanyuan point with the thumb pulp for 2–3 minutes, and then select and apply a cup of appropriate size to the point, retaining the cup for 10–15 minutes.

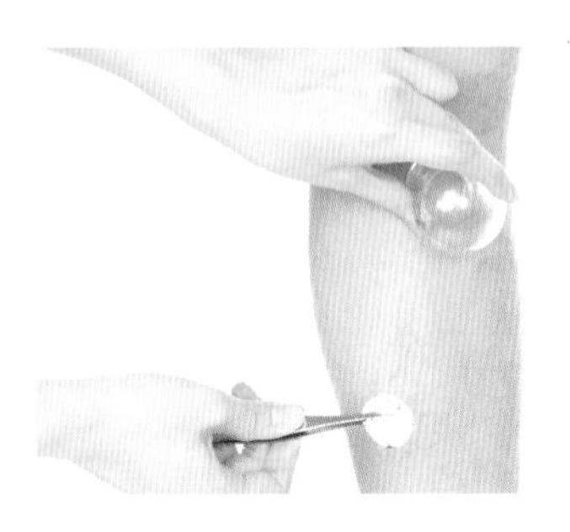

### 9. Yinlingquan Point

**Location:** In the depression on the inner edge of the shinbone below the knee.

**Method:** First knead Yinlingquan point with the thumb pulp for 2–3 minutes, and then cup this point, retaining the cup for 10–15 minutes. With the cup removed, perform moxibustion with a moxa stick for 3–5 minutes.

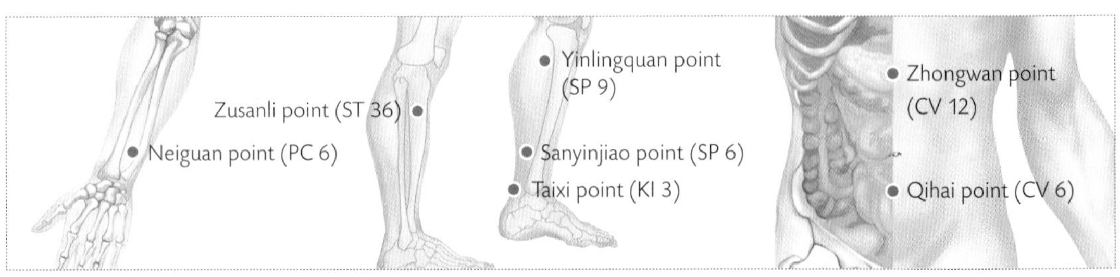

# 3 Hyperlipidemia

The patients of mild symptoms with the disease usually do not feel uncomfortable, and moderate patients may experience dizziness, fatigue, hypodynamia, insomnia, forgetfulness, limb numbness, palpitations, and so on.

The patients should strengthen physical exercise to promote consumption of excessive energy and reduce weight. At the same time, they should have a scientific and controlled diet by reducing the intake of high-fat food and absolutely avoiding fried food. They should eat more fruits and vegetables, drink less coffee, and stop smoking and drinking. They should also actively prevent other diseases caused by hyperlipidemia, such as coronary heart disease and cerebrovascular disease, regularly take physical examination, and pay attention to their physical conditions to receive timely treatment once the problem occurs.

The cupping is mainly applied to Zhongwan, Pishu, Weishu, Fenglong, Qihai, Xuehai, Sanyinjiao, and Taixi points. Select about 5 points from them for operation every day and cup different points in turn each time.

## Cupping Methods

### 1. Zhongwan Point

**Location:** On the upper abdomen, 4 cun above the center of the umbilicus, on the anterior midline.

**Method:** First massage the abdomen above the bellybutton for about 10 circles with the palm or corporately the index finger, the middle finger, and the ring finger. Then select a cup of appropriate size, and apply it to Zhongwan point, retaining the cup for 10–15 minutes. With the cup removed, perform moxibustion with a moxa box for 3–5 minutes until warmth is felt.

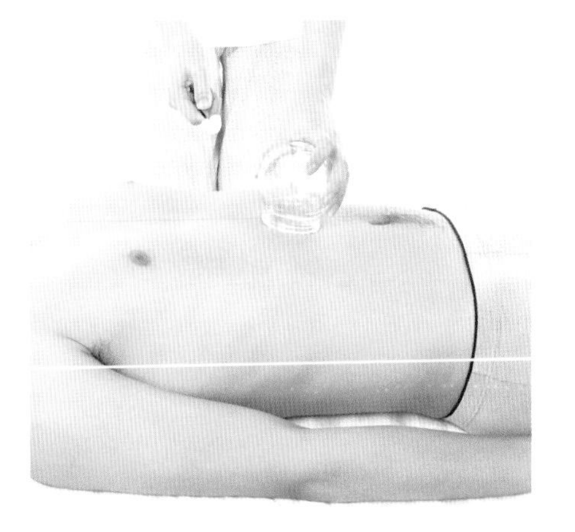

### 2. Qihai Point

**Location:** About 1.5 cun below the navel.

**Method:** First knead Qihai point with the thumb pulp for 2–3 minutes, and then select and apply a cup of appropriate size to the point, retaining the cup for 10–15 minutes. With the cup removed, perform moxibustion with a moxa stick or a moxa box for 3–5 minutes until warmth is felt.

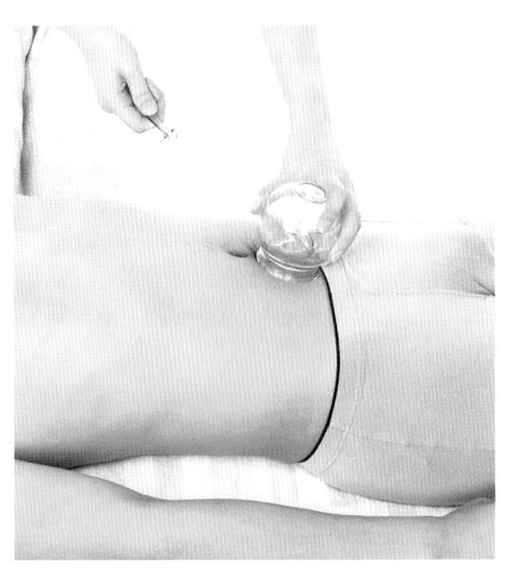

### 3. Pishu and Weishu Points

**Location:** Pishu point is 1.5 cun away horizontally from the eleventh thoracic vertebra; Weishu point is about 1.5 cun below the spinous process of the twelfth thoracic vertebra.

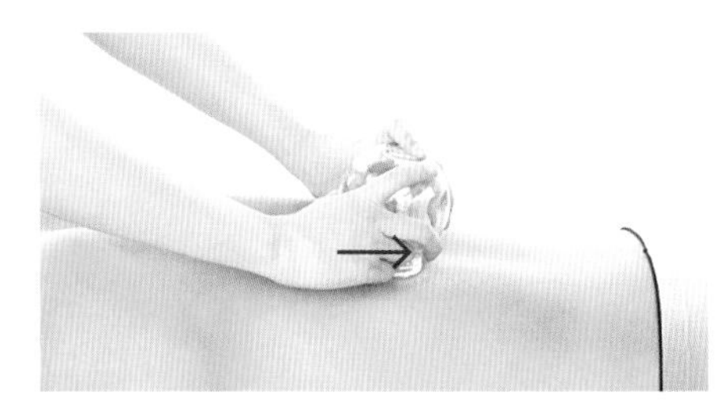

**Method:** Use the moving cupping method by moving the cup on the bladder meridian on the back by segment along the meridian. Move the cup several times mainly on Pishu and Weishu points, and repeatedly push and pull on the points back and forth, until the skin becomes red. The cup may be retained on the abovementioned points for 10–15 minutes after the moving cupping.

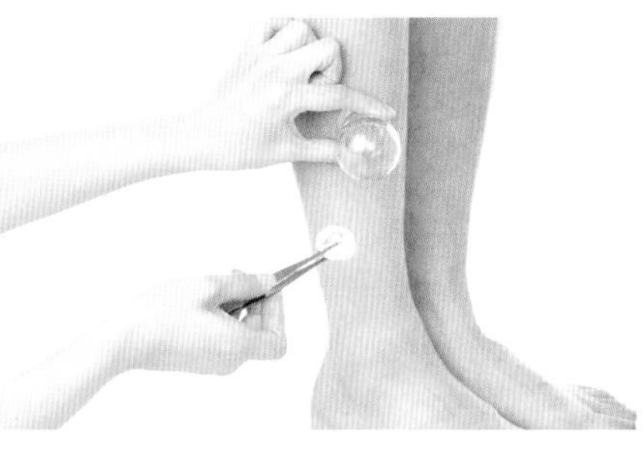

### 4. Fenglong Point

**Location:** 8 cun above the ankle tip.

**Method:** First knead the Fenglong point with the thumb pulp for 2–3 minutes, and then select and apply a cup of appropriate size to the point, retaining the cup for 10–15 minutes.

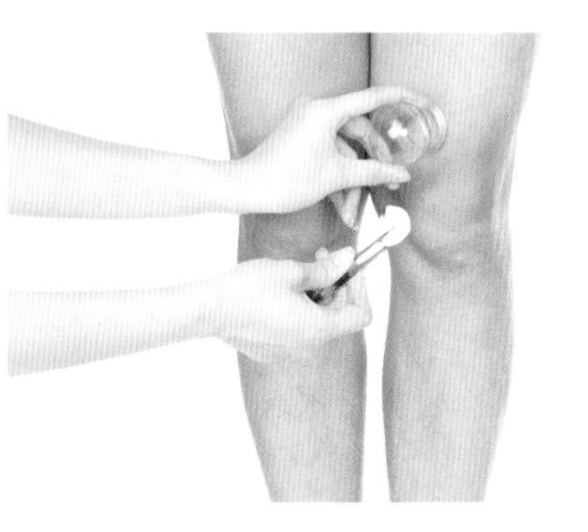

### 5. Xuehai Point

**Location:** In a cavity about 2 cun away from the inner upper corner of the patella, when the knee is bent.

**Method:** First knead Xuehai point with the thumb pulp for 2–3 minutes, and then select and apply a cup of appropriate size to the point, retaining the cup for 10–15 minutes. With the cup removed, perform moxibustion with a moxa stick for 3–5 minutes until warmth is felt.

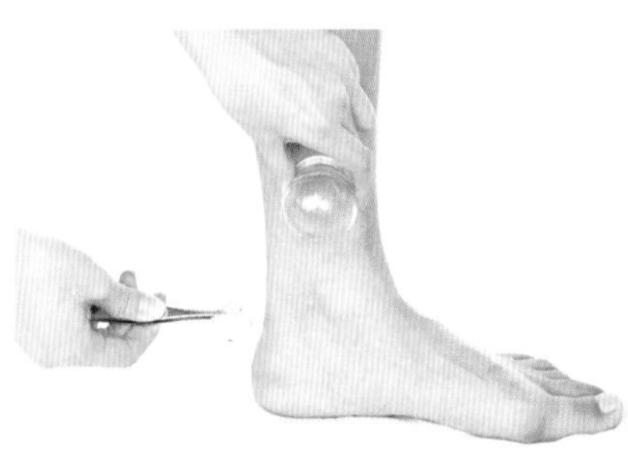

### 6. Sanyinjiao Point

**Location:** At the rear edge of the shinbone, 3 cun above the ankle.

**Method:** First knead Sanyinjiao point with the thumb pulp for 2–3 minutes, until soreness and swelling is felt. Then select and apply a cup of appropriate size to the point, retaining the cup for 10–15 minutes. With the cup removed, perform moxibustion with a moxa stick for 3–5 minutes, until warmth is felt.

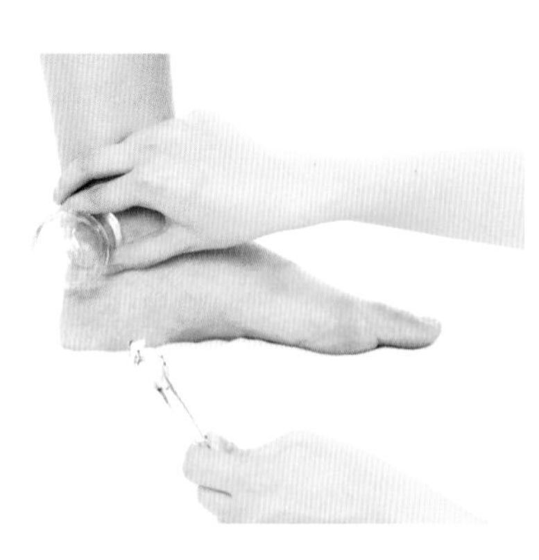

### 7. Taixi Point

**Location:** In a cavity between the medial malleolus and Achilles tendon.

**Method:** First knead Taixi point with the thumb pulp for 2–3 minutes, until soreness and swelling is felt. Then select a cup of appropriate size and apply it to the point, retaining the cup for 10–15 minutes.

# 4 Hypertension

Most people with hypertension initially have fatigue, and occasional dizziness and hypomnesia, which can be relieved after rest, and may have aggravated dizziness, headache and even nausea and vomiting when blood pressure increases obviously.

As the onset of high blood pressure is related to central nervous dysfunction, the patients should pay attention to maintaining a proper balance of work and rest. They should also maintain a good mood, and prevent emotional and mental excitation and nervousness, so as to avoid occurrence of cerebral blood vessel and cardiovascular accidents. They should also have a light diet, avoid spicy food, quit smoking and alcohol consumption, and control obesity. Those who have taken antihypertensive drugs do not need to stop medication suddenly during cupping, but should reduce the amount and time of medication gradually. During the treatment, they should avoid emotional fluctuation, have good rests, and keep bowels open. Patients with serious hypertension should also have treatment of the Traditional Chinese Medicine together with Western medicine.

The cupping can be applied to two groups of points, one group a day and two groups in turn, until the symptoms are alleviated. The first group includes Fengchi, Yongquan, Ganshu, Shenshu, and Zusanli points, and the second group includes Dazhui, Quchi, Fenglong, Taichong, and Taixi points.

## Cupping Methods

### The First Group of Points

#### 1. Fengchi Point

**Location:** In the depression on both sides of the large tendon behind the nape of the neck, next to the lower edge of the skull.

**Method:** First knead Fengchi point with the thumb pulp for 2–3 minutes, until a feeling of soreness and swelling is present. Then select a cup of appropriate size and apply it to the point, retaining the cup for 10–15 minutes.

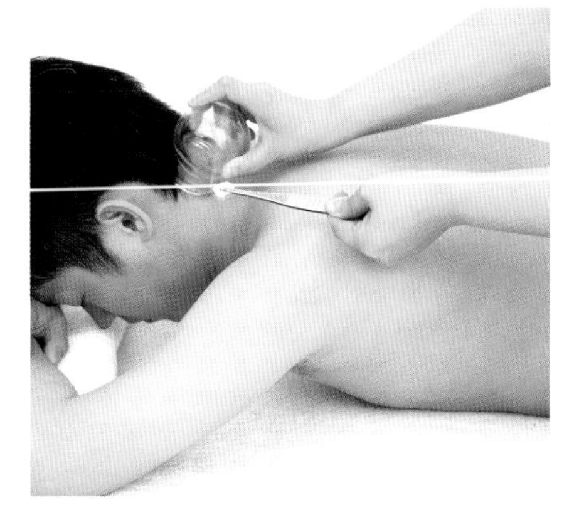

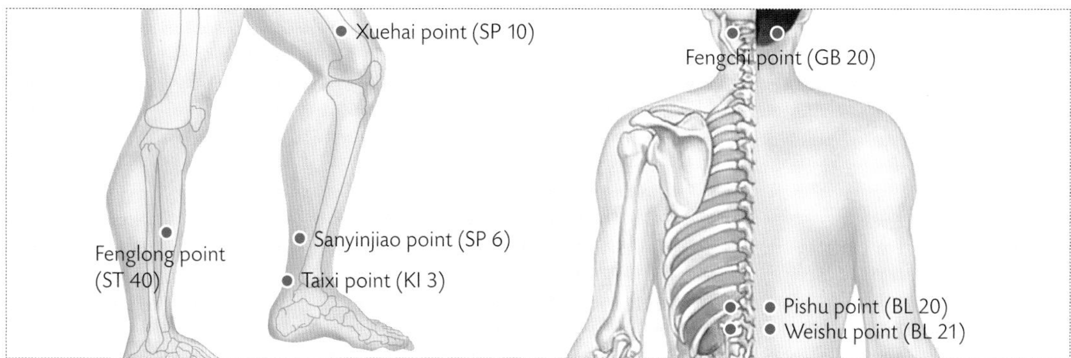

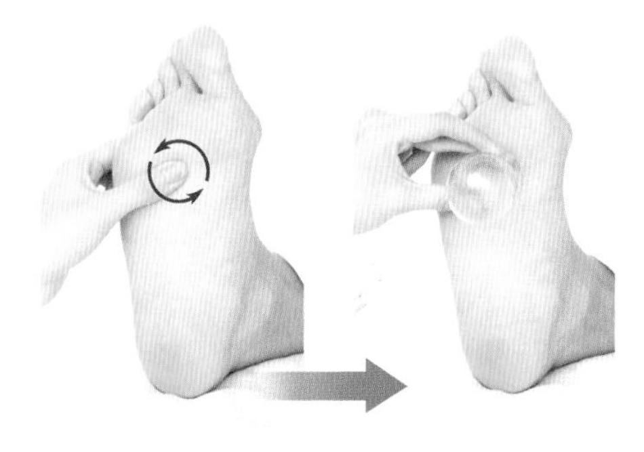

### 2. Yongquan Point

**Location:** In a depression in the front of the sole of the foot, about one-third of the way down from the toes.

**Method:** First knead Yongquan point with the thumb pulp for 2–3 minutes, and then select a cup of appropriate size and apply it to the point, retaining the cup for 10–15 minutes. With the cup removed, perform moxibustion with a moxa stick for 3–5 minutes until warmth is felt.

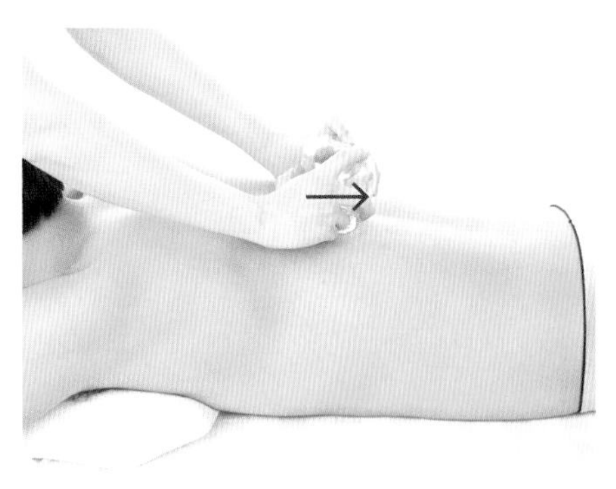

### 3. Ganshu and Shenshu Points

**Location:** Ganshu point is 1.5 cun away from the ninth thoracic spinal process on the inner side of the scapula; Shenshu point is 1.5 cun horizontally from the second lumbar spinal process.

**Method:** Use the moving cupping method by moving the cup on the bladder meridian on the back by segment along the meridian. Move the cup several times mainly on Ganshu and Shenshu points, and repeatedly push and pull on the points back and forth, until the skin becomes red. The cup may be retained on the abovementioned points for 10–15 minutes after the moving cupping.

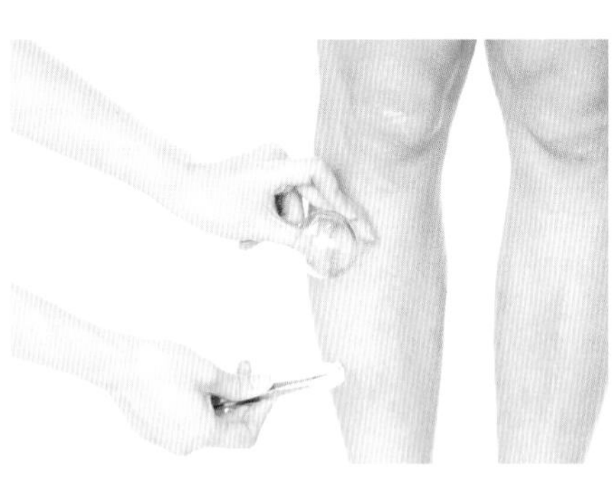

### 4. Zusanli Point

**Location:** About 3 cun below the knee on the outer side of the tibia.

**Method:** First knead Zusanli point with the thumb pulp for 2–3 minutes, and then select a cup of appropriate size and apply it to the point, retaining the cup for 10–15 minutes. With the cup removed, perform moxibustion with a moxa stick for 3–5 minutes until warmth is felt.

## The Second Group of Points

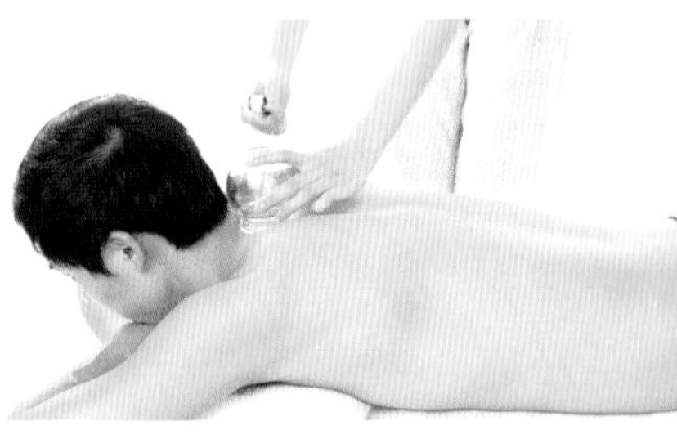

### 1. Dazhui Point

**Location:** Under the spinous process of the seventh cervical vertebrae.

**Method:** Select a cup of appropriate size and apply it to Dazhui point. Retain the cup for 10–15 minutes.

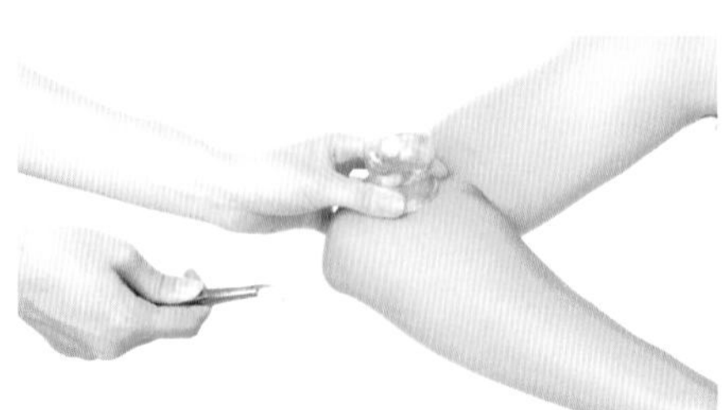

### 2. Quchi Point

**Location:** With the elbow bent halfway, on the outer side of the cubital transverse crease.

**Method:** Select a cup of appropriate size and apply it to Quchi point. Retain the cup for 10–15 minutes.

### 3. Fenglong Point

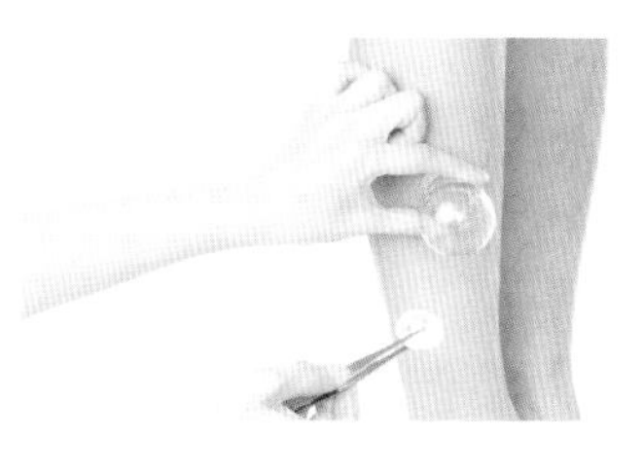

**Location:** 8 cun above the ankle tip.

**Method:** First knead the Fenglong point with the thumb pulp for 2–3 minutes, and then select and apply a cup of appropriate size to the point, retaining the cup for 10–15 minutes.

### 4. Taichong Point

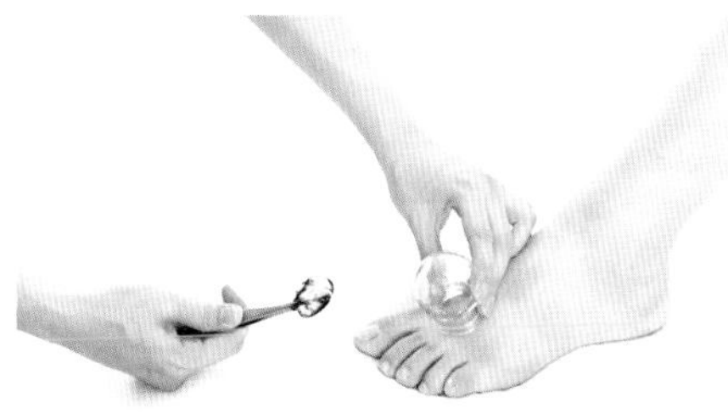

**Location:** On the foot in a notch between the first and second metatarsal bones.

**Method:** First knead Taichong point with the thumb pulp for 2–3 minutes, and then select and apply a cup of appropriate size to the point, retaining the cup for 10–15 minutes.

### 5. Taixi Point

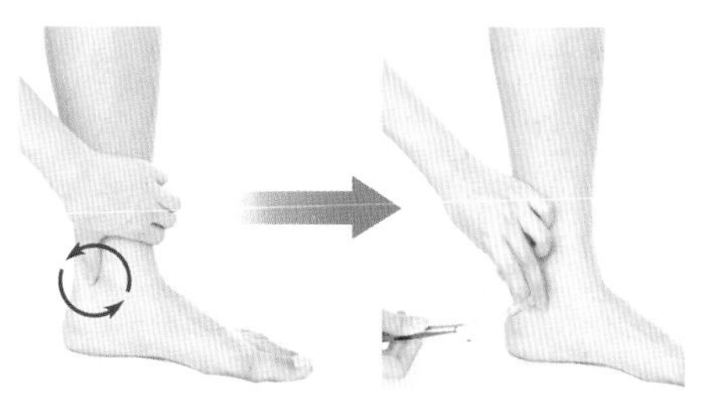

**Location:** In a cavity between the medial malleolus and Achilles tendon.

**Method:** First knead Taixi point with the thumb pulp for 2–3 minutes, and then select a cup of appropriate size and apply it to the point, retaining the cup for 10–15 minutes.

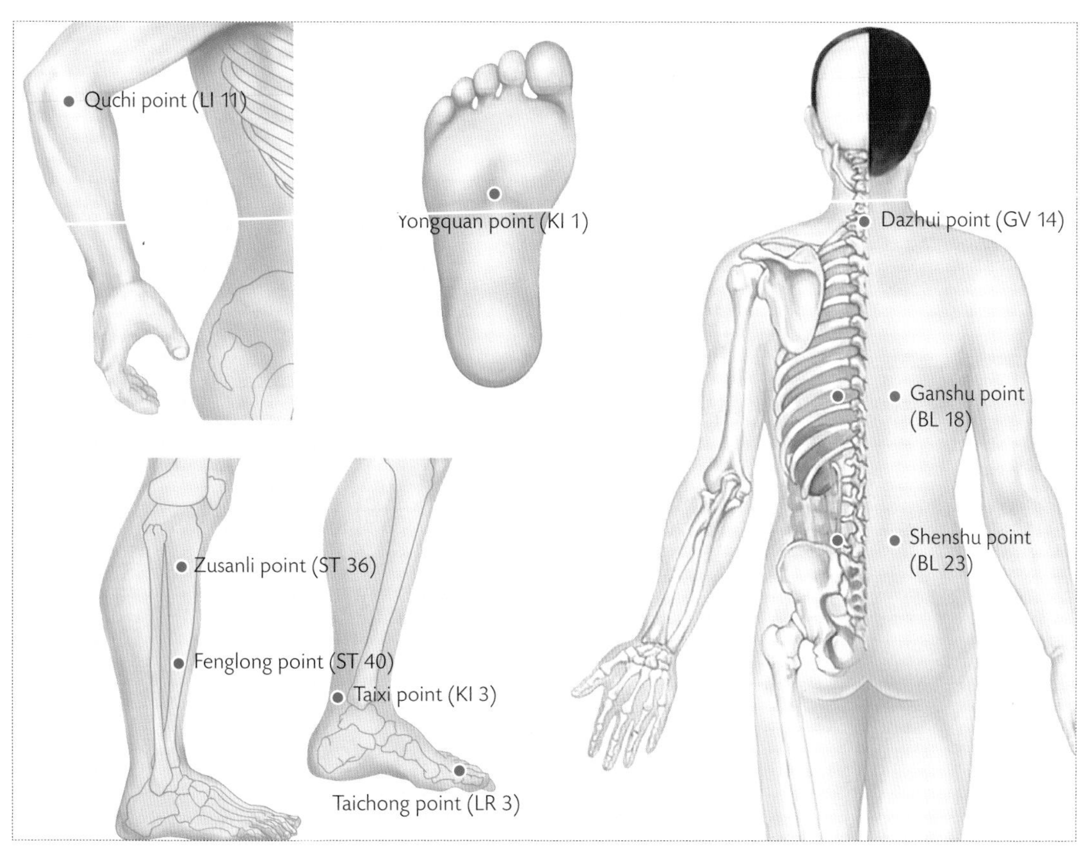

# 5 Hypotension

Patients with hypotension will feel headache, dizziness, loss of weight, tinnitus, palpitation, fatigue, shortness of breath, have sallow or pale complexion, cold hands and feet, spontaneous perspiration, and forgetfulness, as well as frequent occurrence of syncope in a severe case.

Patients should avoid overfatigue, have regular diets, eat more foods with high protein for energy, and quit smoking and alcohol consumption. They may also eat more warm and tonic food like lamb, chicken, leeks, ginger and cinnamon, drink more ginger tea, and avoid eating raw and cold food. They should not participate in strenuous exercise, should get up slowly in the morning, flex and extend limbs slowly, lift heavy objects or stand up after defecation slowly.

The cupping can be applied to two groups of points, one group a day and two groups in turn, until the symptoms are alleviated or disappear. The first group mainly includes Baihui, Xinshu, Pishu, Shenshu, and Sanyinjiao points, and the second group mainly includes Guanyuan, Yongquan, Mingmen, Zusanli, and Taixi points.

## Cupping Methods

### The First Group of Points

#### 1. Baihui Point

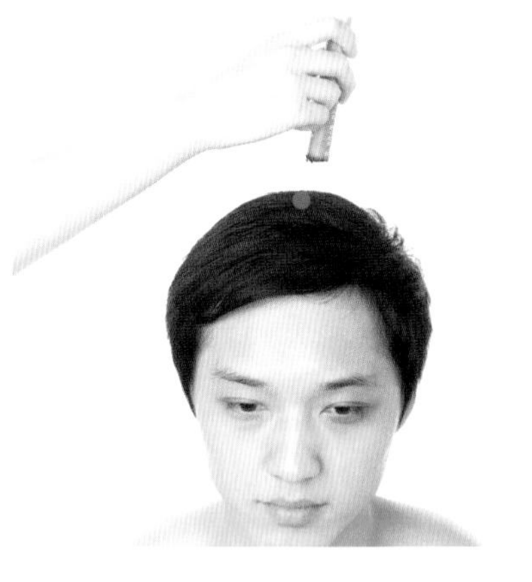

**Location:** On the head, 5 cun superior to the anterior hairline, on the anterior midline.

**Method:** Cup on Baihui point for 10–15 times by using the flash cupping method. Do not retain the cup. Then perform moxibustion with a moxa stick for 3–5 minutes until warmth is felt. If cupping is improper as the hair of the patient is too long, then skip the cupping and do moxibustion directly.

#### 2. Xinshu, Pishu and Shenshu Points

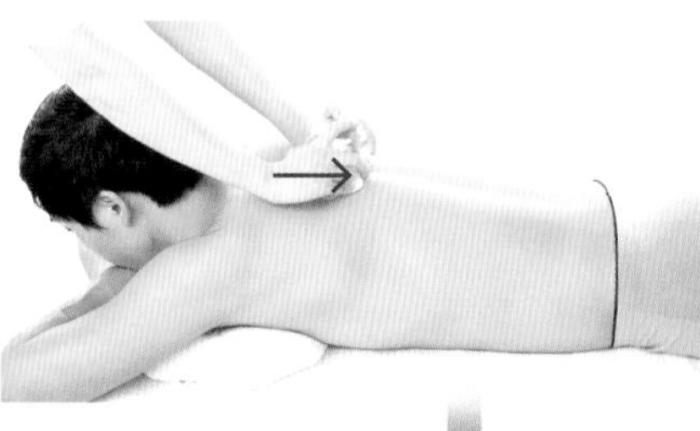

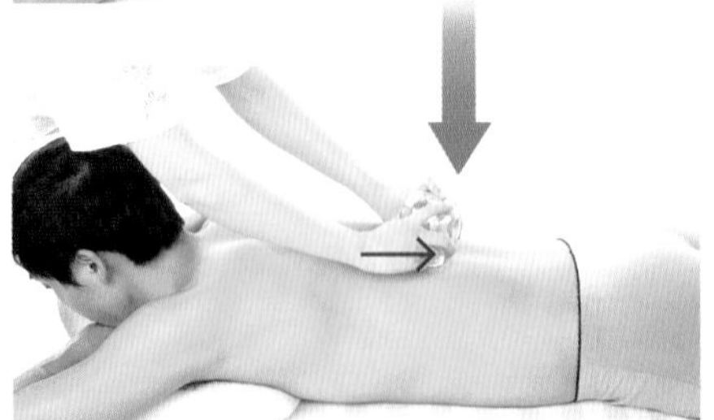

**Location:** Xinshu point is under the fifth thoracic vertebra on the inner side of the scapula, 1.5 cun horizontally away; Pishu point is 1.5 cun away horizontally from the eleventh thoracic vertebra; Shenshu point is 1.5 cun horizontally from the second lumbar spinal process.

**Method:** Use the moving cupping method. Move the cup on the bladder meridian on the back by segment along the meridian, and move the cup several times mainly on the Xinshu, Pishu and Shenshu points. Repeatedly push and pull on the points back and forth, until the skin becomes red. The cup may be retained on the abovementioned points for 10–15 minutes after the moving cupping.

### 3. Sanyinjiao Point

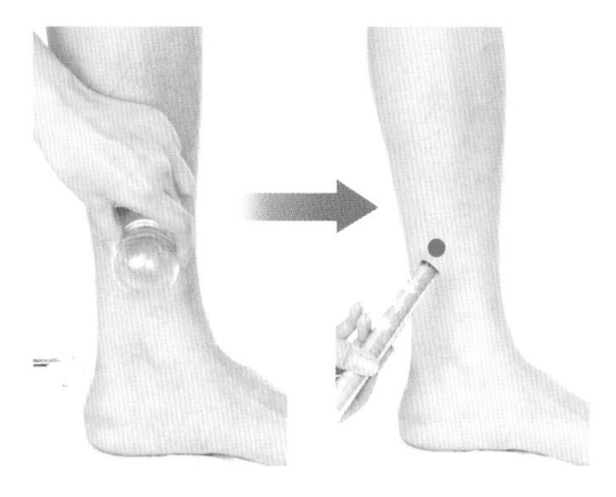

**Location:** At the rear edge of the shinbone, 3 cun above the ankle.

**Method:** First knead Sanyinjiao point with the thumb pulp for 2–3 minutes, until soreness and swelling is felt. Then select and apply a cup of appropriate size to the point, retaining the cup for 10–15 minutes. With the cup removed, perform moxibustion with a moxa stick for 3–5 minutes, until warmth is felt.

## The Second Group of Points

### 1. Guanyuan Point

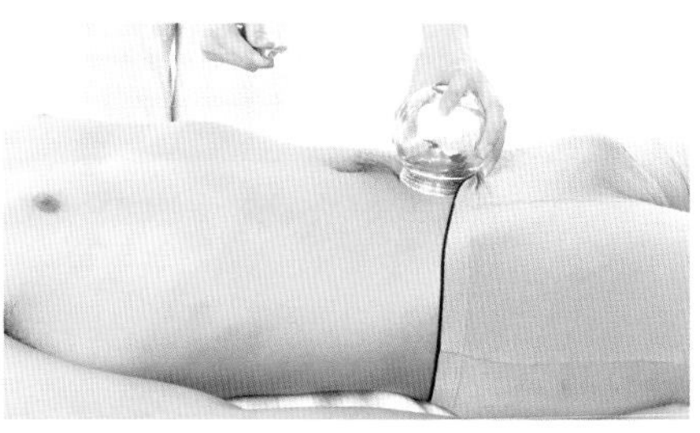

**Location:** About 3 cun below the navel.

**Method:** Cup on Guanyuan point, and retain the cup for 10–15 minutes. After the cup is removed, perform moxibustion with a moxa stick for 3–5 minutes until warmth is felt.

### 2. Yongquan Point

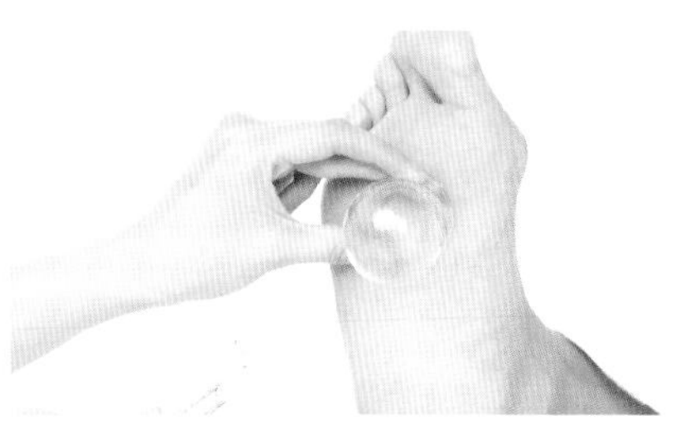

**Location:** In a depression in the front of the sole of the foot, about one-third of the way down from the toes.

**Method:** First, knead Yongquan point with the palm for 2–3 minutes until a feeling of heat is present. Then cup the point, retaining the cup for 10–15 minutes until warmth is felt.

### 3. Mingmen Point

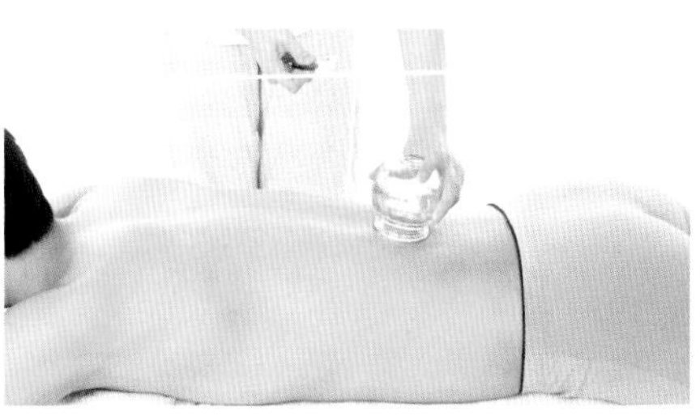

**Location:** In a cavity below the spinous process of the second cervical vertebra.

**Method:** Select and apply a cup of appropriate size to the point, retaining the cup for 10–15 minutes. With the cup removed, perform moxibustion with a moxa stick for 3–5 minutes until warmth is felt.

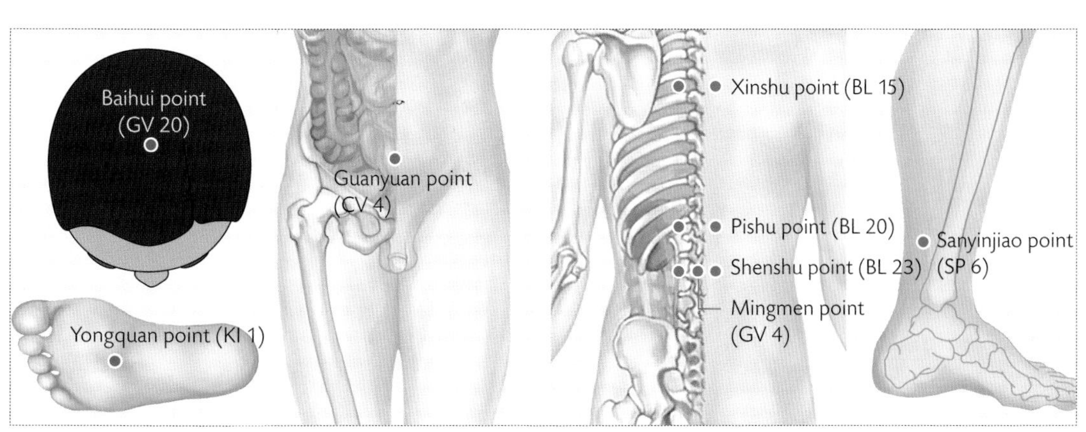

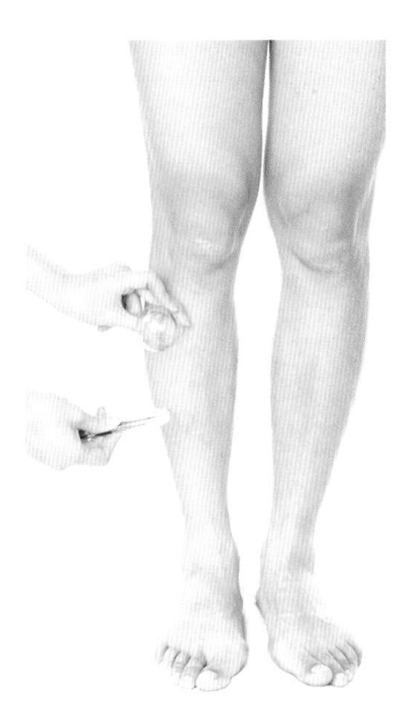

### 4. Zusanli Point

**Location:** About 3 cun below the knee on the outer side of the tibia.

**Method:** First knead Zusanli point with the thumb pulp for 2–3 minutes, and then select a cup of appropriate size and apply it to the point, retaining the cup for 10–15 minutes. With the cup removed, perform moxibustion with a moxa stick for 3–5 minutes until warmth is felt.

### 5. Taixi Point

**Location:** In a cavity between the medial malleolus and Achilles tendon.

**Method:** First knead Taixi point with the thumb pulp for 2–3 minutes, until soreness and swelling is felt. Then select a cup of appropriate size and apply it to the point, retaining the cup for 10–15 minutes.

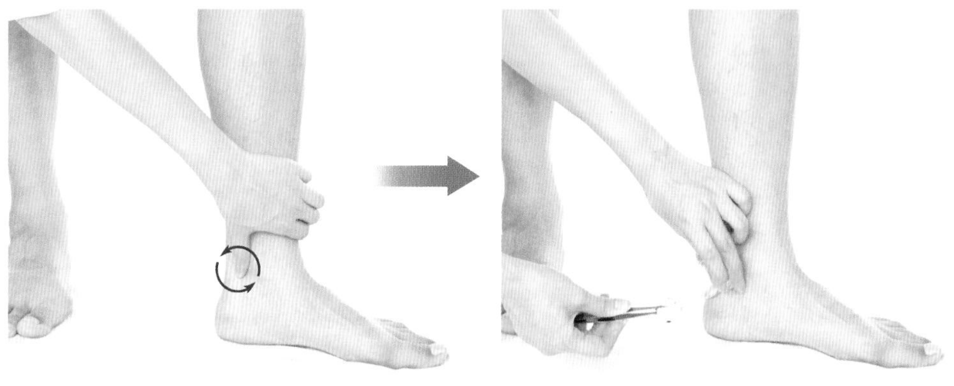

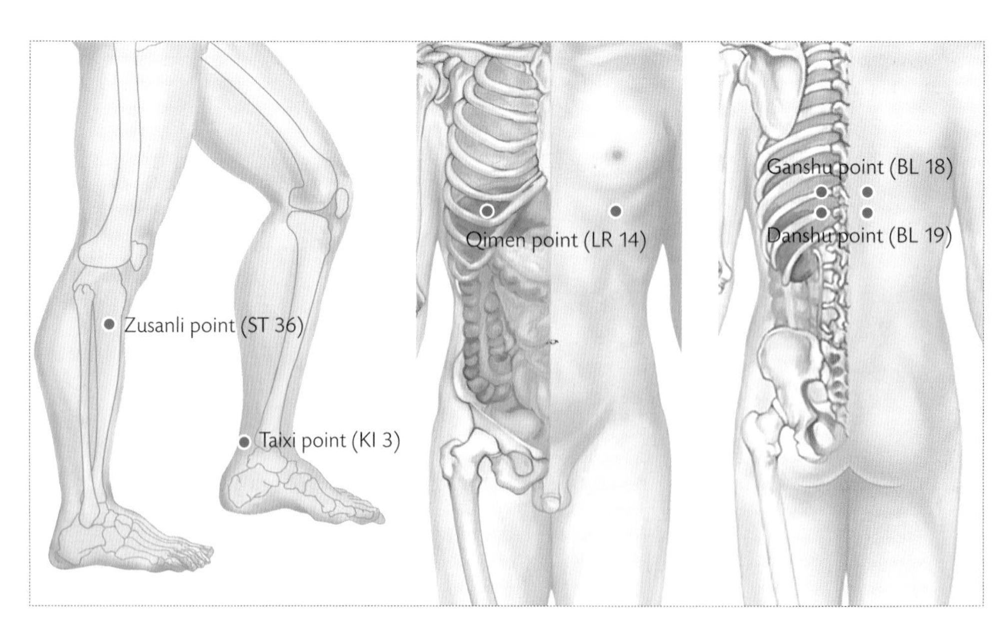

# 6 Liver Disease

The manifestations of liver disease are not obvious under normal circumstances, with main symptoms including fatigue and poor appetite, accompanied by distending pain or discomfort, nausea, aversion to greasy food, fullness after eating, or jaundice.

To promote the repair of liver tissues, one can take in high protein foods like fish, meat, and milk, and eat more fruits and vegetables to increase the intake of vitamins, such as carrot, water spinach, mushroom and white gourd, which are helpful for the recuperation of liver disease. Avoid excessive intake of animal fat and cholesterol, and quit smoking and alcohol consumption.

The cupping should be applied mainly to Ganshu, Danshu, Qimen, Zusanli, and Yanglingquan points, plus Shenshu point for those with fatigue, Zhongwan point for those with poor appetite, and Yinlingquan point for those with dropsical limbs.

## Cupping Methods

### 1. Ganshu Point

**Location:** 1.5 cun away from the ninth thoracic spinal process on the inner side of the scapula.

**Method:** Use the moving cupping method. Move the cup on the bladder meridian on the back by segment along the meridian, and move the cup several times mainly on the Ganshu point. Repeatedly push and pull on the point back and forth, until the skin becomes red. Retain the cup for 10–15 minutes after the moving cupping.

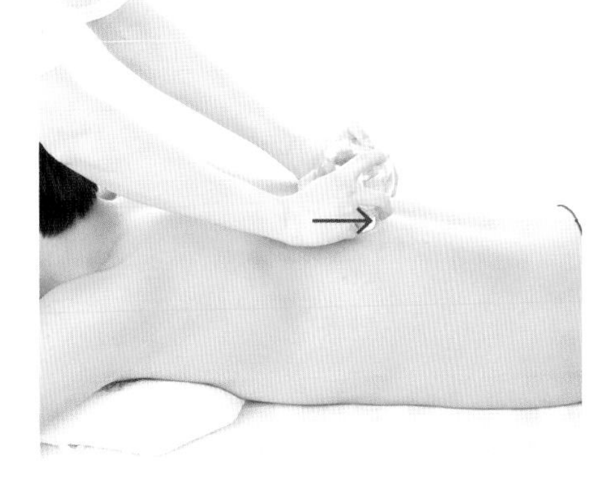

### 2. Danshu Point

**Location:** In the spine area, 1.5 cun lateral to the posterior midline of the lower border of the spinous process of the tenth thoracic vertebra.

**Method:** Use the moving cupping method. Move the cup on the bladder meridian on the back by segment along the meridian, and move the cup several times mainly on the Danshu point. Repeatedly push and pull on the point back and forth, until the skin becomes red. Retain the cup for 10–15 minutes after the moving cupping.

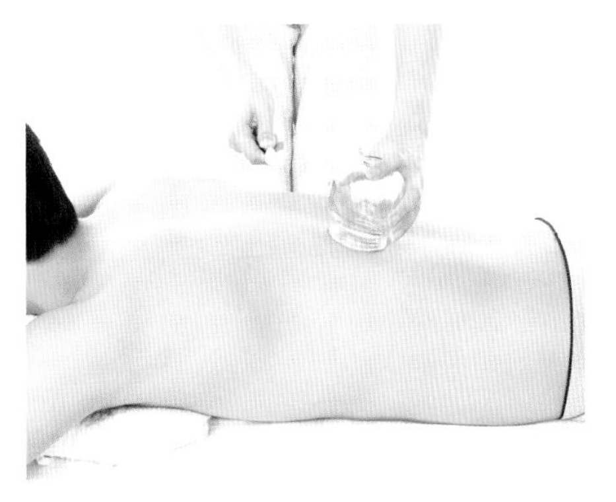

### 3. Qimen Point

**Location:** In the sixth intercostal space directly below the nipple.

**Method:** Select and apply a cup of appropriate size to the point, retaining the cup for 10–15 minutes.

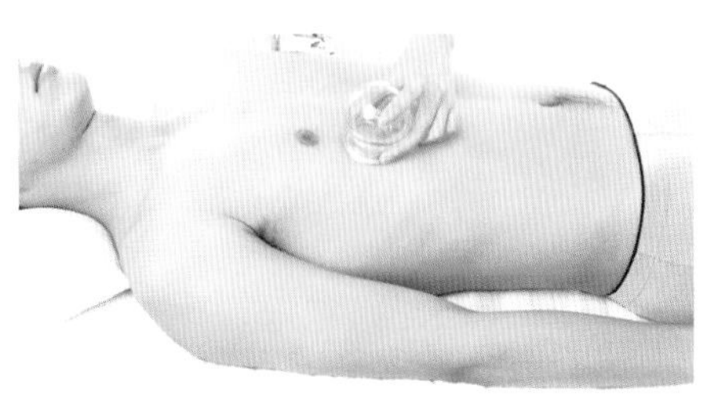

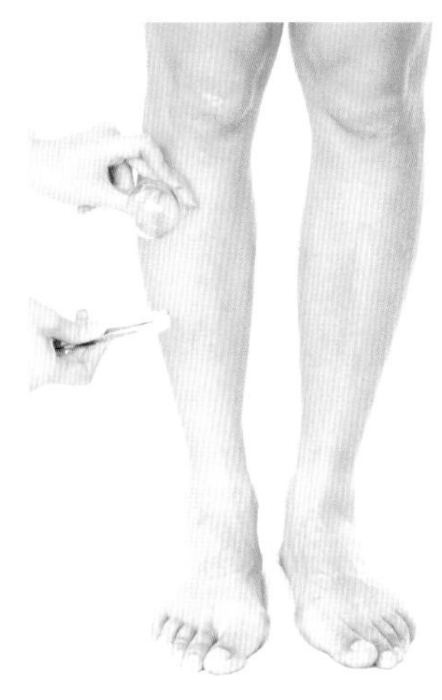

### 4. Zusanli Point

**Location:** About 3 cun below the knee on the outer side of the tibia.

**Method:** First knead Zusanli point with the thumb pulp for 2–3 minutes, and then select a cup of appropriate size and apply it to the point, retaining the cup for 10–15 minutes. With the cup removed, perform moxibustion with a moxa stick for 3–5 minutes until warmth is felt.

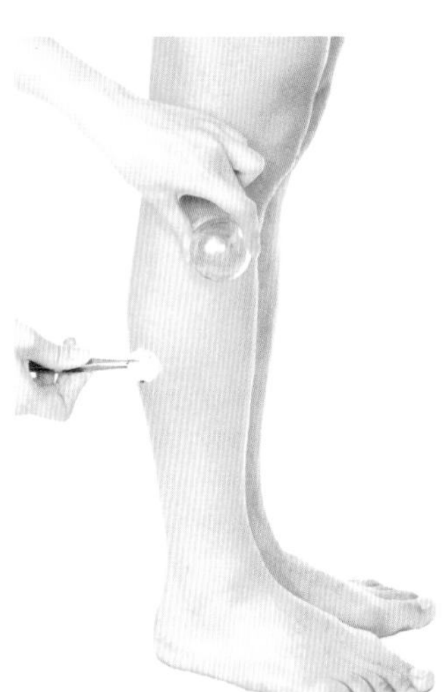

### 5. Yanglingquan Point

**Location:** On the outer side of the shin in a notch at the front lower part of the fibula.

**Method:** First knead Yanglingquan point with the thumb tip for 2–3 minutes. Then apply a cup of appropriate size to the point, and retain the cup for 10–15 minutes. With the cup removed, perform moxibustion with a moxa stick for 3–5 minutes until warmth is felt.

### 6. Shenshu Point

**Location:** 1.5 cun horizontally from the second lumbar spinal process.

**Method:** Use the moving cupping method. Move the cup on the bladder meridian on the back by segment along the meridian, and move it several times mainly on the Shenshu point. Repeatedly push and pull on the point back and forth, until the skin becomes red. The cup may be retained on the abovementioned point for 10–15 minutes after the moving cupping.

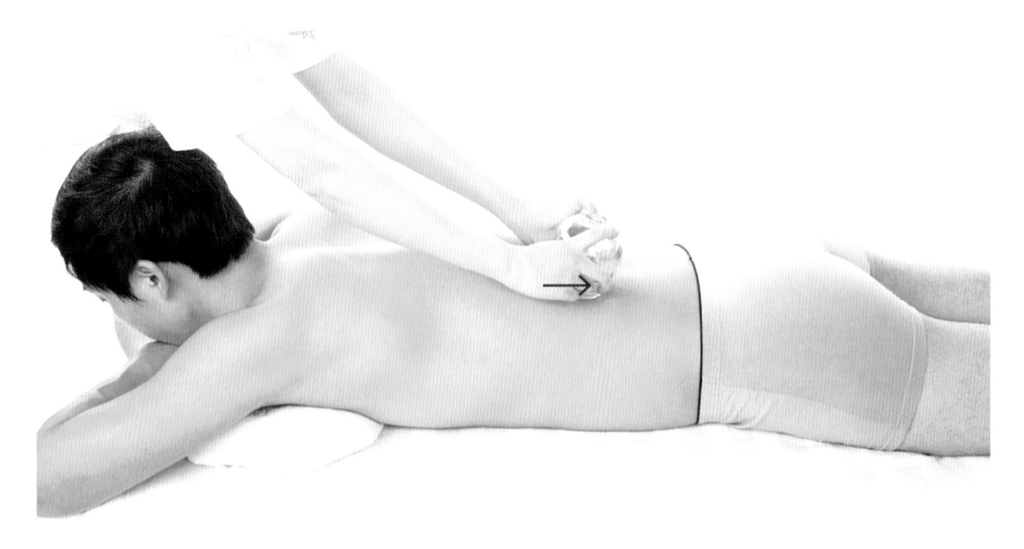

### 7. Zhongwan Point

**Location:** On the upper abdomen, 4 cun above the center of the umbilicus, on the anterior midline.

**Method:** First massage the abdomen above the bellybutton for about 10 circles with the palm or corporately the index finger, the middle finger, and the ring finger. Then select a cup of appropriate size, and apply it to Zhongwan point, retaining the cup for 10–15 minutes. With the cup removed, perform moxibustion with a moxa box for 3–5 minutes until warmth is felt.

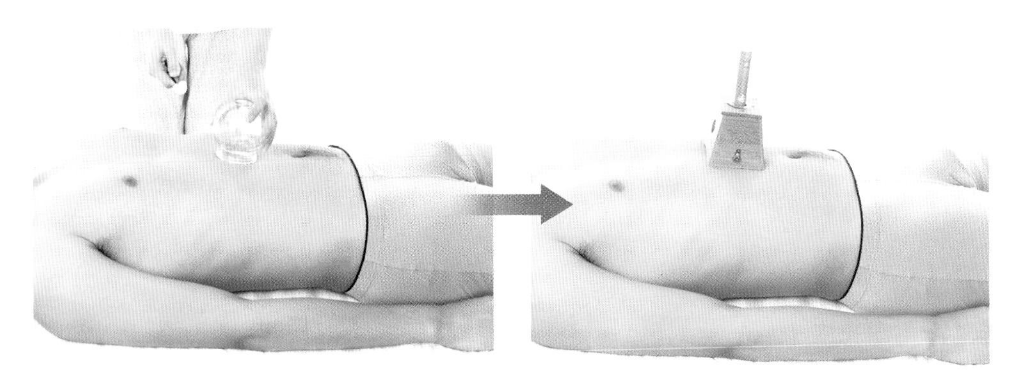

### 8. Yinlingquan Point

**Location:** In the depression on the inner edge of the shinbone below the knee.

**Method:** First knead Yinlingquan point with the thumb pulp for 2–3 minutes, and then cup this point, retaining the cup for 10–15 minutes. With the cup removed, perform moxibustion with a moxa stick for 3–5 minutes.

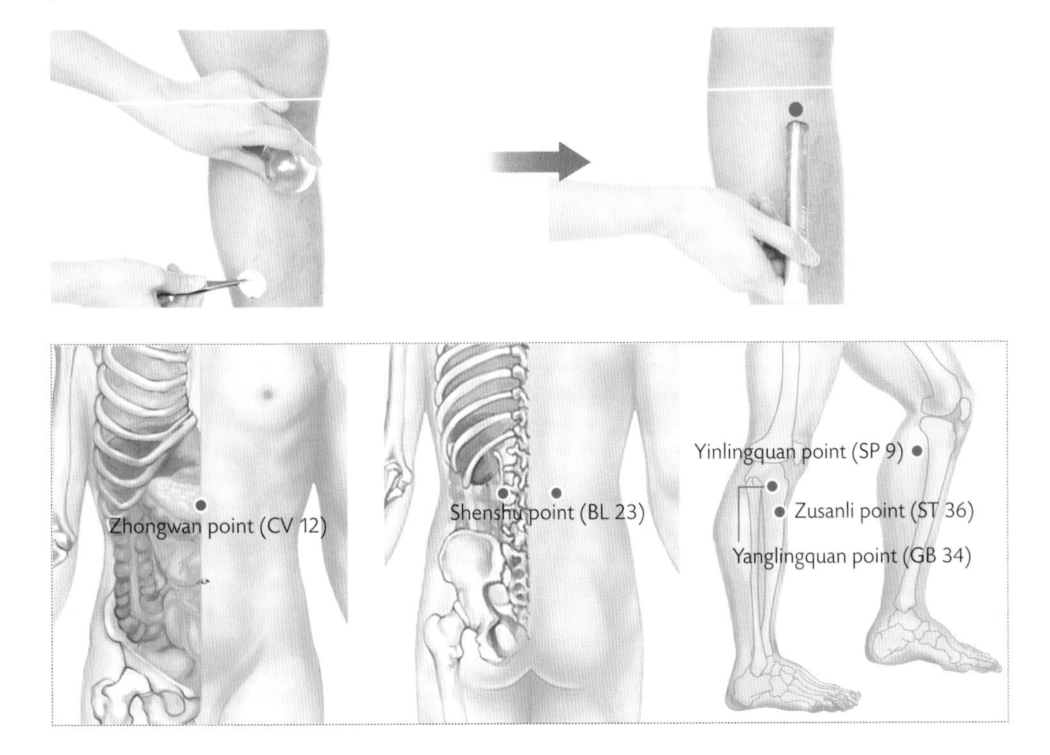

# 7 Stomach Disease

Stomach disease is a general term for many digestive diseases. They have similar symptoms like discomfort and pain of upper abdomen, fullness after a meal, belching, sour regurgitation, and even nausea, vomiting, etc.

Patients with stomach disease should firstly have regular diets, instead of being too hungry or eating too much. Insisting on having dinner at a regular time and at a proper amount can form a conditioned reflex, which is helpful for secretion of digestive glands, and is more conducive to digestion. While eating, they should chew carefully and swallow slowly, and eat less fried, pickled, raw, cold or stimulating food, and quit smoking and alcohol consumption. They should also supplement vitamin C which can protect the stomach. Normal content of vitamin C in the gastric juice can effectively help the stomach function, and protect it and enhance its disease resistance. Moreover, they should pay attention to keeping the stomach warm, without exposure to coldness. The discomfort of the stomach caused by long-term use of drugs can be regulated through Traditional Chinese Medicine.

The cupping can be applied to two groups of points, one group a day and two groups in turn, until the symptoms disappear. The first group includes Zhongwan, Zhangmen, Guanyuan, Jiuwei, and Zusanli points. The second group mainly includes Pishu, Weishu, Neiguan, and Gongsun points.

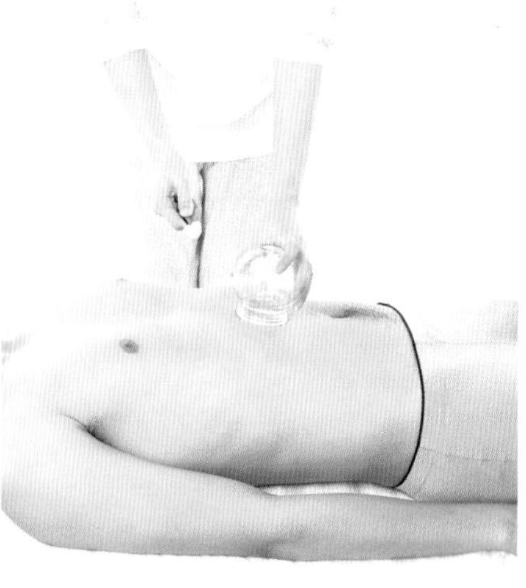

## Cupping Methods

### The First Group of Points

#### 1. Zhongwan Point

**Location:** On the upper abdomen, 4 cun above the center of the umbilicus, on the anterior midline.

**Method:** First massage the abdomen above the bellybutton for about 10 circles with the palm or corporately the index finger, the middle finger, and the ring finger. Then select a cup of appropriate size, and apply it to Zhongwan point, retaining the cup for 10–15 minutes. With the cup removed, perform moxibustion with a moxa box for 3–5 minutes until warmth is felt.

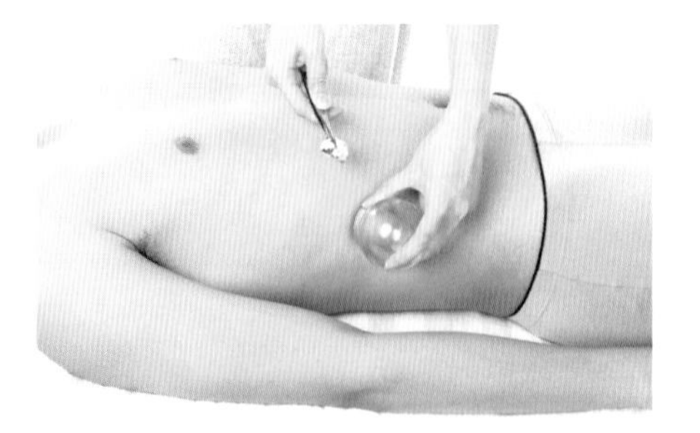

#### 2. Zhangmen Point

**Location:** On the lateral abdomen, below the free extremity of the eleventh rib.

**Method:** Knead Zhangmen point with the thumb pulp for 2–3 minutes, and then cup this point, retaining the cup for 10–15 minutes. With the cup removed, perform moxibustion with a moxa stick for 3–5 minutes until warmth is felt.

### 3. Guanyuan Point

**Location:** About 3 cun below the navel.

**Method:** First knead Guanyuan point with the thumb pulp for 2–3 minutes, and then select and apply a cup of appropriate size to the point, retaining the cup for 10–15 minutes. With the cup removed, perform moxibustion with a moxa stick for 3–5 minutes until warmth is felt.

### 4. Jiuwei Point

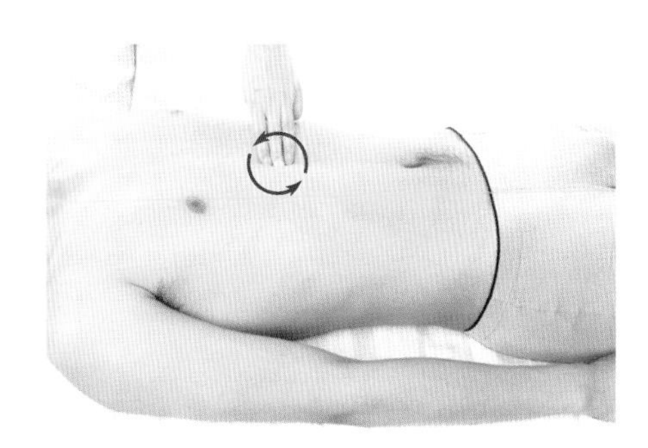

**Location:** On the upper abdomen, 1 cun below the sternocostal angle, on the anterior midline.

**Method:** Kneed Jiuwei point with the palm or with the index finger, the middle finger, and the ring finger together for 3–5 minutes, retaining the cup for 10–15 minutes. With the cup removed, perform moxibustion with a moxa box for 3–5 minutes until warmth is felt.

### 5. Zusanli Point

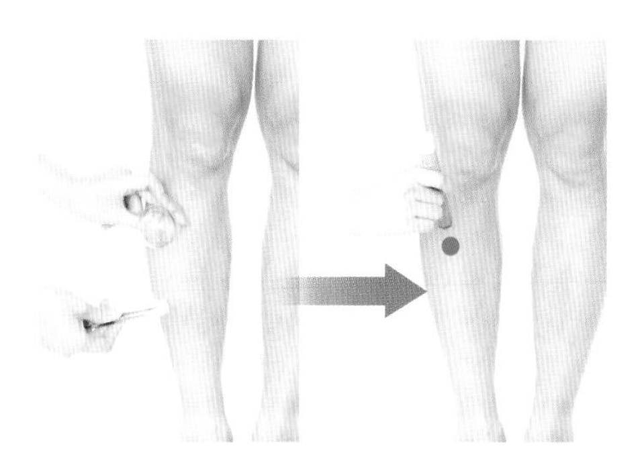

**Location:** About 3 cun below the knee on the outer side of the tibia.

**Method:** First knead Zusanli point with the thumb pulp for 2–3 minutes, and then select a cup of appropriate size and apply it to the point, retaining the cup for 10–15 minutes. With the cup removed, perform moxibustion with a moxa stick for 3–5 minutes until warmth is felt.

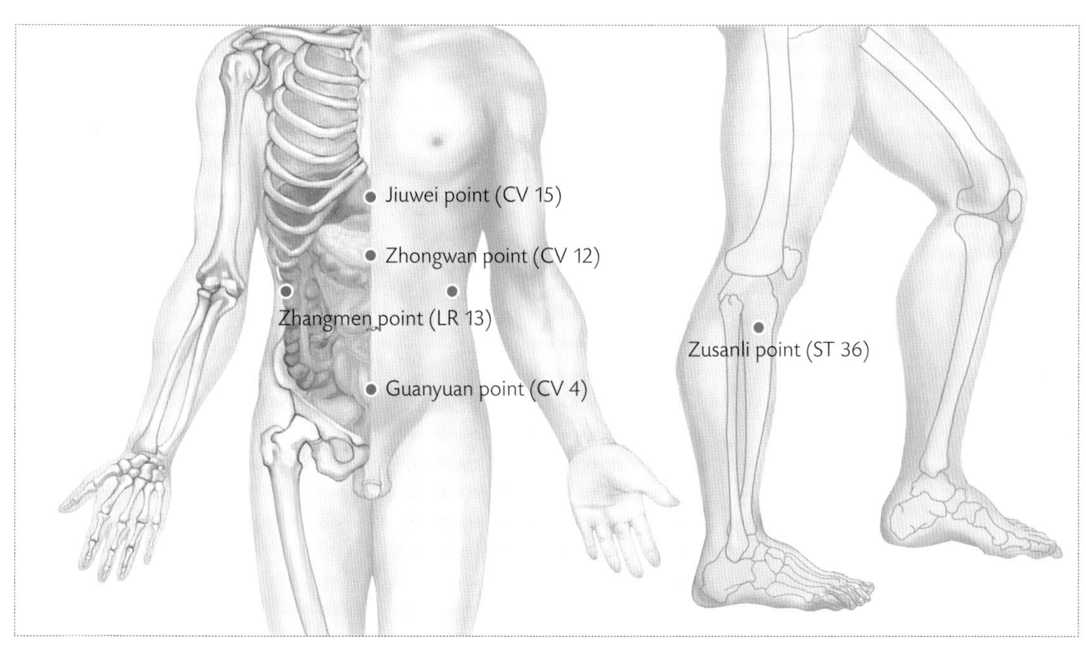

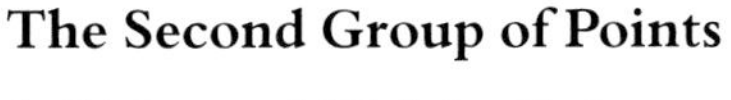

## The Second Group of Points

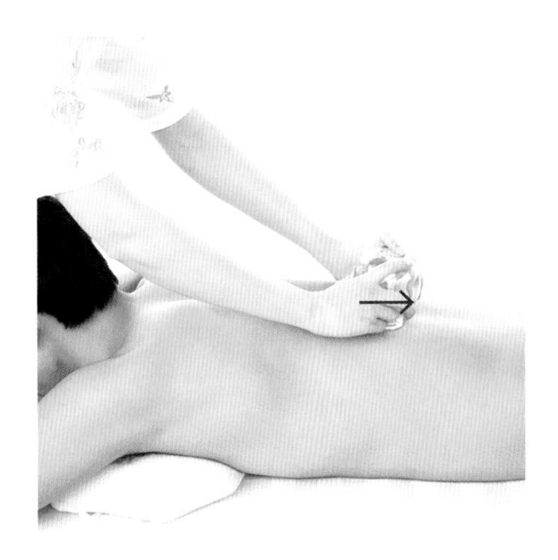

### 1. Pishu and Weishu Points

**Location:** Pishu point is 1.5 cun away horizontally from the eleventh thoracic vertebra; Weishu point is about 1.5 cun below the spinous process of the twelfth thoracic vertebra.

**Method:** Use the moving cupping method. Move the cup on the bladder meridian on the back by segment along the meridian, and move it several times mainly on Pishu and Weishu points. Repeatedly push and pull on the points back and forth, until the skin becomes red. The cup may be retained on the abovementioned points for 10–15 minutes after the moving cupping.

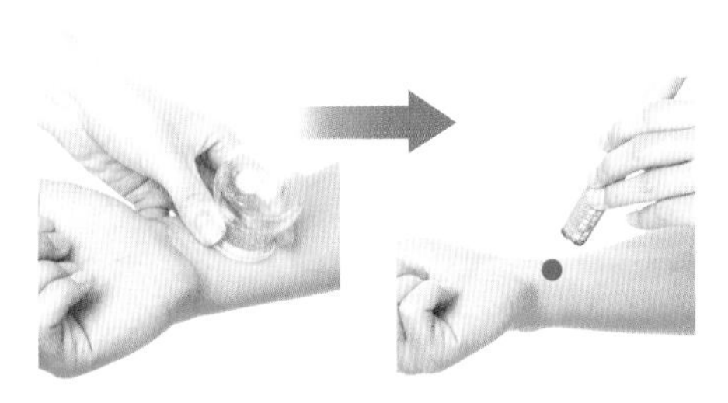

### 2. Neiguan Point

**Location:** Between the two tendons about 2 cun above the wrist joint bend.

**Method:** First knead Guanyuan point with the thumb pulp for 2–3 minutes until soreness and swelling is felt, and then select and apply a cup of appropriate size to the point, retaining the cup for 10–15 minutes. With the cup removed, perform moxibustion with a moxa stick for 3–5 minutes until warmth is felt.

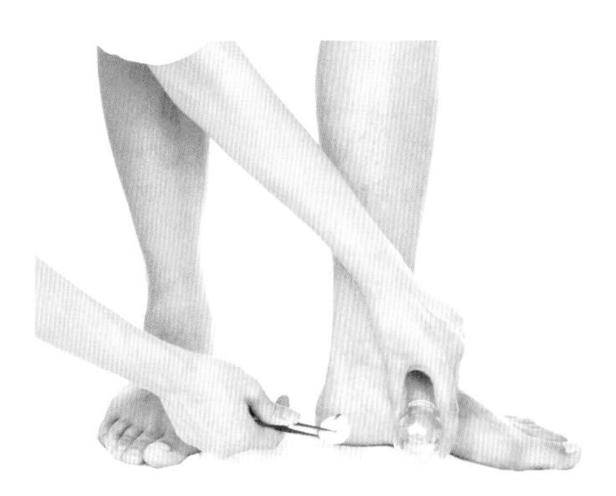

### 3. Gongsun Point

**Location:** In the metatarsal area, at the anterior border of the red and white flesh to the base of the first metatarsal bone.

**Method:** First knead Gongsun point with the thumb pulp for 2–3 minutes until soreness and swelling is felt, and then select and apply a cup of appropriate size to the point, retaining the cup for 10–15 minutes. With the cup removed, perform moxibustion with a moxa stick for 3–5 minutes until warmth is felt.

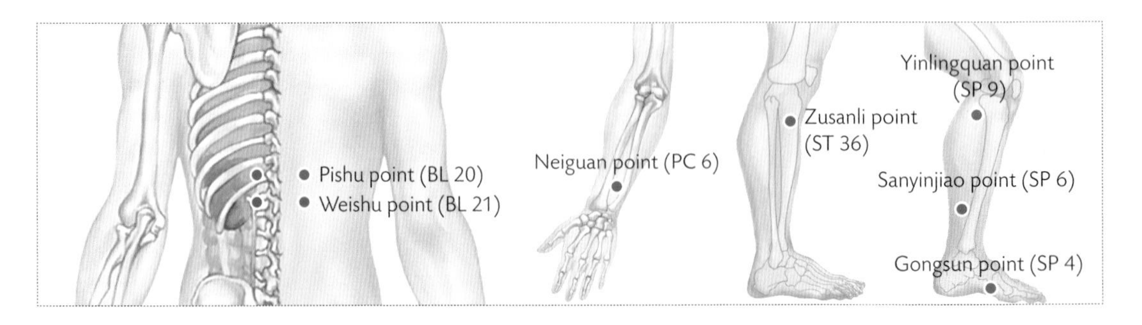

# 8 Kidney Disease

Hypertension, edema, backache, frequent urination, urgency of urination, oliguria, anuria, or proteinuria, male sexual dysfunction (impotence, spermatorrhea, premature ejaculation, infertility), female infertility, are all symptoms of kidney disease.

People with kidney disease should live a moderate life and develop good habits, such as not staying up late or smoking or drinking alcohol. They should participate in aerobic exercise, build up their body, and maintain a good mood. Appropriate regulation of moods and self-pressure can prevent the outbreak of kidney disease. In addition, they should also control the diet structure, avoid intake of excessive acidic substances, and eat more food rich in organic active alkali and more vegetables, but less meat, so as to protect the kidney. Timely seek medical advice to avoid delaying the disease if one is unclear about the specific conditions, or the conditions are found aggravated.

The cupping can be applied to two groups of points, one group a day and two groups in turn. The first group includes Zusanli, Yinlingquan, Sanyinjiao, Guanyuan, and Zhongji points. The second group includes Mingmen, Shenshu, Pishu, Pangguangshu, Sanjiaoshu, Taixi, and Yongquan points.

## Cupping Methods

### The First Group of Points

#### 1. Zusanli Point

**Location:** About 3 cun below the knee on the outer side of the tibia.

**Method:** First knead Zusanli point with the thumb pulp for 2–3 minutes, and then cup this point, retaining the cup for 10–15 minutes. With the cup removed, perform moxibustion with a moxa stick for 3–5 minutes until warmth is felt.

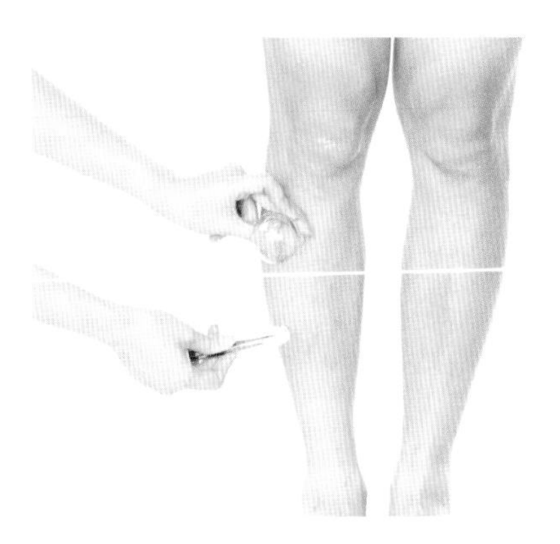

#### 2. Yinlingquan Point

**Location:** In the depression on the inner edge of the shinbone below the knee.

**Method:** First knead Yinlingquan point with the thumb pulp for 2–3 minutes, and then cup this point, retaining the cup for 10–15 minutes. With the cup removed, perform moxibustion with a moxa stick for 3–5 minutes until warmth is felt.

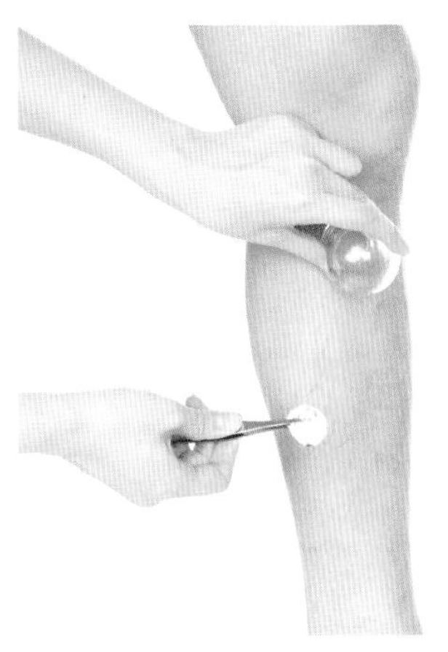

#### 3. Sanyinjiao Point

**Location:** At the rear edge of the shinbone, 3 cun above the ankle.

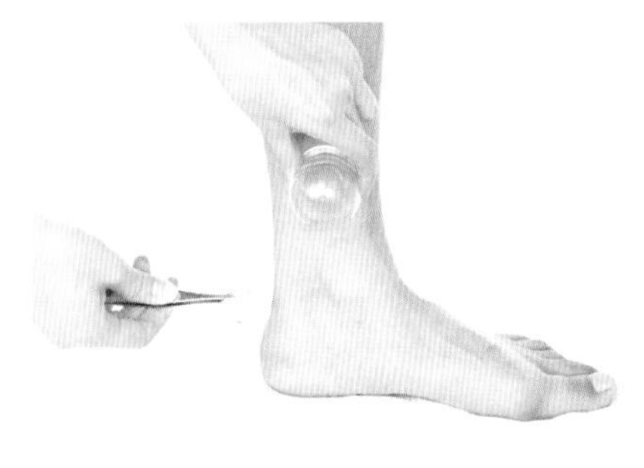

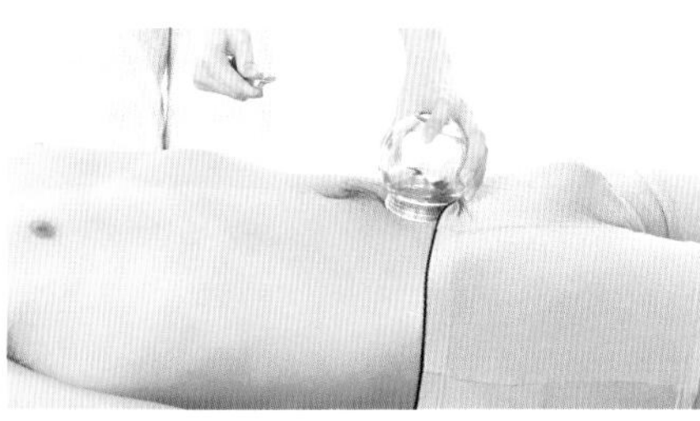

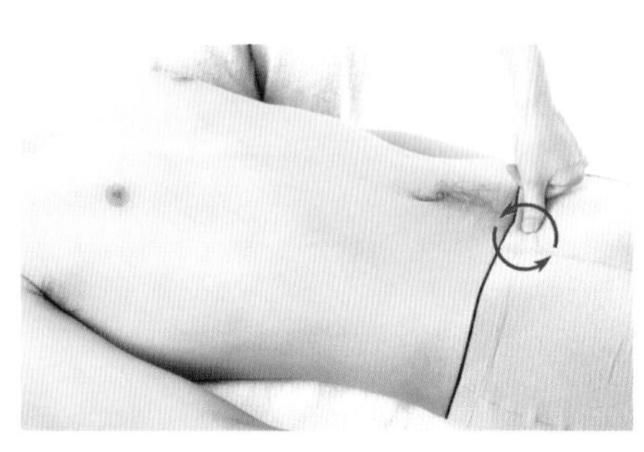

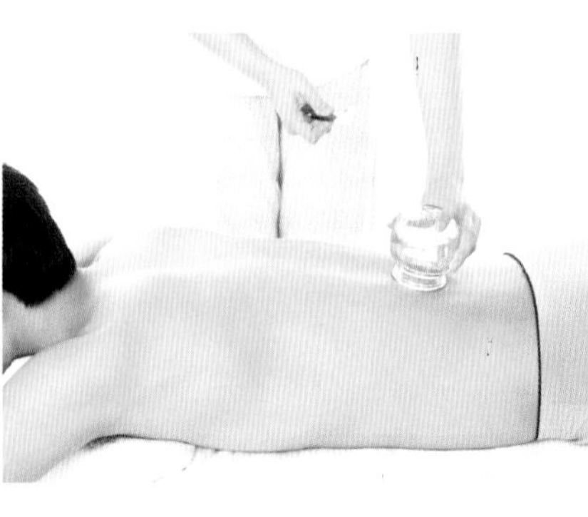

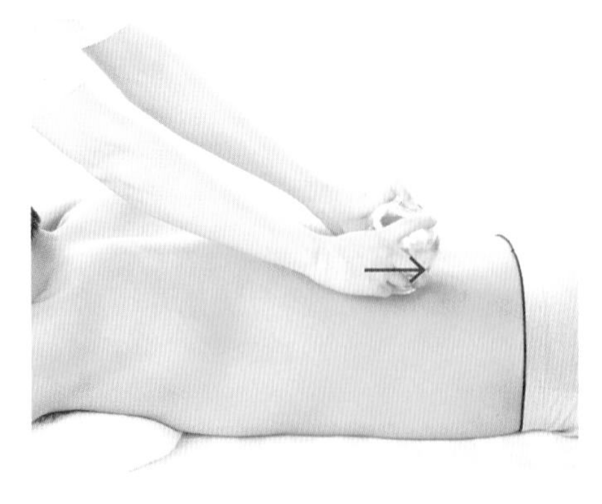

**Method:** First knead Sanyinjiao point with the thumb pulp for 2–3 minutes, and then cup this point, retaining the cup for 10–15 minutes. With the cup removed, perform moxibustion with a moxa stick for 3–5 minutes until warmth is felt.

### 4. Guanyuan Point

**Location:** About 3 cun below the navel.

**Method:** Select and apply a cup of appropriate size to Guanyuan point, retaining the cup for 10–15 minutes. With the cup removed, perform moxibustion with a moxa stick for 3–5 minutes until warmth is felt.

### 5. Zhongji Point

**Location:** On the lower abdomen, 4 cun below the center of the umbilicus, on the anterior midline.

**Method:** First knead Zhongji point with the thumb pulp for 2–3 minutes, and then cup this point, retaining the cup for 10–15 minutes. With the cup removed, perform moxibustion with a moxa stick for 3–5 minutes until warmth is felt.

## The Second Group of Points

### 1. Mingmen Point

**Location:** In a cavity below the spinous process of the second cervical vertebra.

**Method:** Select and apply a cup of appropriate size to Mingmen point, retaining the cup for 10–15 minutes. With the cup removed, perform moxibustion with a moxa stick for 3–5 minutes until warmth is felt.

### 2. Shenshu, Pangguangshu, Pishu and Sanjiaoshu Points

**Location:** Shenshu point is 1.5 cun horizontally from the second lumbar spinal process; Pangguangshu point is in the sacral area, at the same level as the second posterior sacral foramen, 1.5 cun lateral to the median sacral crest; Pishu point is 1.5 cun away horizontally from the eleventh thoracic vertebra; Sanjiaoshu point is 1.5 cun away from the spinous process of the first lumbar vertebra.

**Method:** Use the moving cupping method. Move the cup on the bladder meridian on the back by segment along the meridian, and move it several times mainly on the Shenshu, Pangguangshu, Pishu and Sanjiaoshu points. Repeatedly push and pull on the points back and forth, until the skin becomes red. The cup may be retained on the abovementioned points for 10–15 minutes after the moving cupping.

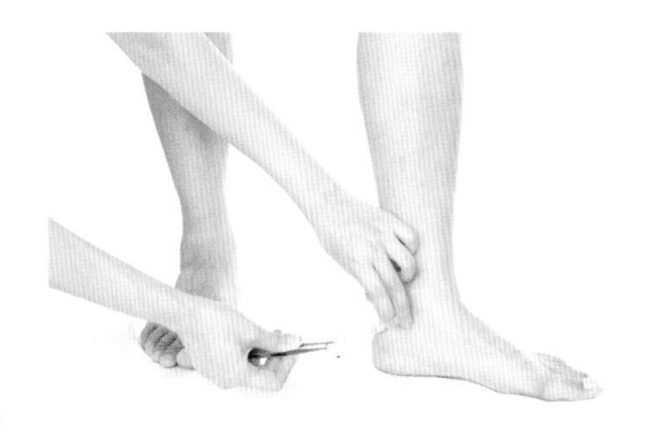

### 3. Taixi Point

**Location:** In a cavity between the medial malleolus and Achilles tendon.

**Method:** First knead Taixi point with the thumb pulp for 2–3 minutes, until soreness and swelling is felt. Then select a cup of appropriate size and apply it to the point, retaining the cup for 10–15 minutes.

### 4. Yongquan Point

**Location:** In a depression in the front of the sole of the foot, about one-third of the way down from the toes.

**Method:** First knead Yongquan point with the palm for 2–3 minutes, until a feeling of heat is present. Then select a cup of appropriate size and apply it to the point, retaining the cup for 10–15 minutes. With the cup removed, perform moxibustion with a moxa stick for 3–5 minutes until warmth is felt.

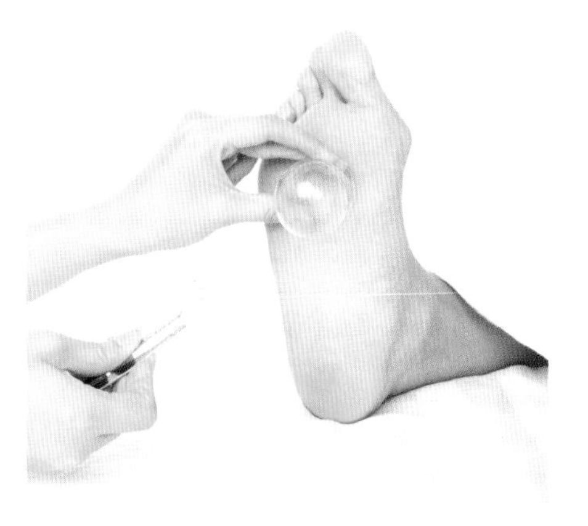

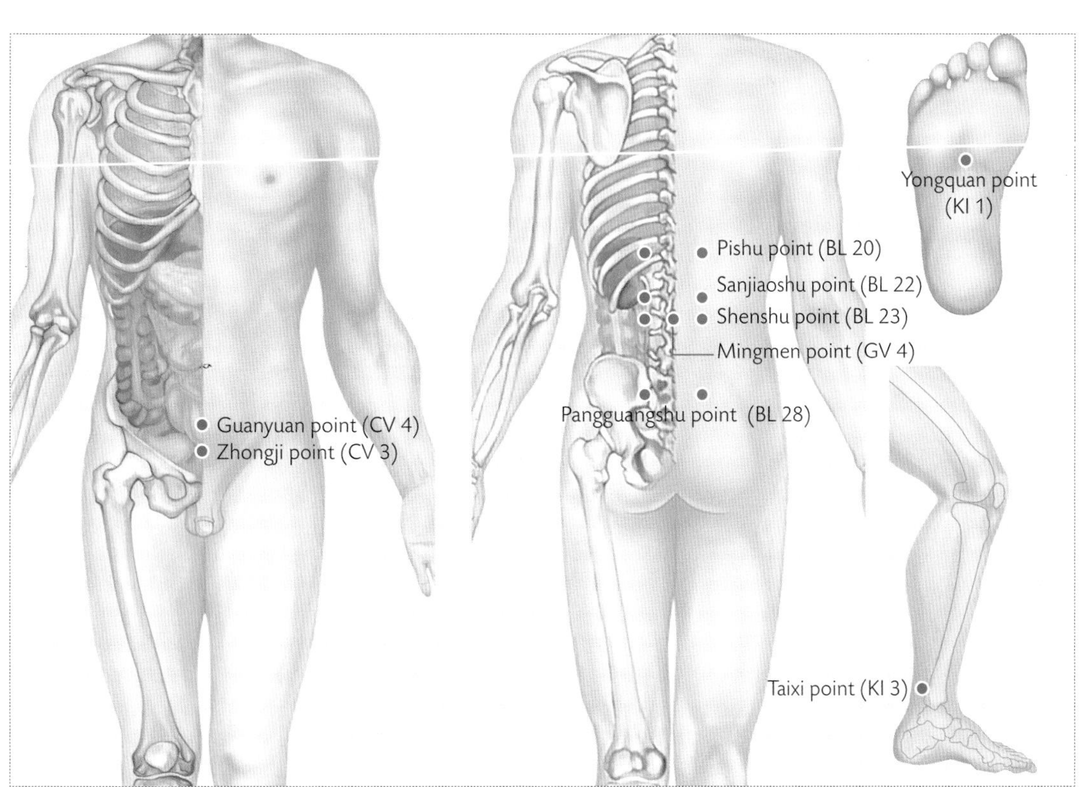

# 9 Headache

As a very common symptom among many diseases, headache can be manifested by distending pain, throbbing pain, stabbing pain, pain with dizziness, dull pain, etc. The headache attack and its duration vary in length, ranging from several minutes to several days.

There are many causes for headache. First, one should rule out other systemic diseases, and take active treatment to relieve the cause if the primary disease is found. During the treatment, the patients should regulate their moods to prevent emotional stress, anxiety and fatigue. They should have a light diet, get plenty of rest, keep sufficient sleep, quit smoking and alcohol consumption, and avoid spicy foods, chocolate, coffee, strong tea, etc.

During the cupping, select Yintang point for frontal headache, Taiyang point for migraine, Baihui point for vertex headache, and Fengchi point for hinder headache. In addition, these acupoints may be cupped in conjunction with Taichong, Hegu, Geshu, and Taixi points.

## Cupping Methods

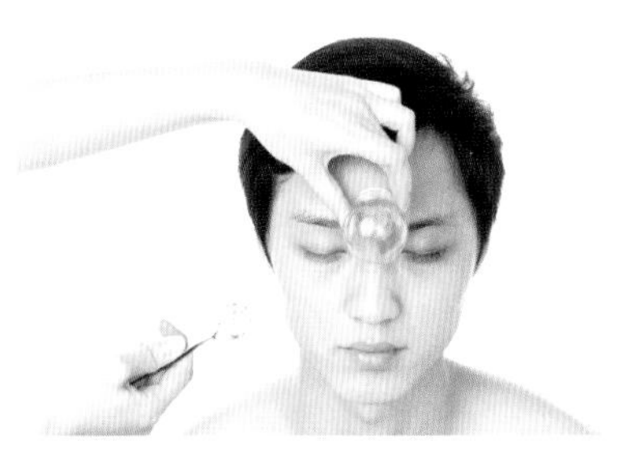

### 1. Yintang Point

**Location:** At the central point right between the eyebrows.

**Method:** First, knead Yintang point with a finger pulp for 2–3 minutes, and then select and apply a small cup to the point, retaining the cup for 5–10 minutes.

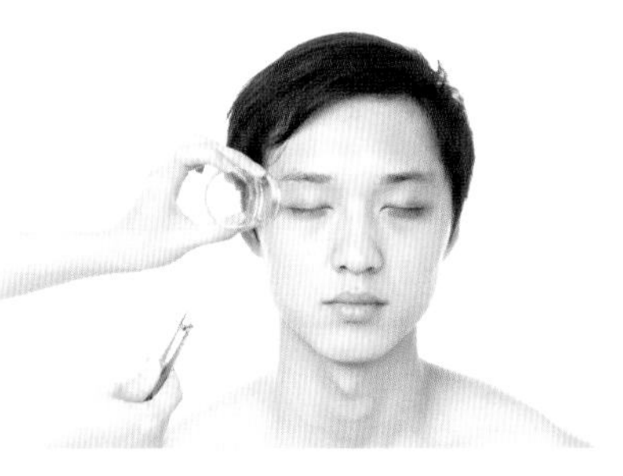

### 2. Taiyang Point

**Location:** In the depression about 1 cun behind the space between the outer tip of the brow and outer eye corner.

**Method:** First, knead Taiyang point with a finger pulp for 2–3 minutes, and then select and apply a small cup to the point, retaining the cup for 5–10 minutes.

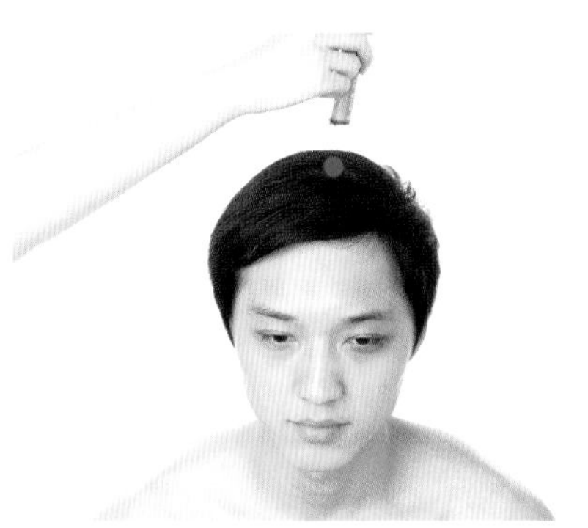

### 3. Baihui Point

**Location:** On the head, 5 cun superior to the anterior hairline, on the anterior midline.

**Method:** Cup Baihui point for 10–15 times by using the flash cupping method. Do not retain the cup. Then perform moxibustion with a moxa stick for 3–5 minutes until warmth is felt.

### 4. Fengchi Point

**Location:** In the depression on both sides of the large

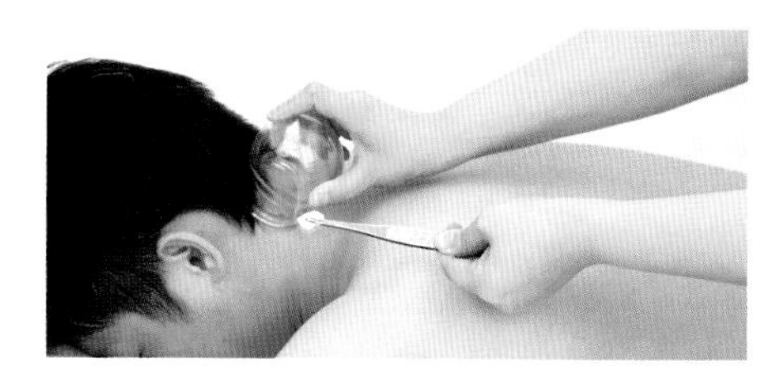

tendon behind the nape of the neck, next to the lower edge of the skull.

**Method:** First knead Fengchi point with the thumb pulp for 2–3 minutes, until a feeling of soreness and swelling is present. Then cup the point, retaining the cup for 10–15 minutes.

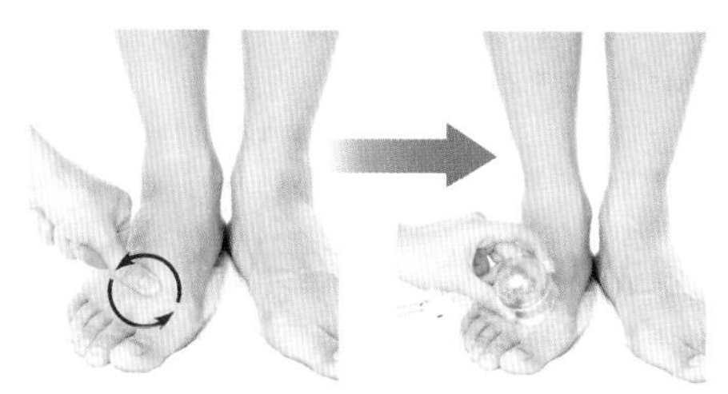

### 5. Taichong Point

**Location:** On the foot in a notch between the first and second metatarsal bones.

**Method:** First knead Taichong point with the thumb pulp for 2–3 minutes until a feeling of soreness and swelling is present, and then select and apply a cup of appropriate size to the point, retaining the cup for 10–15 minutes.

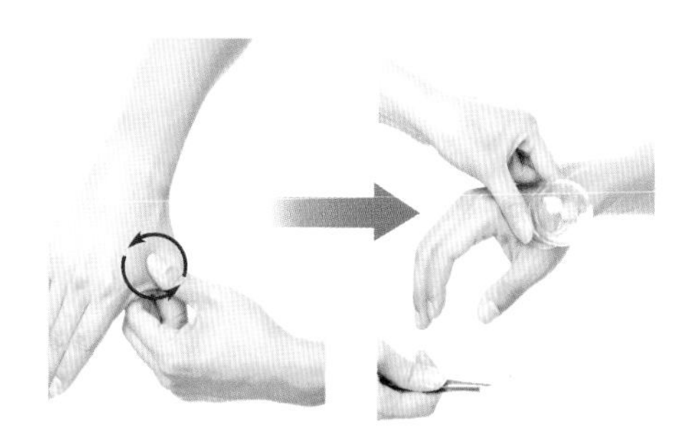

### 6. Hegu Point

**Location:** In the highest point on the back of the hand between the thumb base and the base of the index finger (in the webbing between these two fingers).

**Method:** First knead Hegu point with the thumb pulp for 2–3 minutes until a feeling of soreness and swelling is present, and then select and apply a cup of appropriate size to the point, retaining the cup for 10–15 minutes.

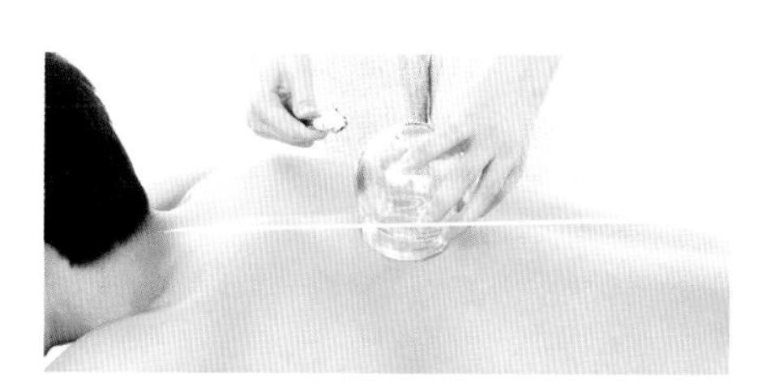

### 7. Geshu Point

**Location:** 1.5 cun away from the spinous process of the seventh thoracic vertebra.

**Method:** Select a cup of appropriate size and apply it to Geshu point. Retain the cup for 10–15 minutes.

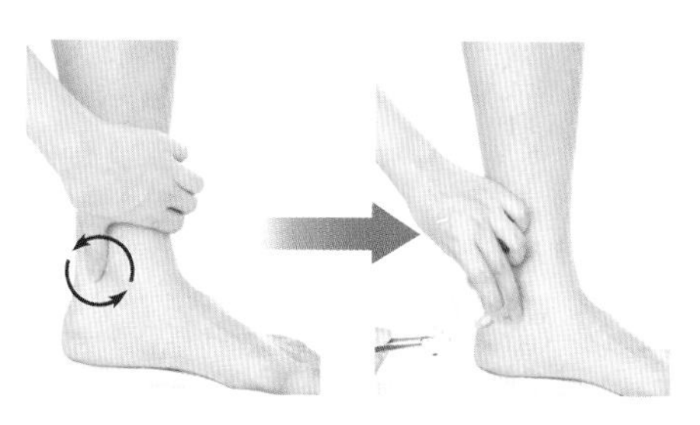

### 8. Taixi Point

**Location:** In a cavity between the medial malleolus and Achilles tendon.

**Method:** First knead Taixi point with the thumb pulp for 2–3 minutes, until soreness and swelling is felt. Then select a cup of appropriate size and apply it to the point, retaining the cup for 10–15 minutes.

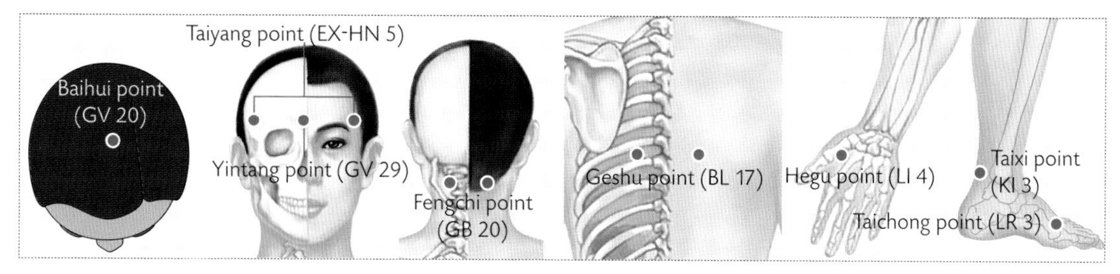

# 10 Cold

The onset of the common cold is acute, with symptoms in the early stages including aversion to cold, dry and itchy throat, sneezing, nasal congestion, runny nose, hoarse voice, dry cough, probably accompanied by sore throat, fever, headache, general malaise, backache, fatigue, and so on.

To prevent colds, one should avoid staying in the places concentrated with people during the flu season, pay attention to personal hygiene, and wear a gauze mask in public places. Patients should keep warm and avoid the cold, keep the indoor air fresh, do more outdoor exercise, and strengthen physical exercise to enhance physique.

The cupping can be applied to Fengchi, Quchi, Dazhui, Feishu, Fengmen, Waiguan, and Hegu points.

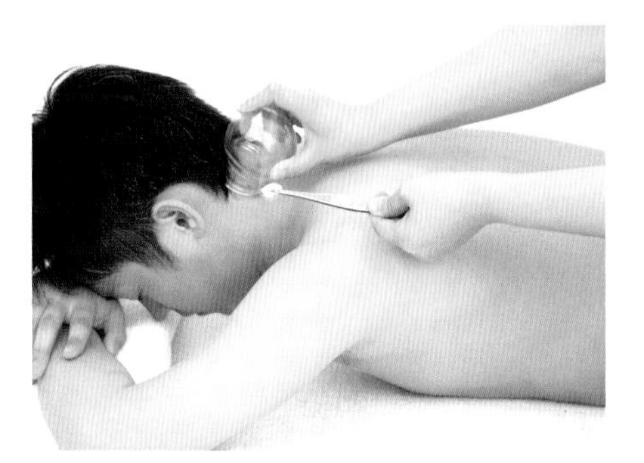

## Cupping Methods

### 1. Fengchi Point

**Location:** In the depression on both sides of the large tendon behind the nape of the neck, next to the lower edge of the skull.

**Method:** First knead Fengchi point with the thumb pulp for 2–3 minutes, until a feeling of soreness and swelling is present. Then cup the point, retaining the cup for 10–15 minutes.

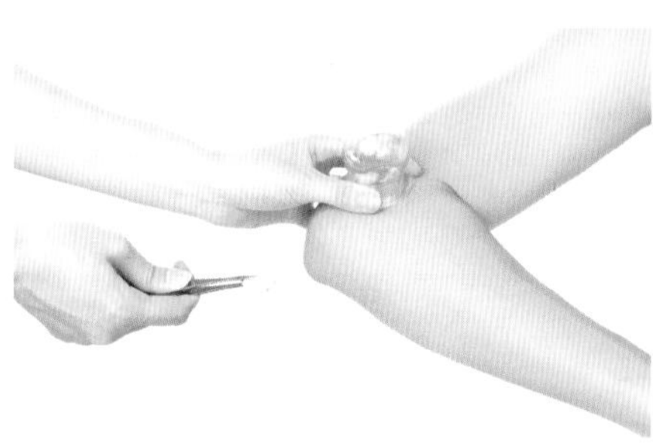

### 2. Quchi Point

**Location:** With the elbow bent halfway, on the outer side of the cubital transverse crease.

**Method:** Select a cup of appropriate size and apply it to Quchi point. Retain the cup for 10–15 minutes.

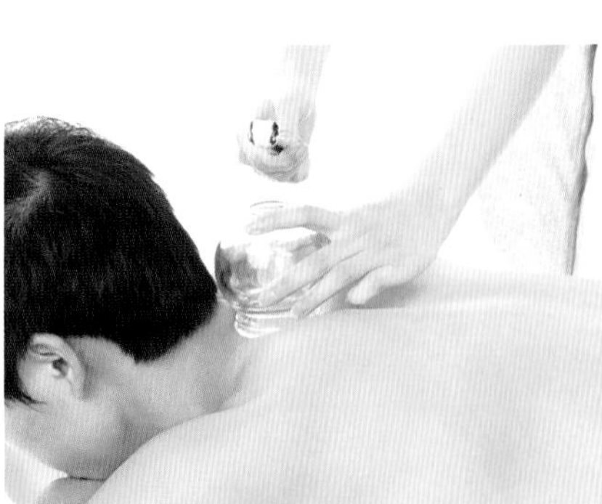

### 3. Dazhui Point

**Location:** Under the spinous process of the seventh cervical vertebrae.

**Method:** Select a cup of appropriate size and apply it to Dazhui point. Retain the cup for 10–15 minutes.

### 4. Feishu Point

**Location:** 1.5 cun beside the third thoracic vertebra on the inner side of the scapula.

**Method:** Use the moving cupping method by moving the cup on the bladder meridian on the back by segment along the meridian. Move the cup several times mainly on Feishu point, and repeatedly push and pull on the point back and forth, until the skin becomes red. The cup may be retained on the abovementioned point for 10–15 minutes after the moving cupping.

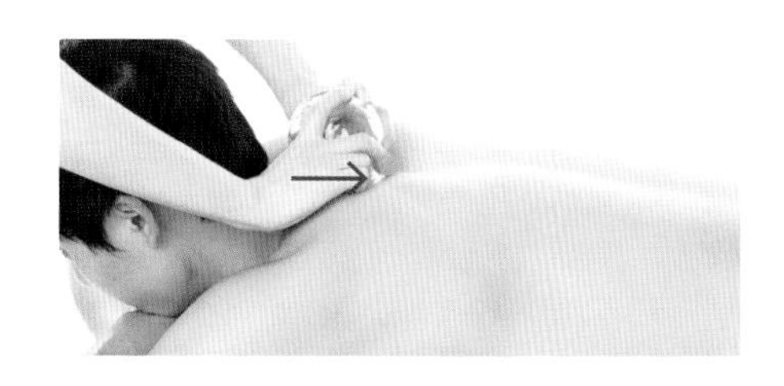

### 5. Fengmen Point

**Location:** In the spine area, 1.5 cun lateral to the posterior midline of the lower border of the spinous process of the second thoracic vertebra.

**Method:** Use the moving cupping method by moving the cup on the bladder meridian on the back by segment along the meridian. Move the cup several times mainly on Fengmen point, and repeatedly push and pull on the point back and forth, until the skin becomes red. The cup may be retained on the abovementioned point for 10–15 minutes after the moving cupping.

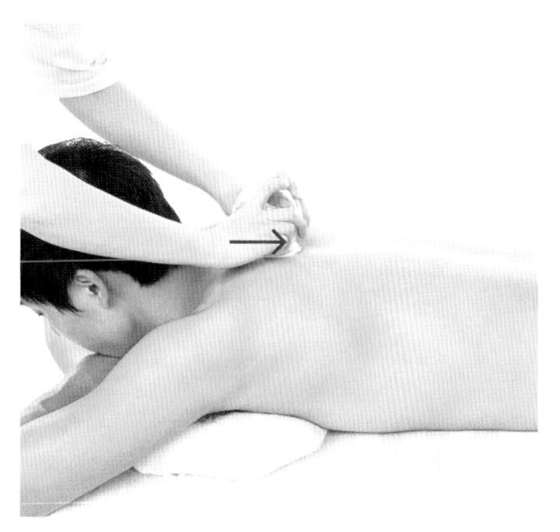

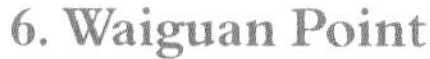

### 6. Waiguan Point

**Location:** The Waiguan point is in the middle on the outside of the arm, between the ulna and radius about 2 cun away from the horizontal line of the wrist joint.

**Method:** First knead Waiguan point with the thumb pulp for 2–3 minutes, until a feeling of soreness and swelling is present, and then select and apply a cup of appropriate size to the point, retaining the cup for 10–15 minutes.

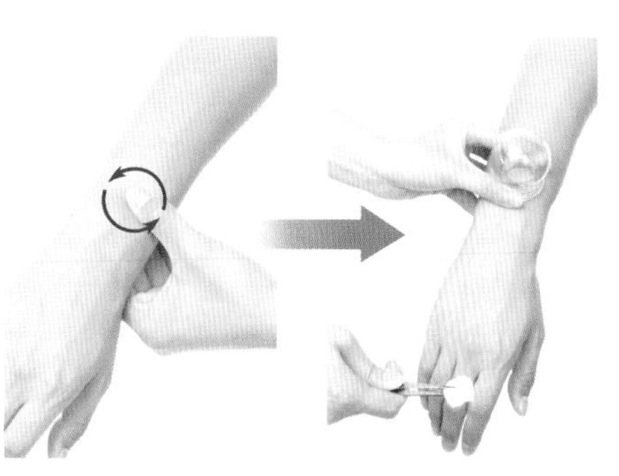

### 7. Hegu Point

**Location:** In the highest point on the back of the hand between the thumb base and the base of the index finger (in the webbing between these two fingers).

**Method:** First knead Hegu point with the thumb pulp for 2–3 minutes, until a feeling of soreness and swelling is present, and then select and apply a cup of appropriate size to the point, retaining the cup for 10–15 minutes.

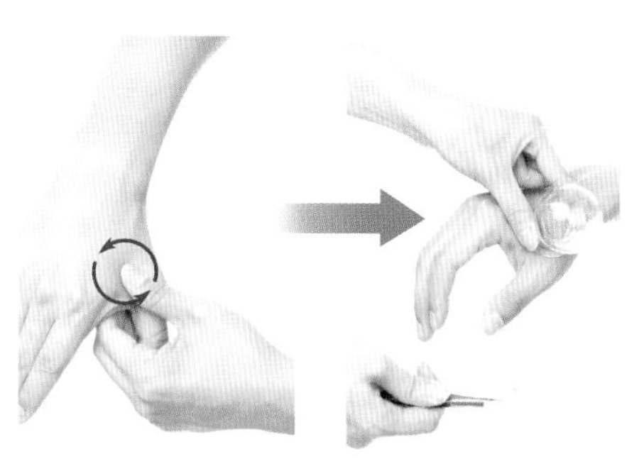

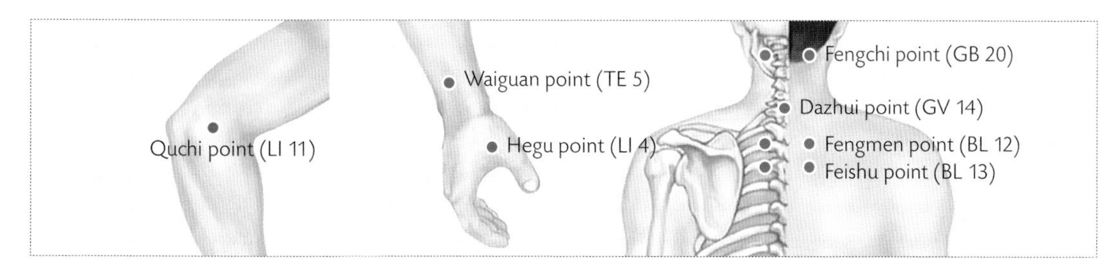

# 11 Cough

Cough is a protective respiratory reflex action by the human body to clear the secretions or foreign substances from the respiratory tract, often accompanied by sputum.

Patients with cough should strengthen exercise and have more outdoor activities to improve the body's resistance to disease. They should promptly put on additional clothes or take off some clothes with the climate change to prevent being too cold or too warm, and often open windows for ventilation to keep the indoor air fresh. Primary disease should be identified for long-term cough, actively cooperating Traditional Chinese Medicine with Western medicine treatment to eliminate the causes.

The cupping should be applied to Dazhui, Chize, Feishu, Fengmen, Tiantu, Zhongfu, and Danzhong points.

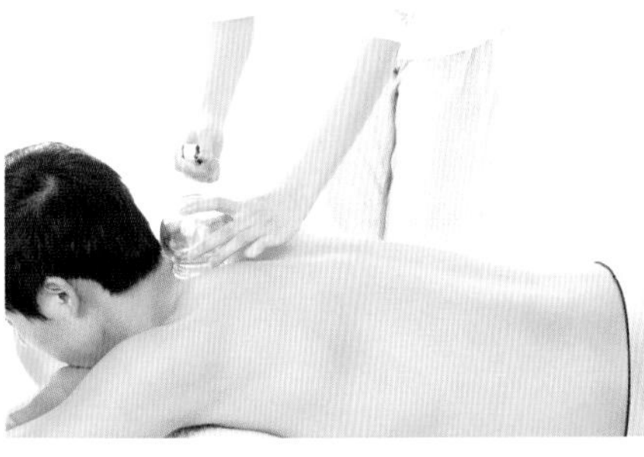

## Cupping Methods

### 1. Dazhui Point

**Location:** Under the spinous process of the seventh cervical vertebrae.

**Method:** Select a cup of appropriate size and apply it to Dazhui point. Retain the cup for 10–15 minutes.

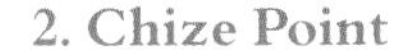

### 2. Chize Point

**Location:** With the elbow bent slightly, in a cavity of the outer side of the biceps brachii on the cubital crease.

**Method:** Select a cup of appropriate size and apply it to Chize point. Retain the cup for 10–15 minutes.

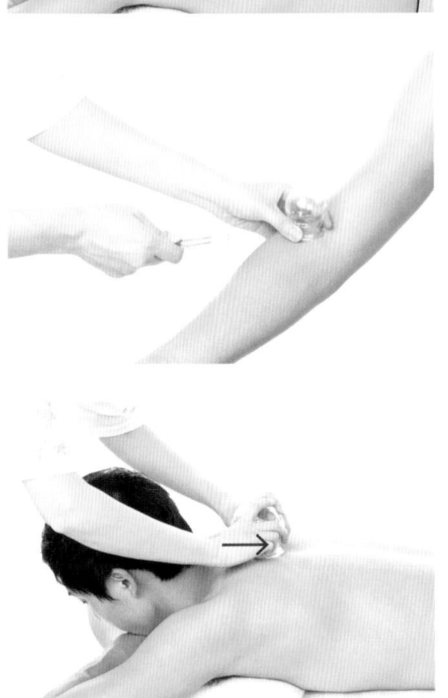

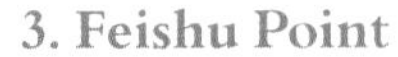

### 3. Feishu Point

**Location:** 1.5 cun beside the third thoracic vertebra on the inner side of the scapula.

**Method:** Use the moving cupping method by moving the cup on the bladder meridian on the back by segment along the meridian. Move the cup several times mainly on Feishu point, and repeatedly push and pull on the point back and forth, until the skin becomes red. The cup may be retained on the abovementioned point for 10–15 minutes after the moving cupping.

### 4. Fengmen Point

**Location:** In the spine area, 1.5 cun lateral to the

posterior midline of the lower border of the spinous process of the second thoracic vertebra.

**Method:** Use the moving cupping method by moving the cup on the bladder meridian on the back by segment along the meridian. Move the cup several times mainly on Fengmen point, and repeatedly push and pull on the point back and forth, until the skin becomes red. The cup may be retained on the abovementioned point for 10–15 minutes after the moving cupping.

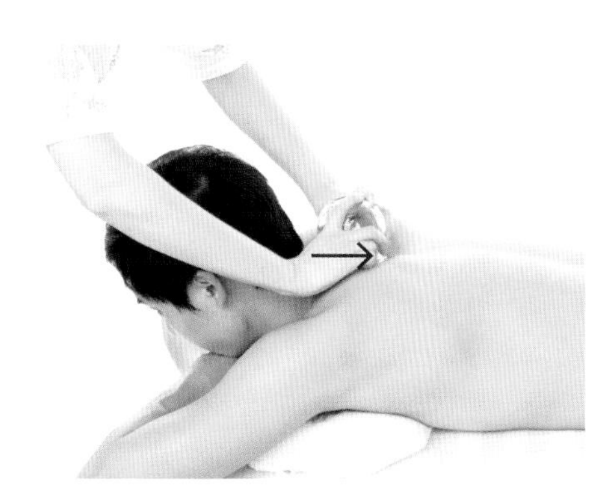

### 5. Tiantu Point

**Location:** Right in the middle of the cavity above the suprasternal fossa, just between the collarbones.

**Method:** Select a cup of appropriate size and apply it to Tiantu point. Retain the cup for 10–15 minutes.

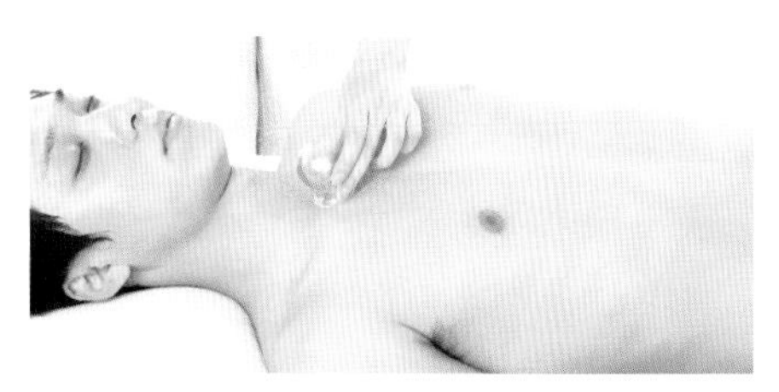

### 6. Zhongfu Point

**Location:** On the chest, 6 cun lateral to the anterior midline, at the same level as the first intercostal space, lateral to the infraclavicular fossae.

**Method:** Select a cup of appropriate size and apply it to Zhongfu point. Retain the cup for 10–15 minutes.

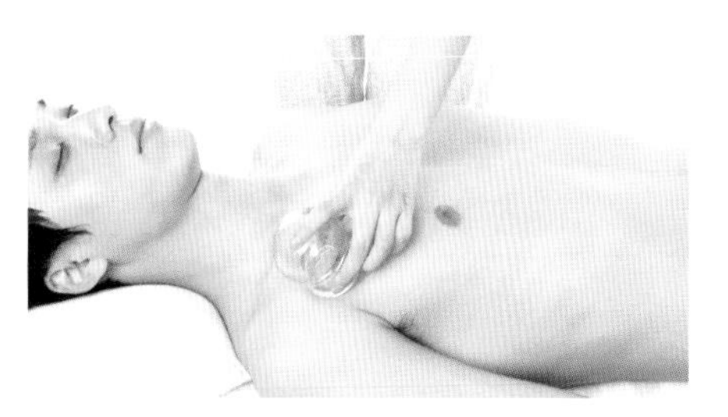

### 7. Danzhong Point

**Location:** Directly in the middle of the chest between the nipples.

**Method:** Use the moving cupping method. Select a cup of appropriate size and move it continuously on the chest along the breastbone from top to bottom, until the skin becomes red. After the moving cupping, retain the cup on the point for 10–15 minutes.

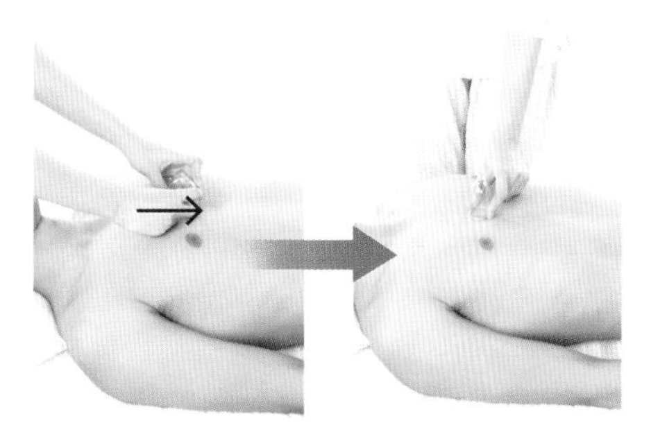

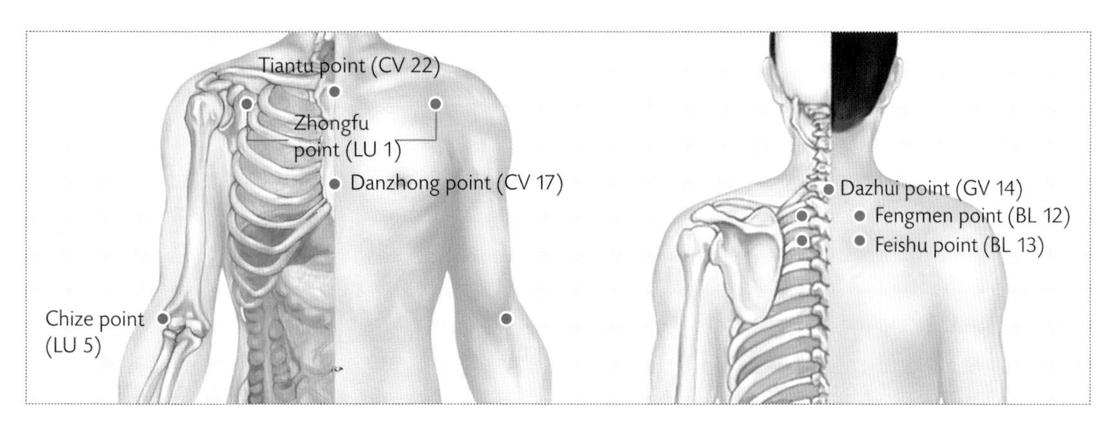

# 12 Bronchial Asthma

The manifestations of the attack of acute bronchial asthma includes sudden outbreak of wheezing, shortness of breath, cough, sputum, difficulty in breathing, and chest tightness, accompanied by expiratory dyspnea with wheezes.

During the attack of asthma, drug therapy should be adopted, and attention should be paid to keeping warm during the alleviation period to prevent inducement. Avoid contact with allergens during treatment. In daily life, one should pay attention to reducing other sources producing allogeneic protein indoors, avoid dampness and darkness indoors to reduce the breeding of molds, and avoid planting flowering plants. Doors and windows should be closed especially in the spring, the peak season when flower powders fly. Do not raise any kind of pet indoors. In terms of diet, avoid eating animal food, greasy or spicy food such as seafood, fat, peppers, garlic, onions, leeks, etc.

The cupping can be applied to two groups of points, one group a day and two groups in turn, until the symptoms are alleviated or disappear. The first group includes Feishu, Dingchuan, Zhongfu, and Danzhong points, and the second group includes Pishu, Shenshu, Mingmen, Fenglong, and Zusanli points.

## Cupping Methods

### The First Group of Points

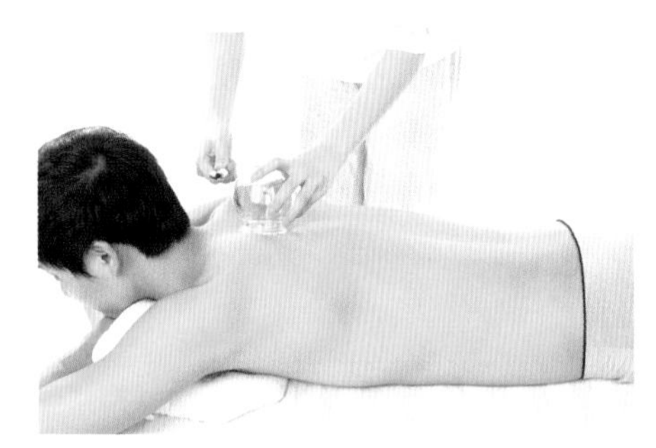

#### 1. Feishu Point

**Location:** 1.5 cun beside the third thoracic vertebra on the inner side of the scapula.

**Method:** Select a cup of appropriate size and apply it to Feishu point. Retain the cup for 10–15 minutes.

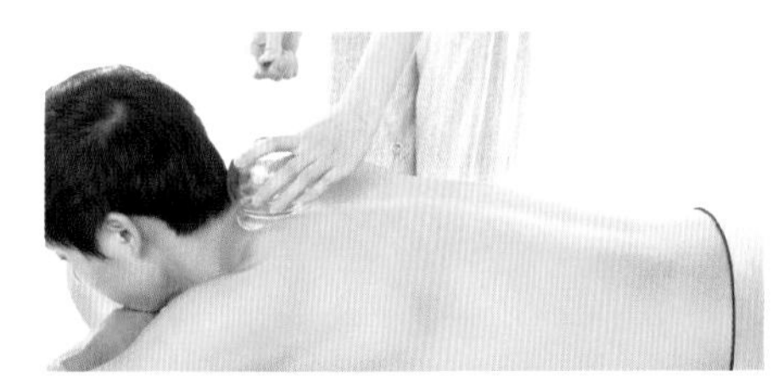

#### 2. Dingchuan Point

**Location:** 0.5 cun away from the spinous process of the seventh cervical vertebra.

**Method:** Select a cup of appropriate size and apply it to Dingchuan point. Retain the cup for 10–15 minutes.

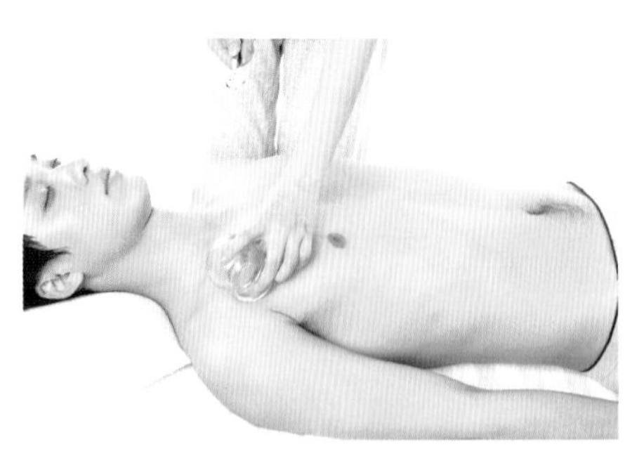

#### 3. Zhongfu Point

**Location:** On the chest, 6 cun lateral to the anterior midline, at the same level as the first intercostal space, lateral to the infraclavicular fossae.

**Method:** Select a cup of appropriate size and apply it to Zhongfu point. Retain the cup for 10–15 minutes.

### 4. Danzhong Point

**Location:** Directly in the middle of the chest between the nipples.

**Method:** Use the moving cupping method. Select a cup of appropriate size and move it continuously on the chest along the breastbone from top to bottom, until the skin becomes red. After the moving cupping, retain the cup on the point for 10–15 minutes.

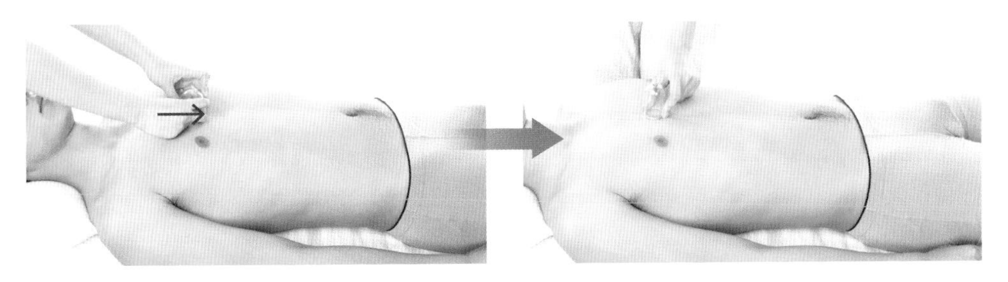

## The Second Group of Points

### 1. Pishu and Shenshu Points

**Location:** Pishu point is 1.5 cun away horizontally from the eleventh thoracic vertebra; Shenshu point is 1.5 cun horizontally from the second lumbar spinal process.

**Method:** Use the moving cupping method. Move the cup on the bladder meridian on the back by segment along the meridian, and move it several times mainly on the Pishu and Shenshu points. Repeatedly push and pull on the points back and forth, until the skin becomes red. The cup may be retained on the abovementioned points for 10–15 minutes after the moving cupping.

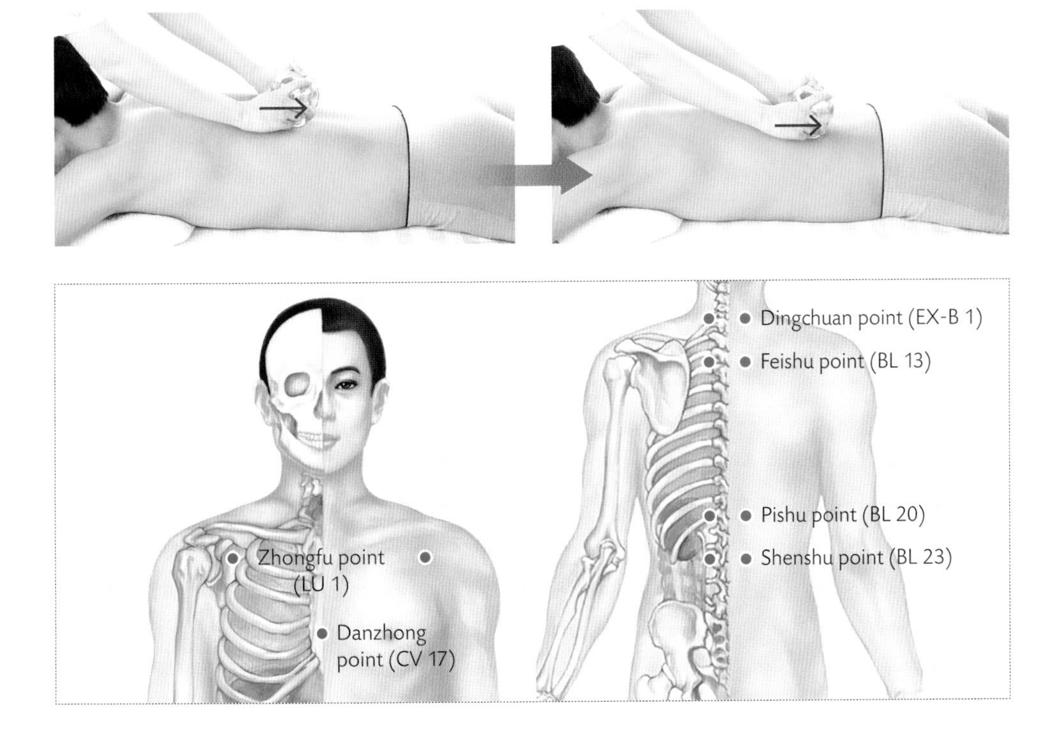

### 2. Mingmen Point

**Location:** In a cavity below the spinous process of the second cervical vertebra.

**Method:** Select a cup of appropriate size and apply it to Mingmen point. Retain the cup for 10–15 minutes.

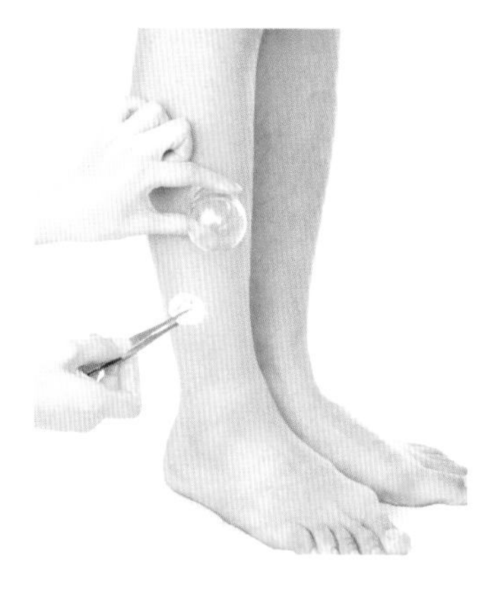

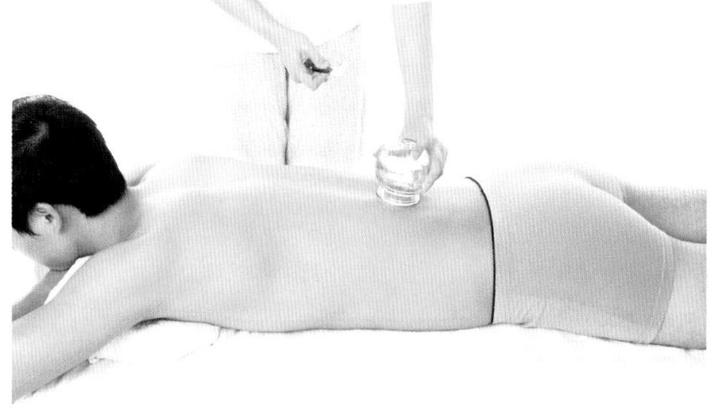

### 3. Fenglong Point

**Location:** 8 cun above the ankle tip.

**Method:** Select a cup of appropriate size and apply it to Fenglong point. Retain the cup for 10–15 minutes.

### 4. Zusanli Point

**Location:** About 3 cun below the knee on the outer side of the tibia.

**Method:** First knead Zusanli point with the thumb pulp for 2–3 minutes, and then select a cup of appropriate size and apply it to the point, retaining the cup for 10–15 minutes.

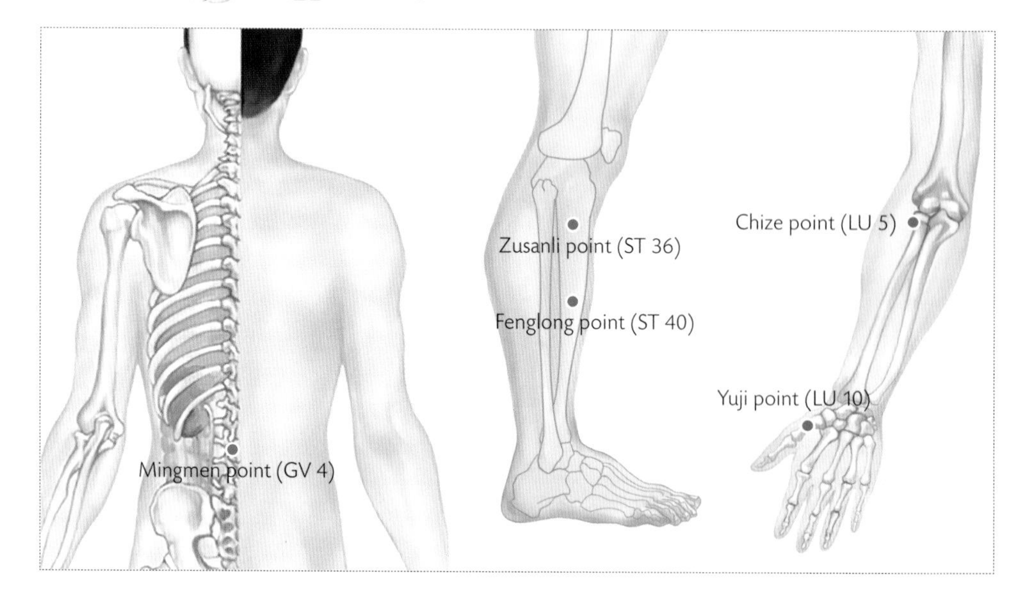

# 13 Bronchitis

Bronchitis is characterized by long-term coughing, sputum, or accompanied by asthma and repeated attacks. Some patients have cough, pharyngitis, and other medical history before their attacks, and later have persistent symptoms and repeated attacks.

Patients who smoke should quit smoking to prevent infection of upper respiratory tract and avoid inhalation of harmful substances. They should stay away from allergens, maintain good household sanitation, keep indoor air circulating, and actively control infections. In the acute phase, they should choose an effective antimicrobial treatment by following medical advice, and meanwhile, use drugs to relieve cough and eliminate phlegm. Old, frail, and weak patients and those coughing phlegm or with much amount of phlegm should be treated mainly for eliminating phlegm. They can also be treated twice a year by adopting the treatment of "triple nine" (i.e., the third nine-day period after the Winter Solstice) in winter and "triple summer" (the hottest days in summer). For the diet, they can eat appropriate amount of lilies, lilyturf roots, loquats etc., which can effectively prevent the attack of bronchitis. They should also strengthen physical exercise to enhance physique and improve respiratory resistance, and dress accordingly during the climate changes and in the cold season to prevent cold and influenza.

The cupping can be applied to two groups of points, one group a day and two groups in turn, until the symptoms are alleviated or disappear. The first group includes Yuji, Zhongfu, Chize, and Danzhong points. The second group includes Dazhu, Dazhui, Feishu, and Dingchuan points.

## Cupping Methods

### The First Group of Points

#### 1. Yuji Point

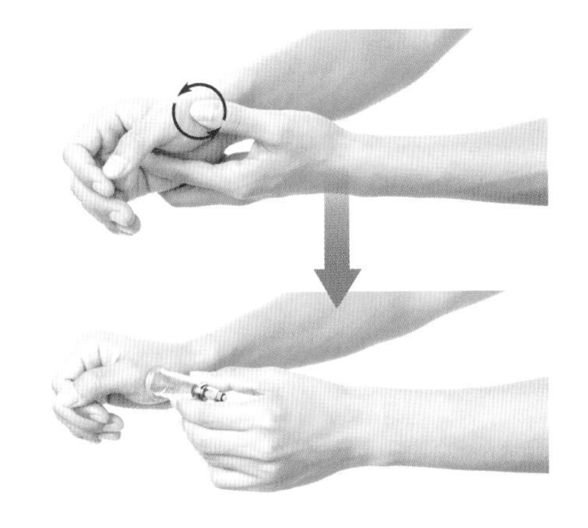

**Location:** With the palm turned upward, in the depression behind the first metacarpophalangeal joint of the thumb.

**Method:** First knead Yuji point with the thumb pulp for 2–3 minutes, until a feeling of soreness is present. Then select a cup of appropriate size and apply it to the point, retaining the cup for 10–15 minutes.

#### 2. Chize Point

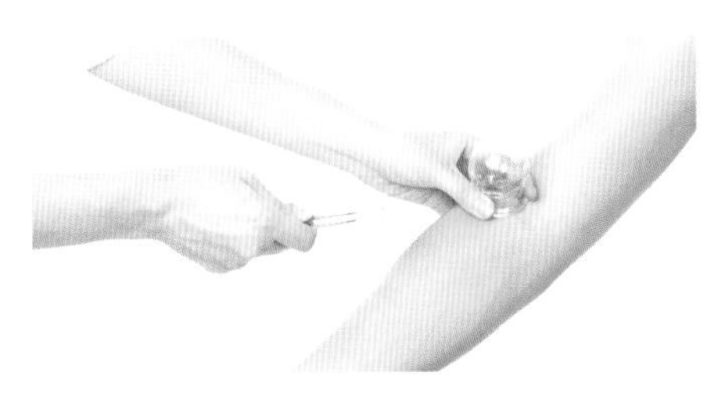

**Location:** With the elbow bent slightly, in a cavity of the outer side of the biceps brachii on the cubital crease.

**Method:** Select a cup of appropriate size and apply it to Chize point. Retain the cup for 10–15 minutes.

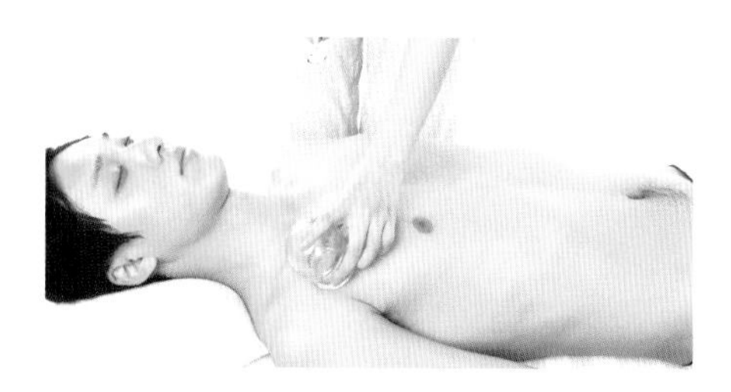

### 3. Zhongfu Point

**Location:** On the chest, 6 cun lateral to the anterior midline, at the same level as the first intercostal space, lateral to the infraclavicular fossae.

**Method:** Select a cup of appropriate size and apply it to Zhongfu point. Retain the cup for 10–15 minutes.

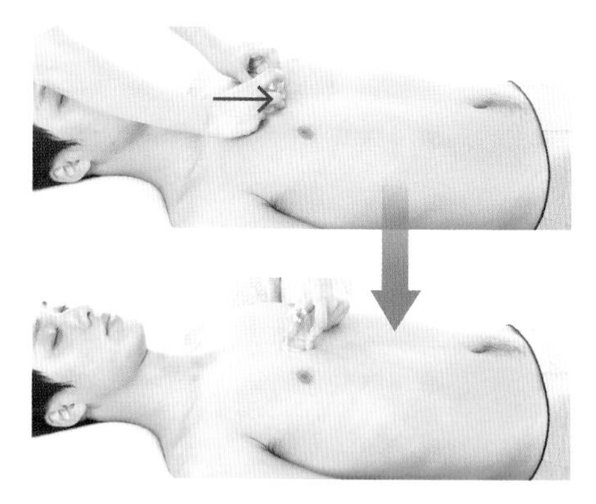

### 4. Danzhong Point

**Location:** Directly in the middle of the chest between the nipples.

**Method:** Use the moving cupping method. Select a cup of appropriate size and move it continuously on the chest along the breastbone from top to bottom, until the skin becomes red. After the moving cupping, retain the cup on the point for 10–15 minutes.

## The Second Group of Points

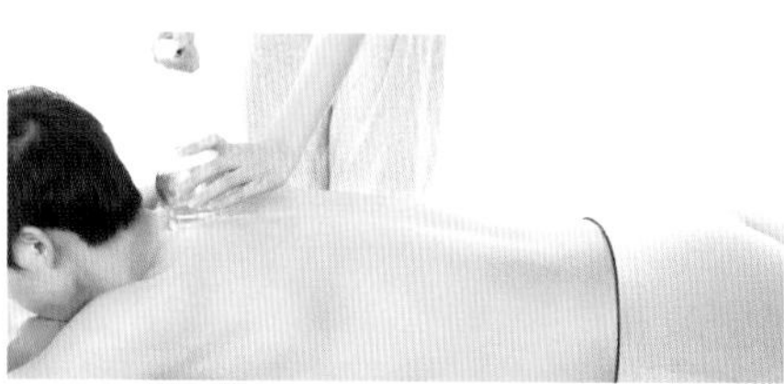

### 1. Dazhu Point

**Location:** In the spine area, 1.5 cun lateral to the posterior midline of the lower border of the spinous process of the first thoracic vertebra.

**Method:** Select a cup of appropriate size and apply it to Dazhu point. Retain the cup for 10–15 minutes.

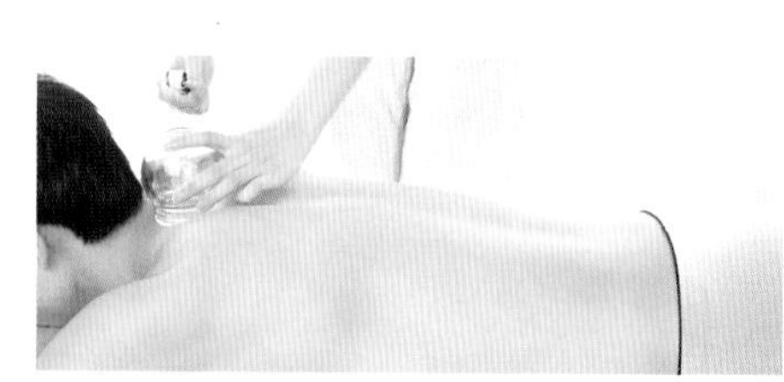

### 2. Dazhui Point

**Location:** Under the spinous process of the seventh cervical vertebrae.

**Method:** Select a cup of appropriate size and apply it to Dazhui point. Retain the cup for 10–15 minutes.

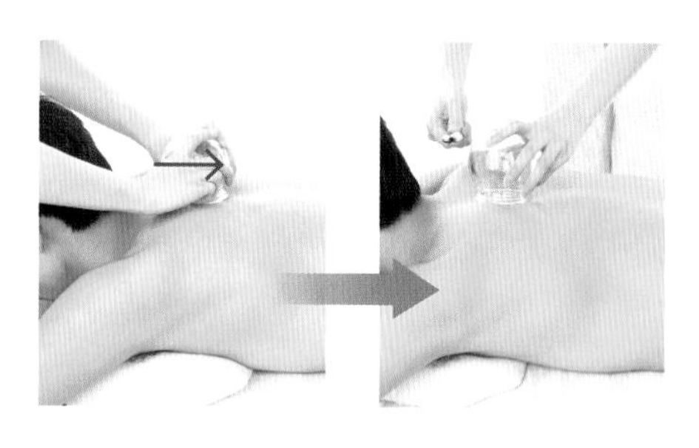

### 3. Feishu Point

**Location:** 1.5 cun beside the third thoracic vertebra on the inner side of the scapula.

**Method:** Use the moving cupping method. Select a cup of appropriate size and move it continuously from the neck to Feishu point, until the skin becomes red. After the moving cupping, retain the cup on the point for 10–15 minutes.

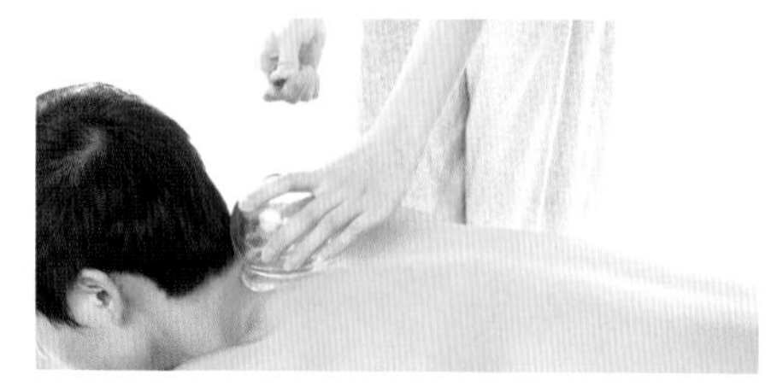

### 4. Dingchuan Point

**Location:** 0.5 cun away from the spinous process of the seventh cervical vertebra.

**Method:** Select a cup of appropriate size and apply it to Dingchuan point. Retain the cup for 10–15 minutes.

# 14 Diarrhea

Diarrhea, a common symptom, means the frequency of defecation are significantly higher than usual, with thin and even water-like stool.

Patients with acute diarrhea should drink soft rice soup, or have gruel and noodles with little oil, weak tea, or juice to facilitate digestion and absorption. Patients with chronic diarrhea should eat yams, coix seeds, lotus root starch, and timely supplement water to prevent dehydration. Patients with serious dehydration should adopt fluid infusion treatment (i.e. a treatment method by letting saline, sugar, blood, electrolytes, and other liquids flow into human body through infusion, oral administration, or other methods, which is medically known as fluid therapy), and supplement electrolytes. To avoid diarrhea, patients should pay attention to food hygiene, and should not drink or eat too much, and not drink or eat cool food.

The cupping for acute diarrhea should be applied to Shenque, Tianshu, Zhongwan, Shangjuxu, Dachangshu, and other points. The cupping for chronic diarrhea should be applied to Yinlingquan, Zusanli, Guanyuan, Pishu, Shenshu, Xiaochangshu and Baliao points.

## Cupping Methods

### 1. Shenque Point

**Location:** At the center of the navel.

**Method:** Centered on the umbilicus, massage the abdomen with the palm counterclockwise for around twenty circles, which should be performed gently, until the abdomen feels warm. Select and apply a cup of appropriate size to Shenque point, retaining the cup for 5–10 minutes. After the cup is removed, perform moxibustion with a moxa stick for 3–5 minutes until warmth is felt.

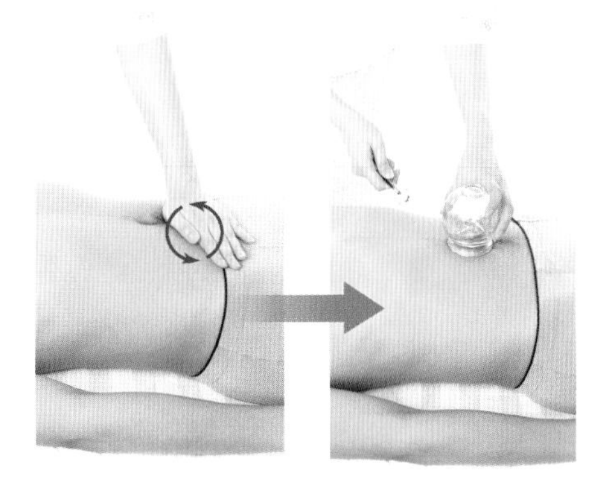

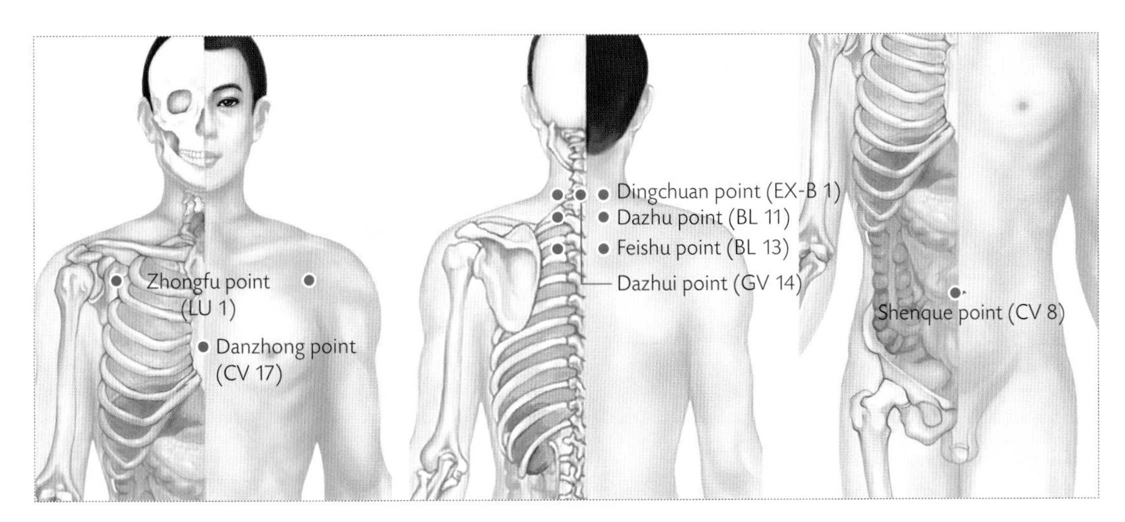

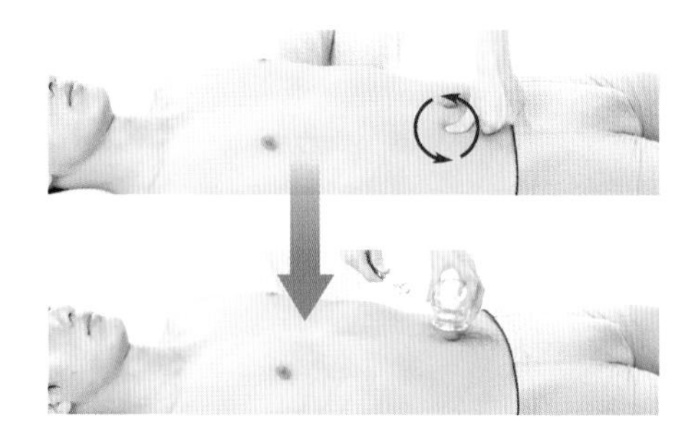

### 2. Tianshu Point

**Location:** About 2 cun horizontally away from the navel.

**Method:** First, press Tianshu point with the thumb tip for 2–3 minutes, until a feeling of soreness and swelling is present. Then select a cup of appropriate size and apply it to the point, retaining the cup for 5–10 minutes.

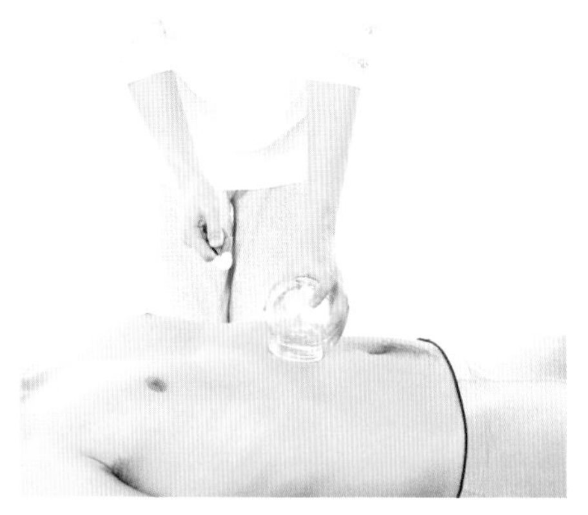

### 3. Zhongwan Point

**Location:** On the upper abdomen, 4 cun above the center of the umbilicus, on the anterior midline.

**Method:** First, massage the upper abdomen above the belly button for about ten circles with the palm or together with the index finger, the middle finger, and the ring finger. This should be performed gently. Then select a cup of appropriate size, and apply it to Zhongwan point, retaining the cup for 10–15 minutes. With the cup removed, perform moxibustion with a moxa box for 3–5 minutes.

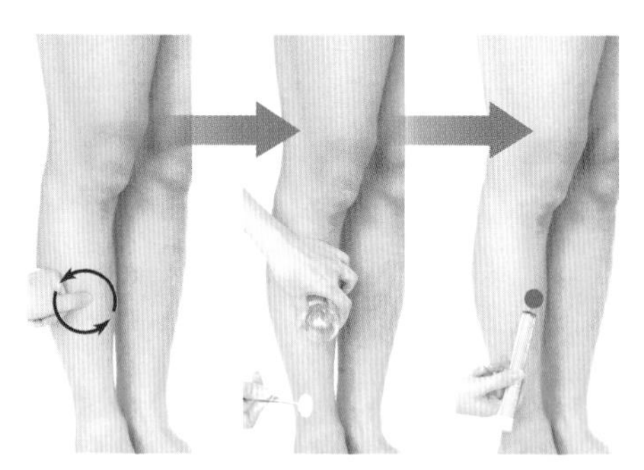

### 4. Shangjuxu Point

**Location:** One middle finger cun (the length of the second section of the middle finger) on the outside of the tibial crest, 3 cun below the Zusanli point.

**Method:** First knead Shangjuxu point with the thumb pulp for 2–3 minutes, and then cup this point, retaining the cup for 10–15 minutes. With the cup removed, perform moxibustion with a moxa stick for 3–5 minutes until warmth is felt.

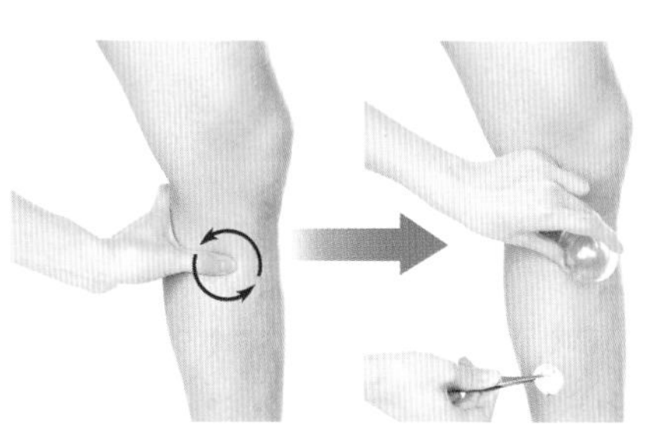

### 5. Yinlingquan Point

**Location:** In the depression on the inner edge of the shinbone below the knee.

**Method:** First knead Yinlingquan point with the thumb pulp for 2–3 minutes, and then cup this point, retaining the cup for 10–15 minutes. With the cup removed, perform moxibustion with a moxa stick for 3–5 minutes.

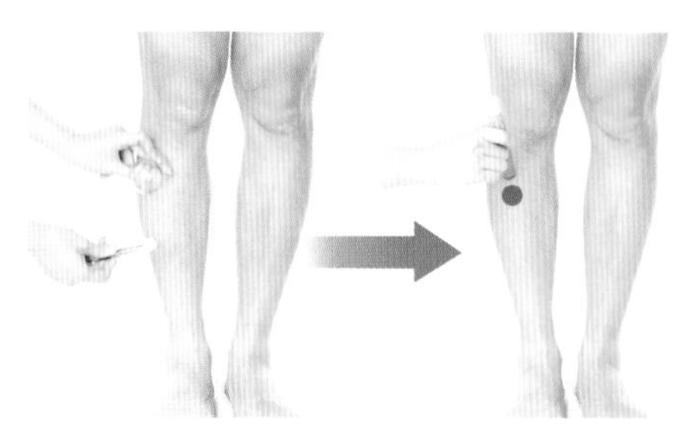

### 6. Zusanli Point

**Location:** About 3 cun below the knee on the outer side of the tibia.

**Method:** First knead Zusanli point with the thumb pulp for 2–3 minutes, and then cup this point, retaining the cup for 10–15 minutes. With the cup removed, perform moxibustion with a moxa stick for 3–5 minutes until warmth is felt.

### 7. Guanyuan Point

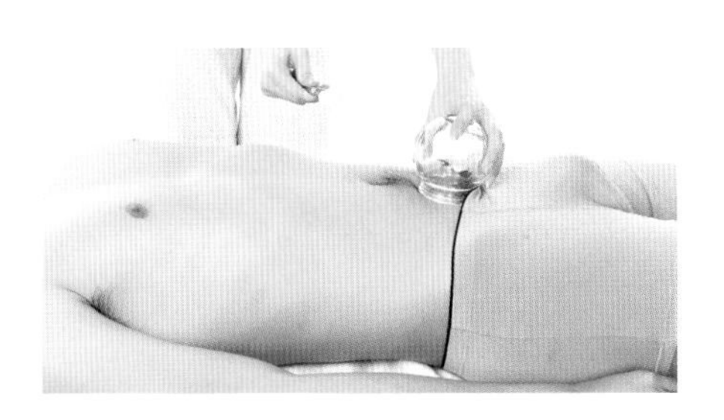

**Location:** About 3 cun below the navel.

**Method:** First knead Guanyuan point with the thumb pulp for 2–3 minutes, and then cup this point, retaining the cup for 10–15 minutes. With the cup removed, perform moxibustion with a moxa stick for 3–5 minutes until warmth is felt.

### 8. Pishu, Shenshu, Xiaochangshu, Dachangshu and Baliao Points

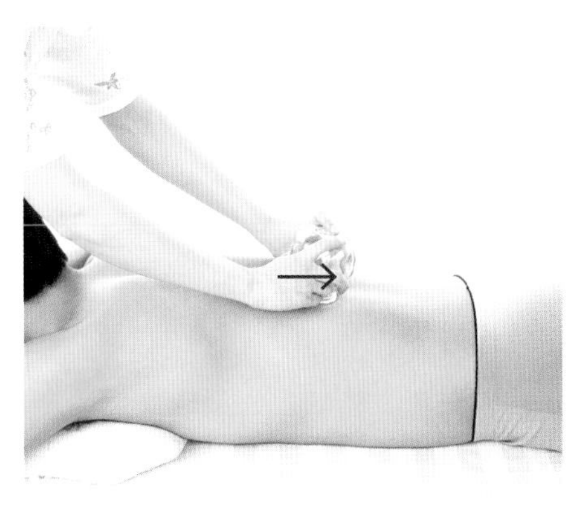

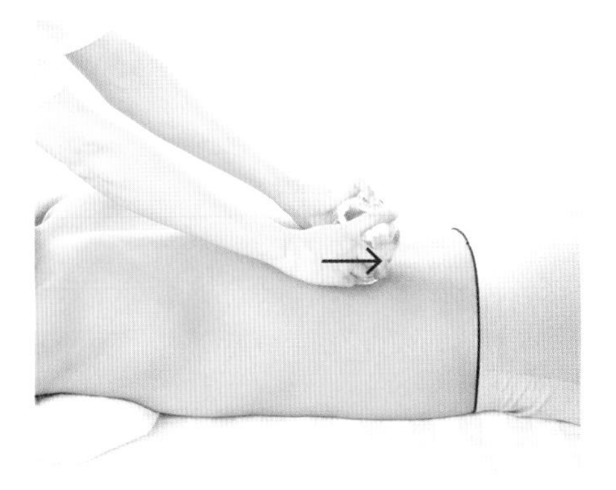

**Location:** Pishu point is 1.5 cun away horizontally from the eleventh thoracic vertebra; Shenshu point is 1.5 cun horizontally from the second lumbar spinal process; Xiaochangshu point is in the sacral area, at the same level as the first sacral foramen, 1.5 cun lateral to the median sacral crest; Dachangshu point is about 1.5 cun away from the fourth lumbar vertebra on two sides; There are eight Baliao points in total, four on each side of the sacral spine. These are the upper, secondary, middle and lower Baliao points. They are located respectively in the first, second, third and fourth posterior sacral foramina (opening between vertebrae).

**Method:** Use the moving cupping method by moving the cup on the bladder meridian on the back by segment along the meridian. Move the cup several times mainly on Pishu, Shenshu, Xiaochangshu, Dachangshu and Baliao points, and repeatedly push and pull on the points back and forth, until the skin becomes red. The cup may be retained on the abovementioned points for 10–15 minutes after the moving cupping.

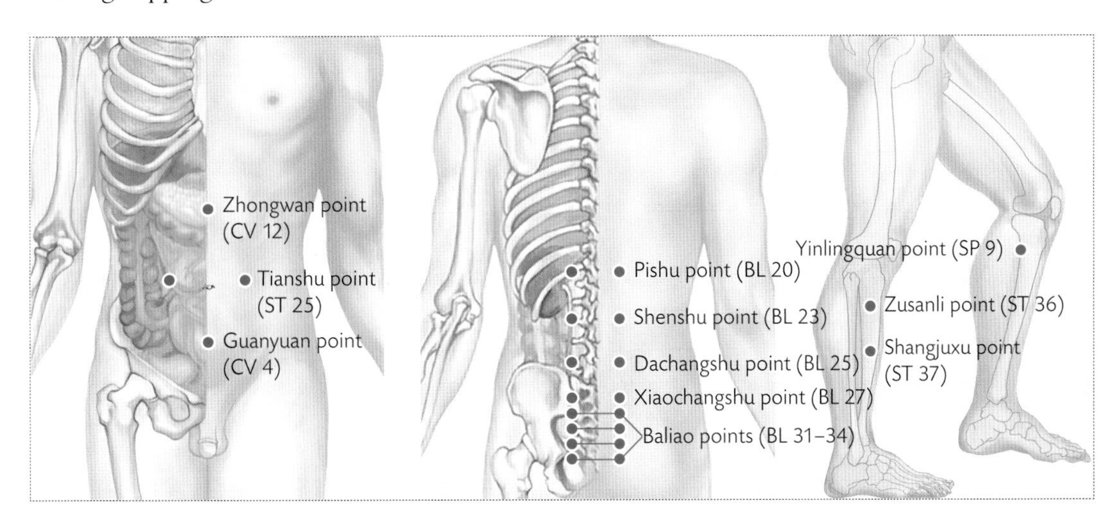

# 15 Stomachache

This type of patients will feel abdominal distension, stomachache, cold pain, burning pain, and other discomforts in the upper abdomen, probably accompanied by flatulence, nausea, vomiting, diarrhea, chest tightness, and other symptoms. Patients with severe pain may suffer from acute and chronic gastritis, gastrointestinal ulcers, and other diseases.

Kneading points on the stomach, spleen, and liver meridians every day may prevent attack of stomachache In daily life, people with stomach troubles should have regular diets, prevent drinking and eating too much, eat digestible food, avoid raw, cold, rough, hard, sour, spicy, and stimulating food. They should try to avoid worries and anxiety, and maintain an optimistic attitude.

The cupping should be applied to Zhongwan, Tianshu, Zusanli, Liangqiu, and Hegu points for acute stomachache, and to Weishu, Pishu, Ganshu, Qihai, Neiguan, and Gongsun points for chronic stomachache.

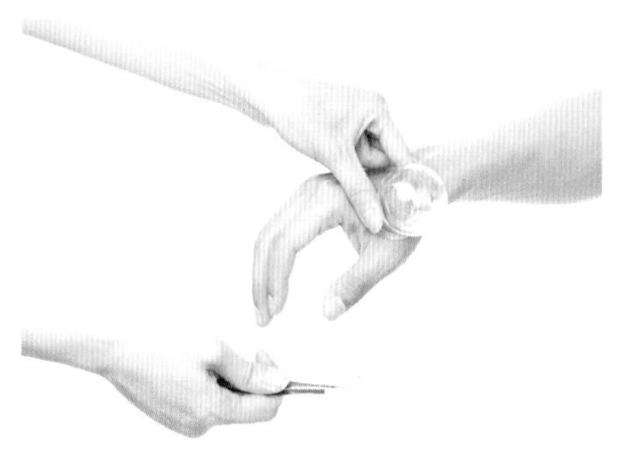

## Cupping Methods

### 1. Hegu Point

**Location:** In the highest point on the back of the hand between the thumb base and the base of the index finger (in the webbing between these two fingers).

**Method:** First knead Hegu point with the thumb pulp for 2–3 minutes, and then select and apply a cup of appropriate size to the point, retaining the cup for 10–15 minutes.

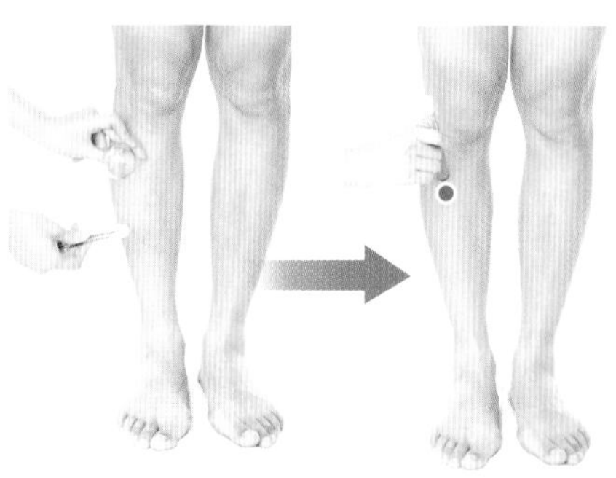

### 2. Zusanli Point

**Location:** About 3 cun below the knee on the outer side of the tibia.

**Method:** First knead Zusanli point with the thumb pulp for 2–3 minutes, and then select a cup of appropriate size and apply it to the point, retaining the cup for 10–15 minutes. With the cup removed, perform moxibustion with a moxa stick for 3–5 minutes until warmth is felt.

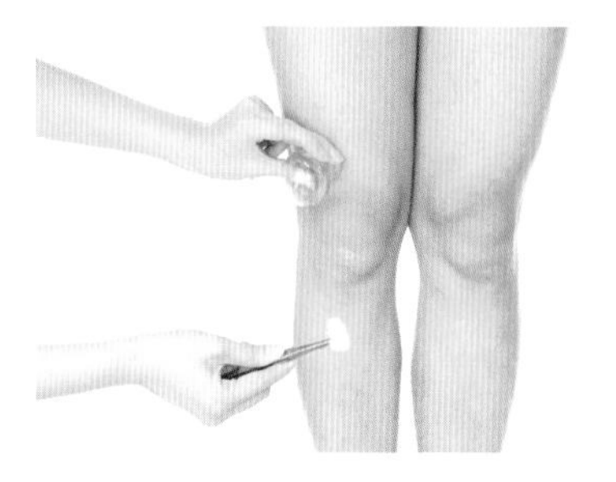

### 3. Liangqiu Point

**Location:** In the anterior region of the thigh, 2 cun above the base of the patella, and between vastus lateralis muscle and the lateral border of the rectus femoris tendon.

**Method:** First knead Liangqiu point with the thumb pulp for 2–3 minutes, and then select a cup of appropriate size and apply it to the point, retaining for 10–15 minutes. With the cup removed, perform moxibustion with a moxa stick for 3–5 minutes until warmth is felt.

### 4. Zhongwan Point

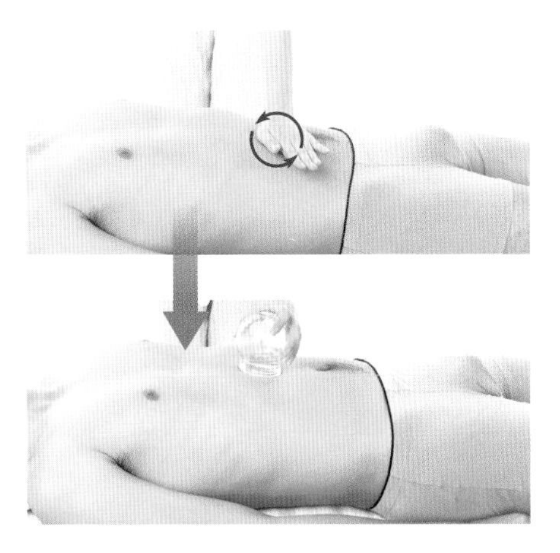

**Location:** On the upper abdomen, 4 cun above the center of the umbilicus, on the anterior midline.

**Method:** First massage the abdomen above the bellybutton for about ten circles with the palm or corporately the index finger, the middle finger, and the ring finger. Then select a cup of appropriate size, and apply it to Zhongwan point, retaining the cup for 10–15 minutes. With the cup removed, perform moxibustion with a moxa box for 3–5 minutes until warmth is felt.

### 5. Tianshu Point

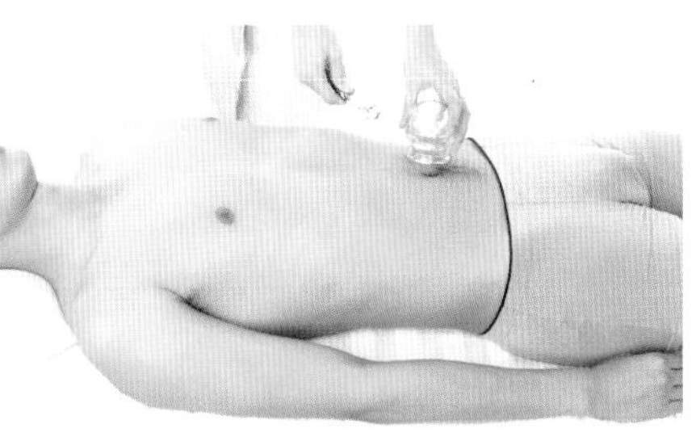

**Location:** About 2 cun horizontally away from the navel.

**Method:** First, press Tianshu point with a fingertip for 2–3 minutes, until a feeling of soreness and swelling is present. Then select a cup of appropriate size and apply it to the point, retaining the cup for 5–10 minutes.

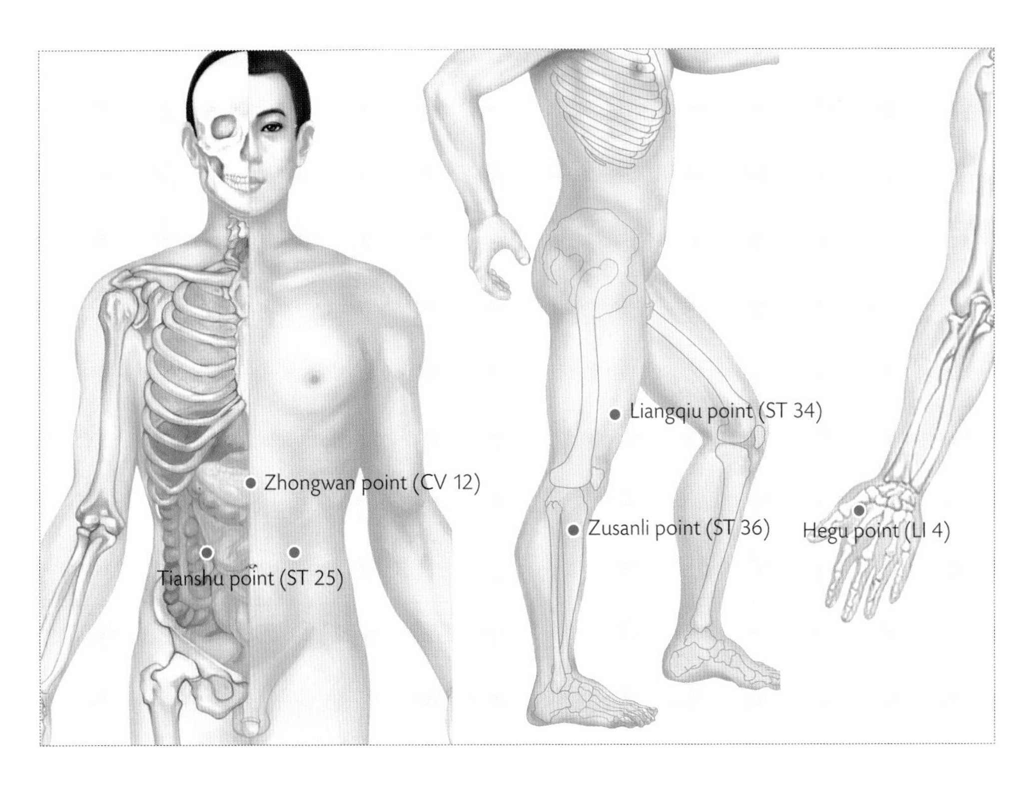

### 6. Weishu, Pishu and Ganshu Points

**Location:** Weishu point is about 1.5 cun below the spinous process of the twelfth thoracic vertebra; Pishu point is 1.5 cun away horizontally from the eleventh thoracic vertebra; Ganshu point is 1.5 cun away from the ninth thoracic spinal process on the inner side of the scapula.

**Method:** Use the moving cupping method by moving the cup on the bladder meridian on the back by segment along the meridian. Move the cup several times mainly on Weishu, Pishu and Ganshu points, and repeatedly push and pull on the points back and forth, until the skin becomes red. The cup may be retained on the abovementioned points for 10–15 minutes after the moving cupping.

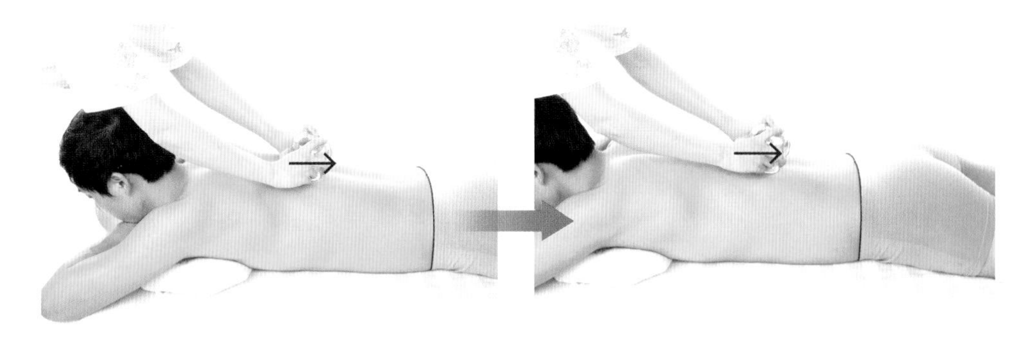

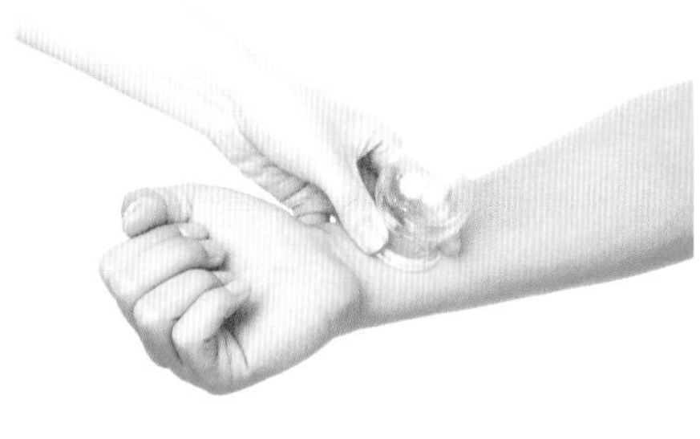

### 7. Neiguan Point

**Location:** Between the two tendons about 2 cun above the wrist joint bend.

**Method:** First knead Neiguan point with the thumb pulp for 2–3 minutes until soreness and swelling is felt, and then select and apply a cup of appropriate size to the point, retaining the cup for 10–15 minutes.

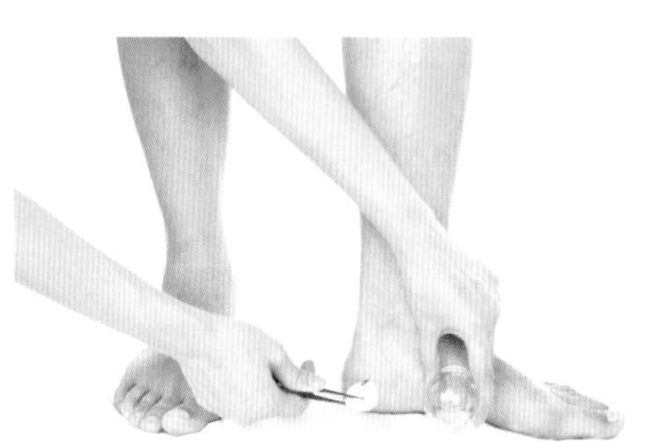

### 8. Gongsun Point

**Location:** In the metatarsal area, at the anterior border of the red and white flesh to the base of the first metatarsal bone.

**Method:** First knead Gongsun point with the thumb pulp for 2–3 minutes until soreness and swelling is felt, and then select and apply a cup of appropriate size to the point, retaining the cup for 10–15 minutes.

### 9. Qihai Point

**Location:** About 1.5 cun below the navel.

**Method:** First knead Qihai point with the thumb pulp for 2–3 minutes, and then select and apply a cup of appropriate size to the point, retaining the cup for 10–15 minutes. With the cup removed, perform moxibustion with a moxa stick for 3–5 minutes until warmth is felt.

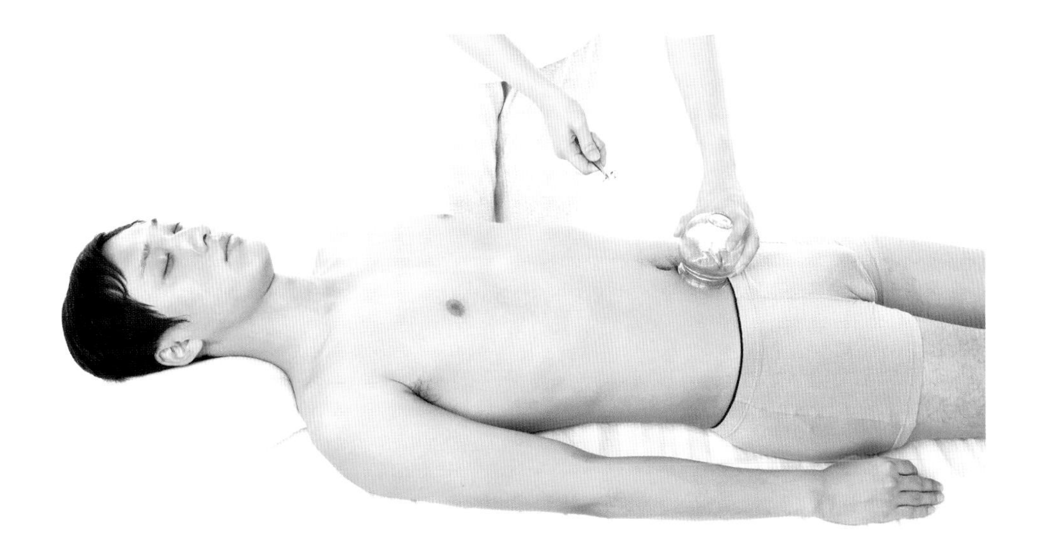

**Stomach, Spleen and Liver Meridians**

Each of the stomach, spleen, and liver meridians is one of twelve meridians of human body. The stomach meridian near the nose links with the large intestine meridian, and connects with the internal organs, including nose, eyes, upper teeth, lips, throat, and breast. It belongs to the stomach, collateral to the spleen, and connects, on the big toe, with the spleen. The spleen meridian connects with the internal organs, including the pharynx and tongue, belonging to the spleen, collateral to the stomach, infusing into the heart, and linking, in the chest, with the heart meridian. The collaterals start from the meridian, descend to the meridian of the foot-yang ming, enter the abdominal cavity, and make contact with the intestine and the stomach. The liver meridian on the big toe nail links with the gall meridian, connecting with the internal organs, including the external genitals, eye system, back part of the throat, nasopharynx, inner surface of the lips, stomach, and lungs. It belongs to the liver, collateral to the gall, and connecting, in the lungs, with the lung meridian.

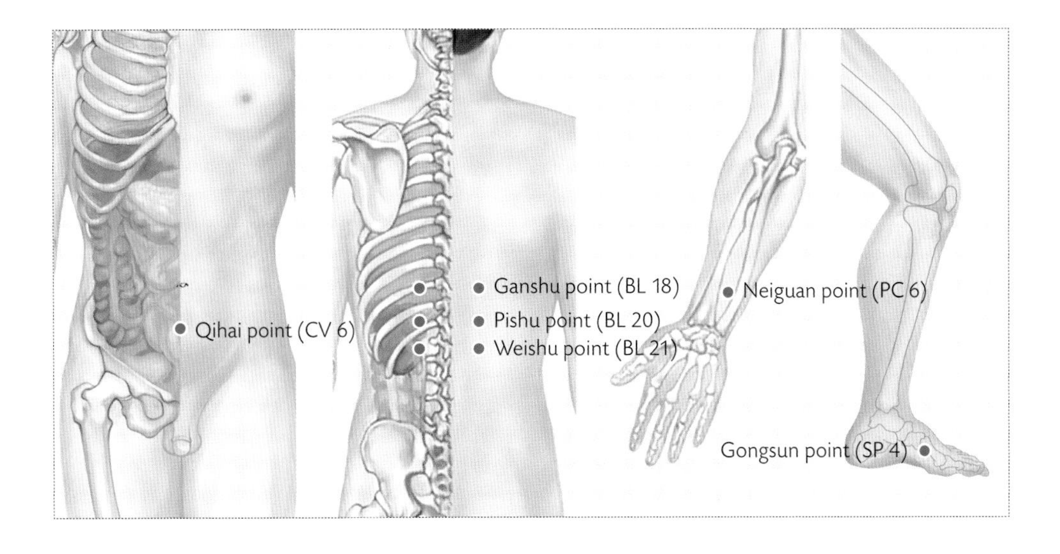

# 16 Chronic Gastritis

Patients with chronic gastritis often have no obvious symptoms or have different levels of indigestion symptoms, such as dull pain in the upper abdomen, loss of appetite, fullness after meal, sour regurgitation, etc. Severe patients may have hematemesis, melena, dehydration, and so on.

In daily life, patients should maintain lighthearted, quit smoking and alcohol consumption, avoid eating too sour, spicy, irritating, raw, cold, and indigestible food. Be cautious in using drugs. Long-term abuse of this type of drugs will injure the gastric mucosa, thus inducing chronic gastritis and ulcers. Patients with atrophic gastritis can eat yogurt and acidic food for a long time, which will help the treatment of atrophic gastritis.

The cupping can be applied to two groups of points, one group a day and two groups in turn. The first group includes Weishu, Pishu, Zhongwan, and Zusanli points. The second group includes Neiguan, Jiuwei, Zhangmen, and Gongsun points.

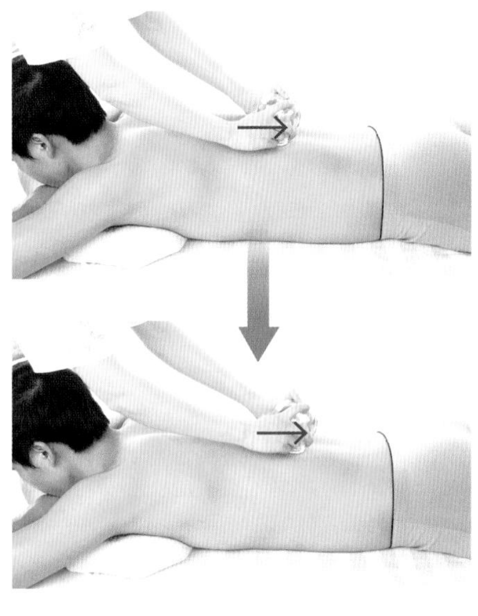

## Cupping Methods

### The First Group of Points

#### 1. Pishu and Weishu Points

**Location:** Pishu point is 1.5 cun away horizontally from the eleventh thoracic vertebra; Weishu point is about 1.5 cun below the spinous process of the twelfth thoracic vertebra.

**Method:** Use the moving cupping method by moving the cup on the bladder meridian on the back by segment along the meridian. Move the cup several times mainly on Pishu and Weishu points, and repeatedly push and pull on the points back and forth, until the skin becomes red. The cup may be retained on the abovementioned points for 10–15 minutes after the moving cupping.

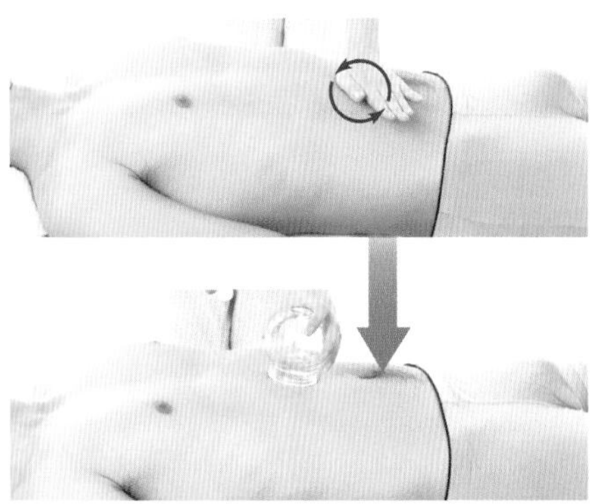

#### 2. Zhongwan Point

**Location:** On the upper abdomen, 4 cun above the center of the umbilicus, on the anterior midline.

**Method:** First, massage the upper abdomen above the belly button for about ten circles with the palm or together with the index finger, the middle finger, and the ring finger. This should be performed gently. Then select a cup of appropriate size, and apply it to Zhongwan point, retaining the cup for 10–15 minutes. With the cup removed, perform moxibustion with a moxa box for 3–5 minutes until warmth is felt.

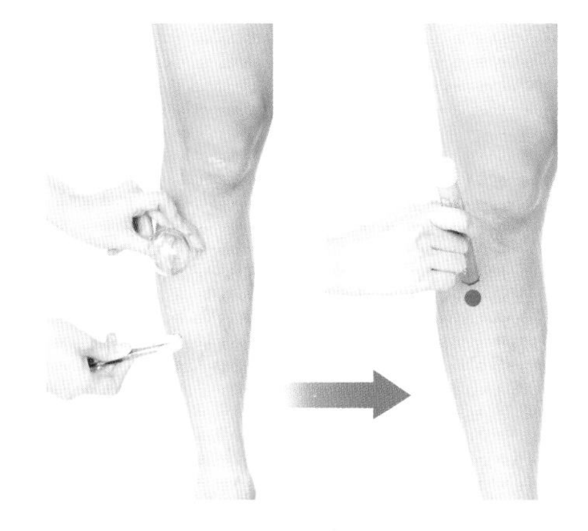

### 3. Zusanli Point

**Location:** About 3 cun below the knee on the outer side of the tibia.

**Method:** First knead Zusanli point with the thumb pulp for 2–3 minutes, and then select a cup of appropriate size and apply it to the point, retaining the cup for 10–15 minutes. With the cup removed, perform moxibustion with a moxa stick for 3–5 minutes until warmth is felt.

## The Second Group of Points

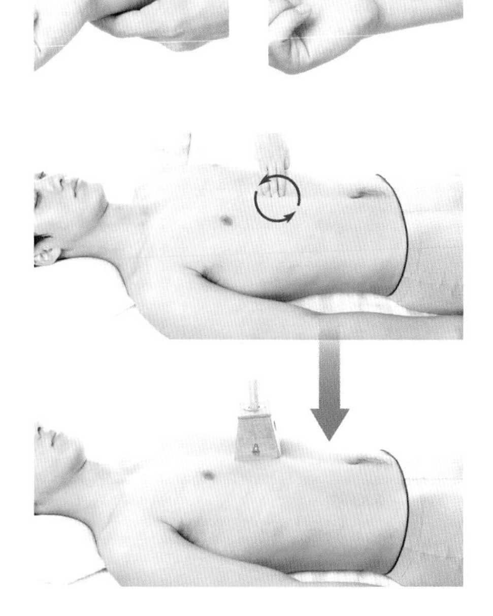

### 1. Neiguan Point

**Location:** Between the two tendons about 2 cun above the wrist joint bend.

**Method:** First knead Neiguan point with the thumb pulp for 2–3 minutes until soreness and swelling is felt, and then select and apply a cup of appropriate size to the point, retaining the cup for 10–15 minutes.

### 2. Jiuwei Point

**Location:** On the upper abdomen, 1 cun below the sternocostal angle, on the anterior midline.

**Method:** First, massage the upper abdomen above the belly button for about 3–5 minutes with the palm or together with the index finger, the middle finger, and the ring finger. Then select a cup of appropriate size, and apply it to Jiuwei point, retaining the cup for 10–15 minutes. With the cup removed, perform moxibustion with a moxa box for 3–5 minutes until warmth is felt.

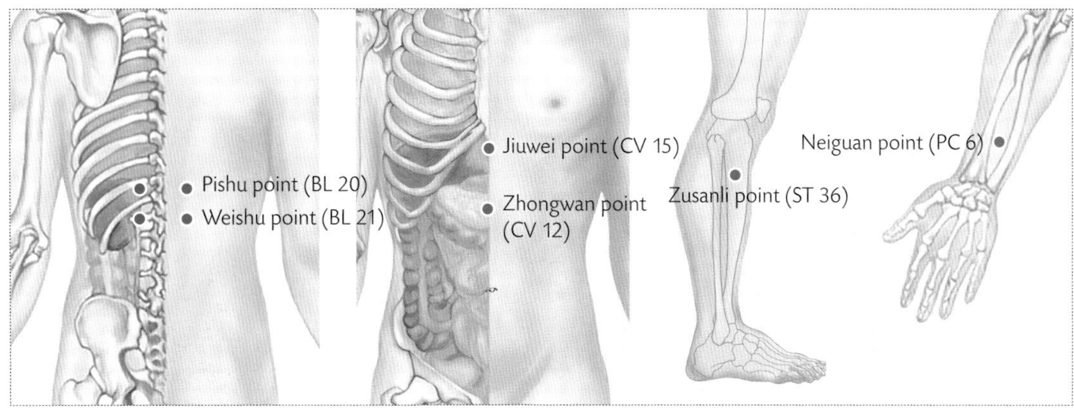

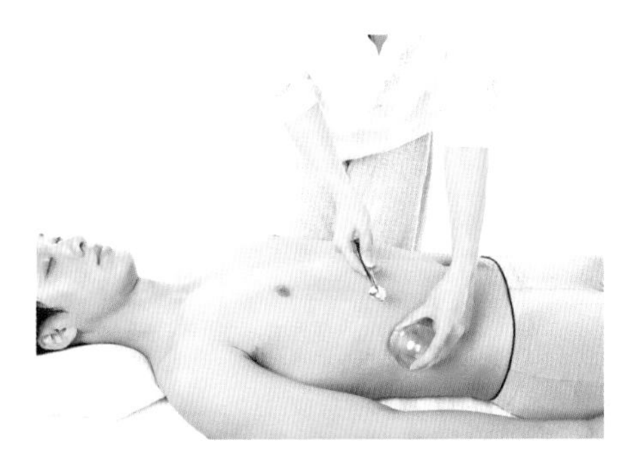

### 3. Zhangmen Point

**Location:** On the lateral abdomen, below the free extremity of the eleventh rib.

**Method:** Knead Zhangmen point with the thumb pulp for 2–3 minutes, and then select a cup of appropriate size and apply it to the point, retaining the cup for 10–15 minutes. With the cup removed, perform moxibustion with a moxa stick for 3–5 minutes until warmth is felt.

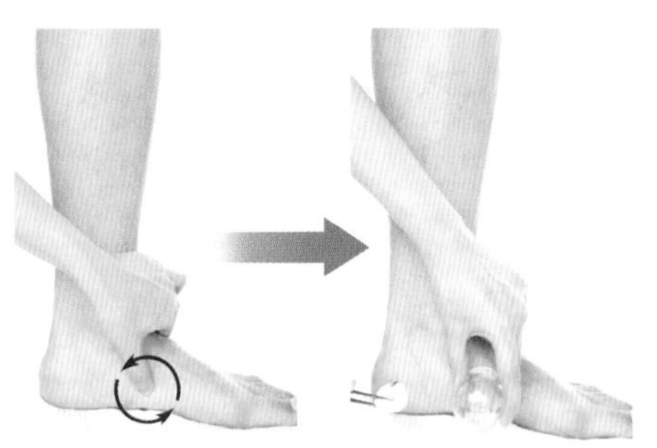

### 4. Gongsun Point

**Location:** In the metatarsal area, at the anterior border of the red and white flesh to the base of the first metatarsal bone.

**Method:** First knead Gongsun point with the thumb pulp for 2–3 minutes until soreness and swelling is felt, and then select and apply a cup of appropriate size to the point, retaining the cup for 10–15 minutes.

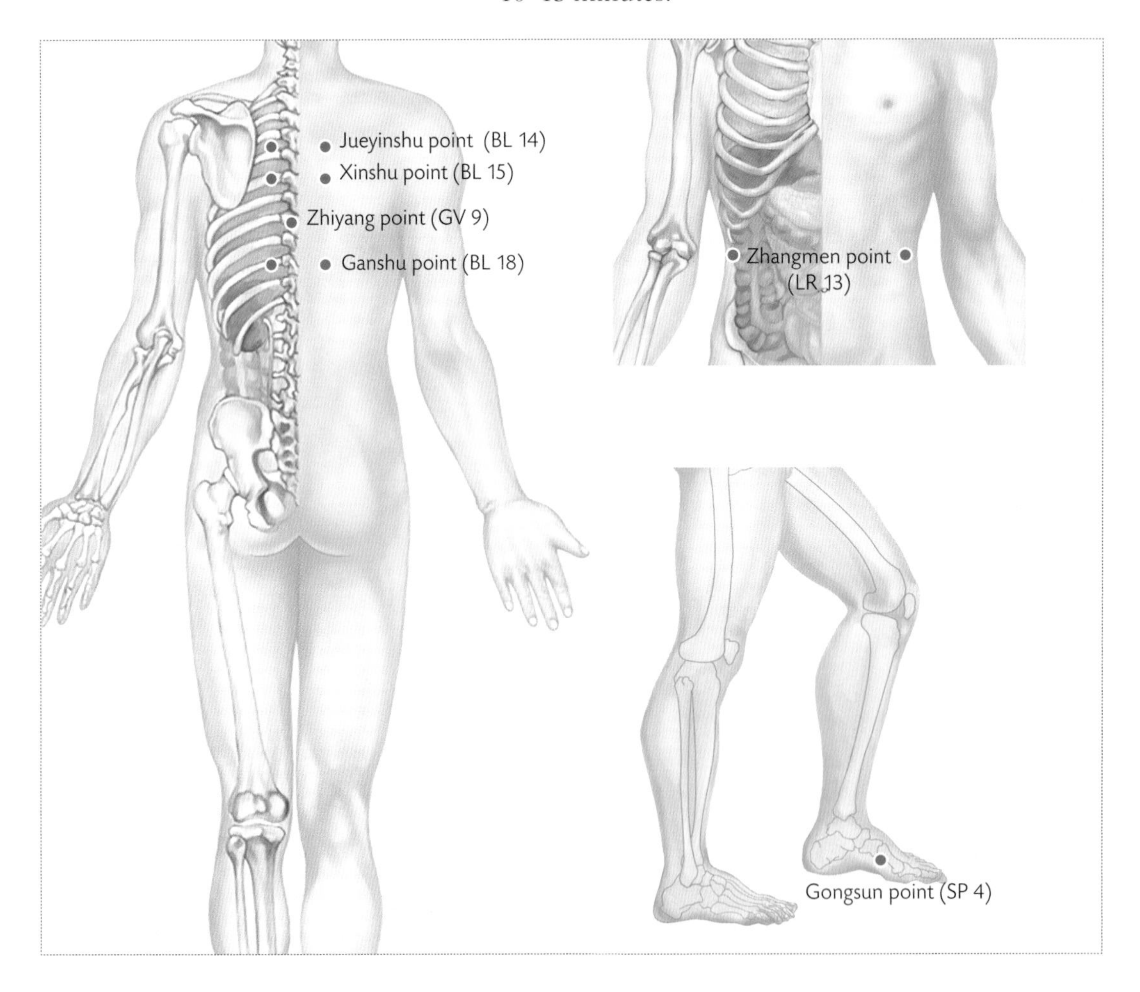

# 17 Palpitations

Patients with palpitations will have such symptoms as conscious uneasiness, violent heartbeats, nervousness, inability to control themselves, distraction, fast or slow heartbeats, which may attack in a paroxysmal or sustained manner, or accompanied by shortness of breath, tiredness, dizziness, insomnia, forgetfulness, etc.

When the conditions are serious, patients should stay in bed, and receive combined therapy of Traditional Chinese Medicine and Western medicine, supported by the cupping therapy under close observation. During treatment, they should pay attention to rest, avoid fatigue and emotional fluctuation, eat light food, and abstain themselves from smoking and alcohol drinking. Pay attention that although cupping can alleviate the attack of palpitations and reduce the frequency of seizure, it cannot completely substitute other therapeutic methods.

The cupping can be applied to two groups of points, one group a day and two groups in turn, until the symptoms disappear. The first group includes Xinshu, Jueyinshu, Ganshu, Zhiyang, and Danzhong points. The second group includes Taixi, Neiguan, Shenmen, Zusanli, and Yongquan points.

## Cupping Methods

### The First Group of Points

#### 1. Xinshu, Jueyinshu and Ganshu Points

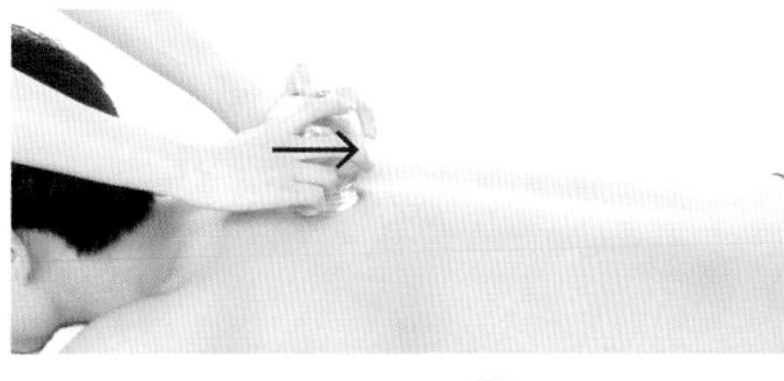

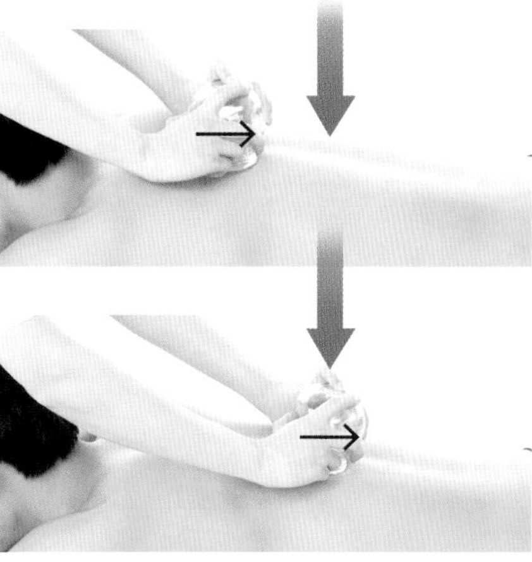

**Location:** Xinshu point is under the fifth thoracic vertebra on the inner side of the scapula, 1.5 cun horizontally away; Jueyinshu point is in the spine area, 1.5 cun lateral to the posterior midline of the lower border of the spinous process of the fourth thoracic vertebra; Ganshu point is 1.5 cun away from the ninth thoracic spinal process on the inner side of the scapula.

**Method:** Use the moving cupping method. Move the cup on the bladder meridian on the back by segment along the meridian, and move the cup several times mainly on Xinshu, Jueyinshu and Ganshu points. Repeatedly push and pull on the points back and forth, until the skin becomes red. The cup may be retained on the abovementioned points for 10–15 minutes after the moving cupping.

#### 2. Zhiyang Point

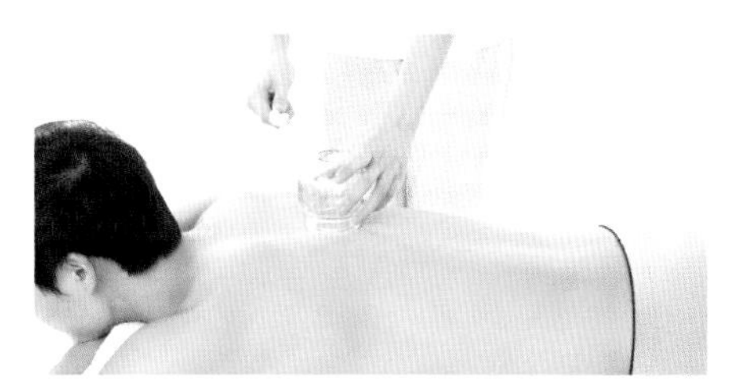

**Location:** In a cavity below the spinous process of the seventh thoracic vertebra on the midline of the back.

**Method:** Select a cup of appropriate size and apply it to Zhiyang point. Retain the cup for 10–15 minutes.

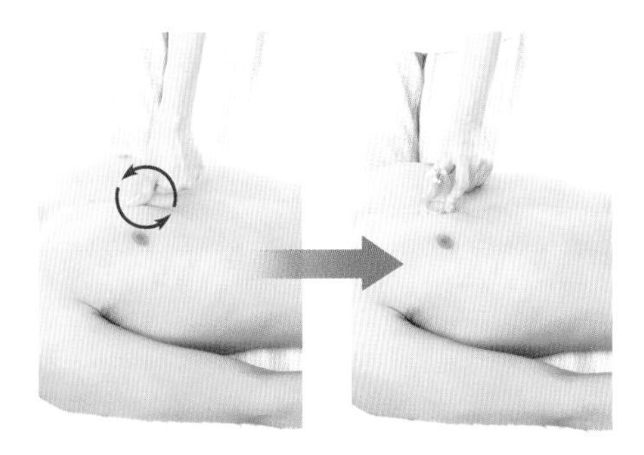

### 3. Danzhong Point

**Location:** Directly in the middle of the chest between the nipples.

**Method:** First knead Danzhong point with the thumb pulp for 2–3 minutes, and then select and apply a cup of appropriate size to the point, retaining the cup for 10–15 minutes. After the cup is removed, perform moxibustion with a moxa stick for 3–5 minutes until warmth is felt.

## The Second Group of Points

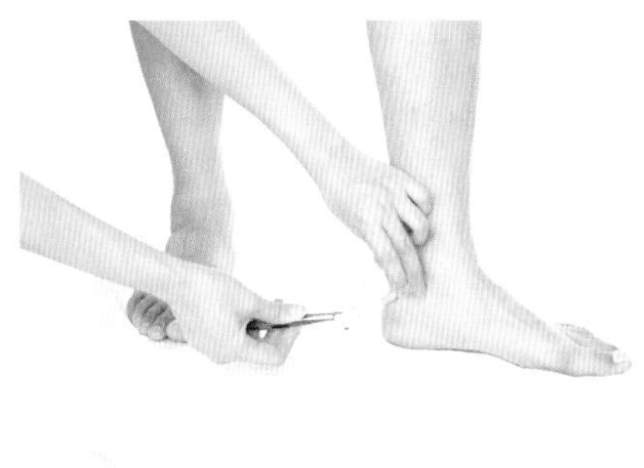

### 1. Taixi Point

**Location:** In a cavity between the medial malleolus and Achilles tendon.

**Method:** Select a cup of appropriate size and apply it to the point, retaining the cup for 10–15 minutes.

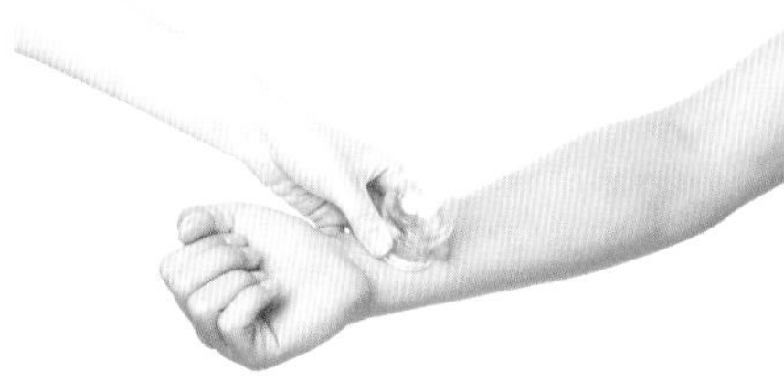

### 2. Neiguan Point

**Location:** Between the two tendons about 2 cun above the wrist joint bend.

**Method:** First knead Neiguan point with the thumb pulp for 2–3 minutes, until soreness and swelling is felt. Then retain the cup on the point for 10–15 minutes.

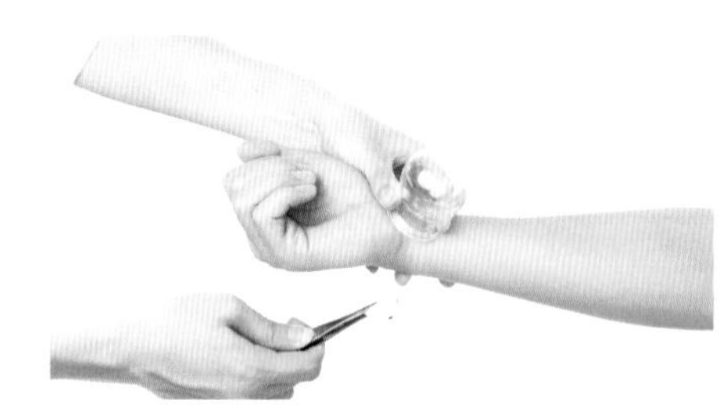

### 3. Shenmen Point

**Location:** On the inner wrist near the small finger when the palm is turned upward.

**Method:** First knead Shenmen point with the thumb pulp for 2–3 minutes, and then select and apply a small cup to the point, retaining the cup for 5–10 minutes.

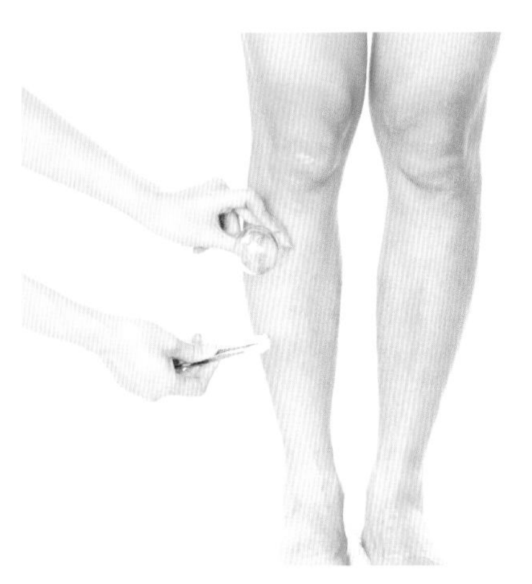

### 4. Zusanli Point

**Location:** About 3 cun below the knee on the outer side of the tibia.

**Method:** First knead Zusanli point with the thumb pulp for 2–3 minutes, and then cup the point, retaining the cup for 10–15 minutes.

### 5. Yongquan Point

**Location:** In a depression in the front of the sole of the foot, about one-third of the way down from the toes.

**Method:** First knead Yongquan point with

the palm for 2–3 minutes, until a feeling of heat is present. Then select a cup of appropriate size and apply it to the point, retaining the cup for 10–15 minutes. With the cup removed, perform moxibustion with a moxa stick for 3–5 minutes until warmth is felt.

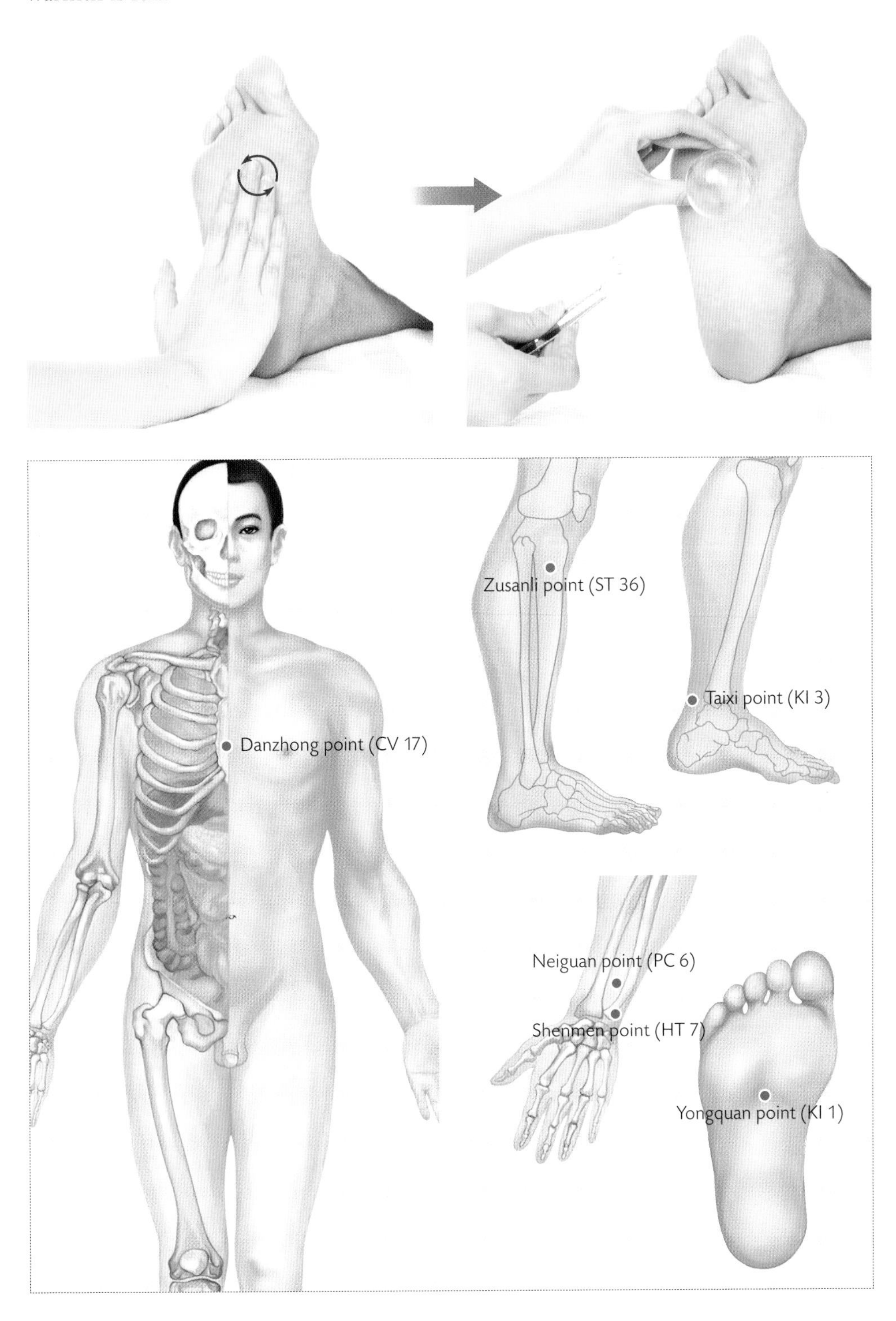

# 18 Stroke Hemiplegia

The manifestations of this disease mainly include "three hemis," i.e., hemiparalysis, hemi-sensation, and hemianopia, as well as speech disorder, dysphagia, cognitive disorder, daily activity disorder, disorder in urinary and fecal discharge, etc.

Patients may have combined cupping therapy and rehabilitation training to restore various functions as soon as possible. They should actively treat the primary diseases inducing stroke, such as hypertension, to prevent another stroke. They can also receive massage therapy.

The cupping is mainly applied to the affected parts. Cup mainly Waiguan, Shousanli, Hegu, and Jianliao points for upper limb paralysis, and mainly Huantiao, Piguan, Weizhong, Yanglingquan, Xuanzhong, and Jiexi points for lower limb paralysis. Massage the treated parts after the cup is removed to help the movement of the affected limbs.

## Cupping Methods

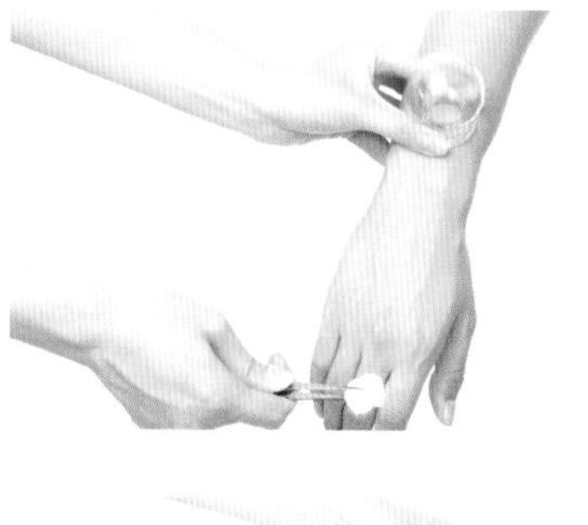

### 1. Waiguan Point

**Location:** In the middle on the outside of the arm, between the ulna and radius about 2 cun away from the horizontal line of the wrist joint.

**Method:** Select an appropriate cup and apply it to Waiguan point, retaining the cup for 10–15 minutes.

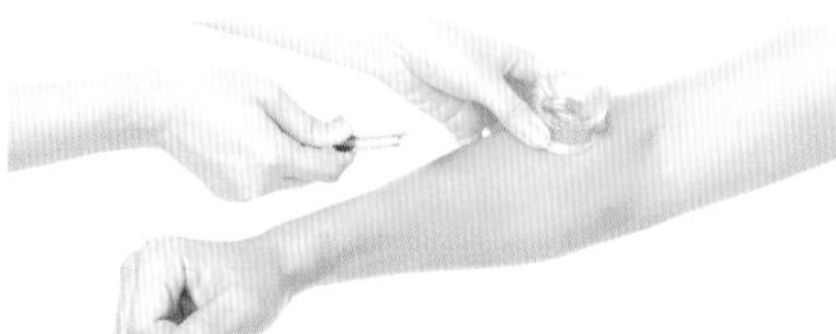

### 2. Shousanli Point

**Location:** 2 cun below the Quchi point.

**Method:** Select an appropriate cup and apply it to Shousanli point, retaining the cup for 10–15 minutes.

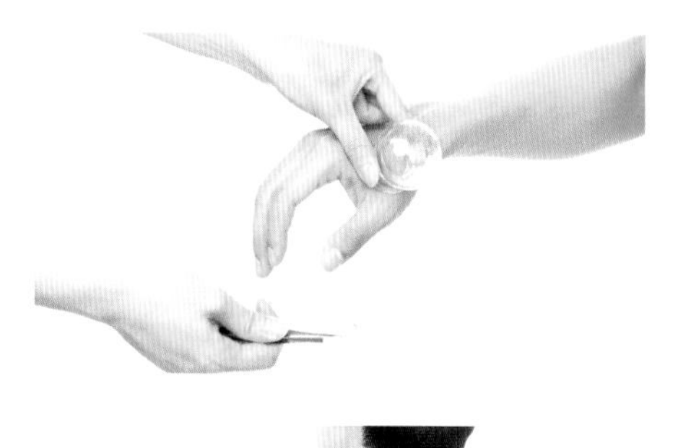

### 3. Hegu Point

**Location:** In the highest point on the back of the hand between the thumb base and the base of the index finger (in the webbing between these two fingers).

**Method:** Select an appropriate cup and apply it to Hegu point, retaining the cup for 10–15 minutes.

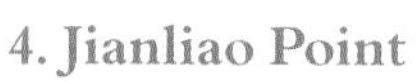

### 4. Jianliao Point

**Location:** In the deltoid muscle area, in the depression between acromial angle and the greater tubercle of humerus.

**Method:** Select an appropriate cup and apply it to Jianliao point, retaining the cup for 10–15 minutes.

### 5. Huantiao Point

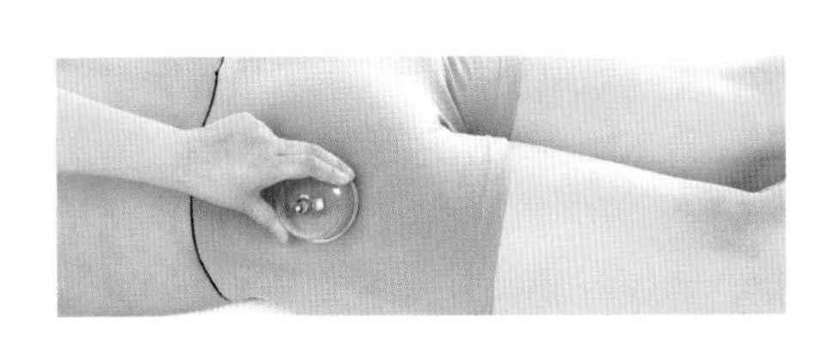

**Location:** In the depression on the outer side of the gluteus maximus, on both sides when standing.

**Method:** Retaine the cup on Huantiao point for 10–15 minutes.

### 6. Biguan Point

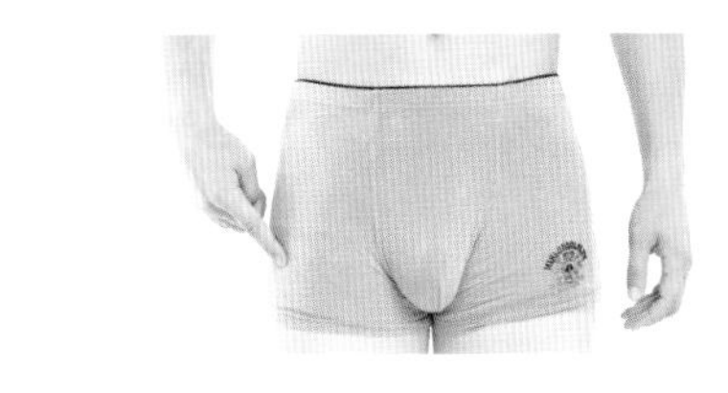

**Location:** In the anterior region of thigh, in the depression among three muscles: the proximal portion of the rectus femoris muscle, the sartorius muscle, and the tensor fasciae latae muscle.

**Method:** First, massage Biguan point with index finger or middle finger, and then select a cup of appropriate size and apply it to Biguan point. Retain the cup for 10–15 minutes.

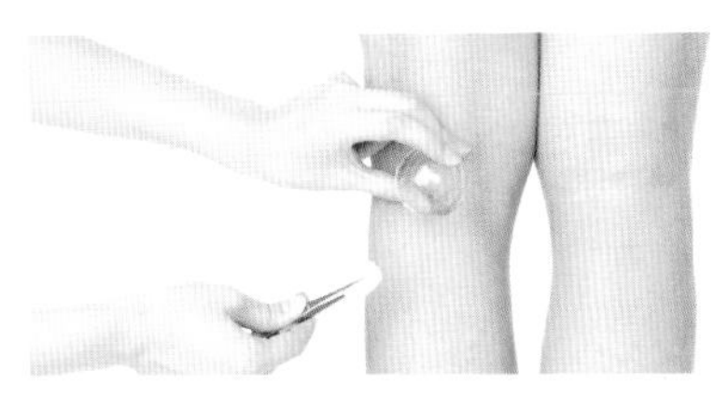

### 7. Weizhong Point

**Location:** Right in the middle of popliteal crease (at the back of the knee).

**Method:** Select an appropriate cup and apply it to Weizhong point, retaining the cup for 10–15 minutes.

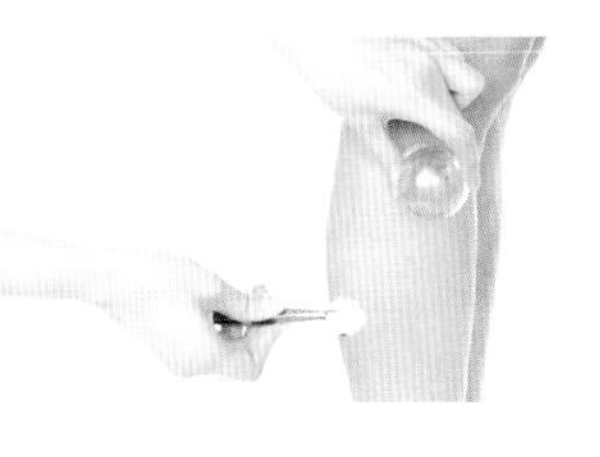

### 8. Yanglingquan Point

**Location:** On the outer side of the shin in a notch at the front lower part of the fibula.

**Method:** Select an appropriate cup and apply it to Yanglingquan point, retaining the cup for 10–15 minutes.

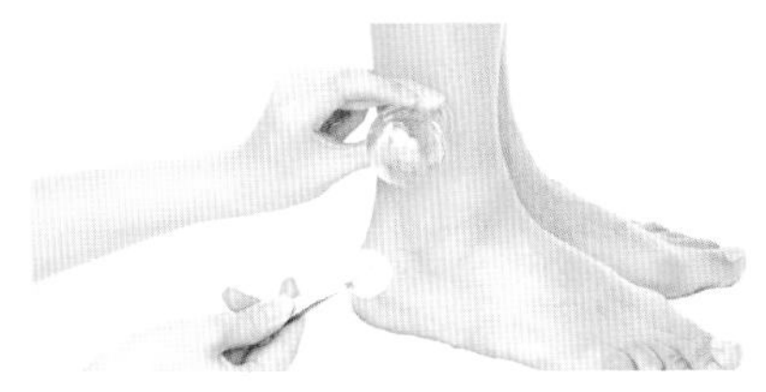

### 9. Xuanzhong Point

**Location:** In a cavity 3 cun above the outer ankle tip.

**Method:** Select an appropriate cup and apply it to Xuanzhong point, retaining the cup for 10–15 minutes.

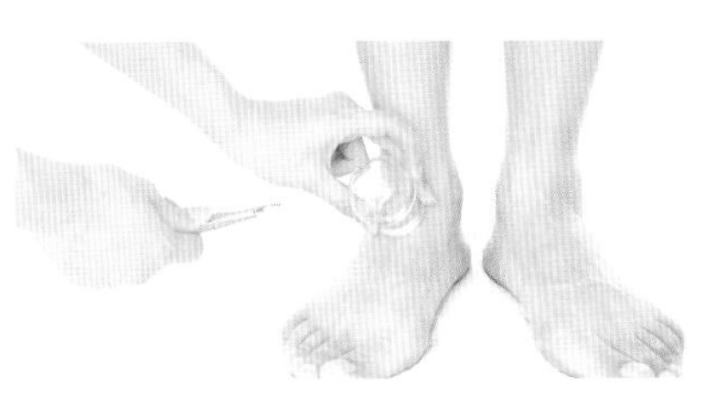

### 10. Jiexi Point

**Location:** In the middle at the front of the ankle.

**Method:** Select an appropriate cup and apply it to Jiexi point, retaining the cup for 10–15 minutes.

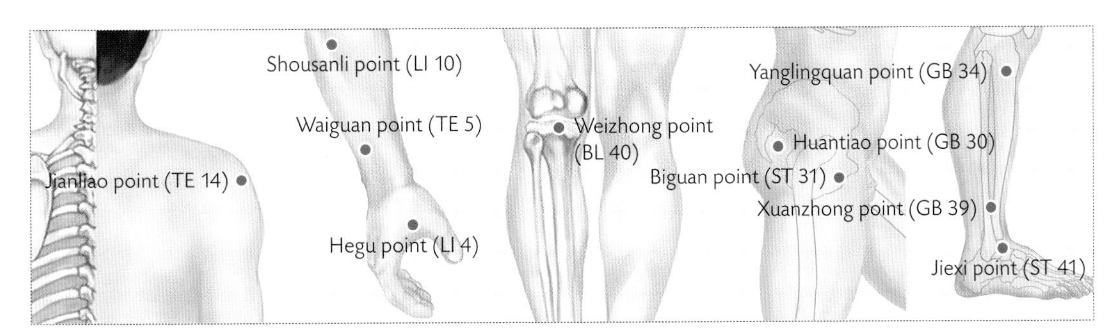

# 19 Urinary Retention

Urinary retention means inability to discharge a large amount of urine accumulated in the bladder. Acute urinary retention breaks out suddenly, and the urine cannot be discharged out of the bladder, leading to unbearable pain. Chronic urinary retention is characterized by poor urination ability and frequent urination.

Patients with acute urinary retention should pay attention to receive treatment combined with uriniferous measures. During treatment, patients should relieve their nervousness and repeatedly do alternative abdominal muscles tensing and relaxing exercise.

The cupping should be applied mainly to Zhongji, Guanyuan, Qihai, Yinlingquan, Shenshu, Pishu, Pangguangshu, Sanyinjiao, and Taixi points.

## Cupping Methods

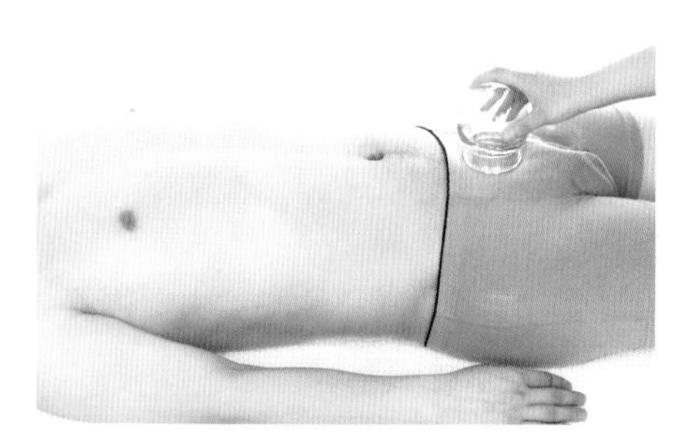

### 1. Zhongji Point

**Location:** On the lower abdomen, 4 cun below the center of the umbilicus, on the anterior midline.

**Method:** Select and apply a cup of appropriate size to the point, retaining the cup for 10–15 minutes. With the cup removed, perform moxibustion with a moxa stick for 3–5 minutes until warmth is felt.

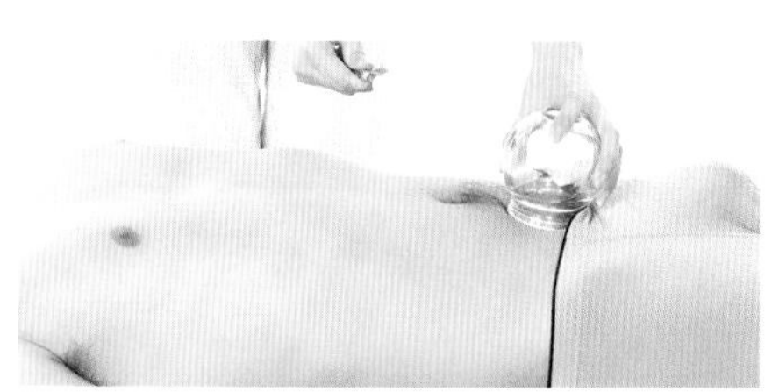

### 2. Guanyuan Point

**Location:** About 3 cun below the navel.

**Method:** Select and apply a cup of appropriate size to the point, retaining the cup for 10–15 minutes. With the cup removed, perform moxibustion with a moxa stick for 3–5 minutes until warmth is felt.

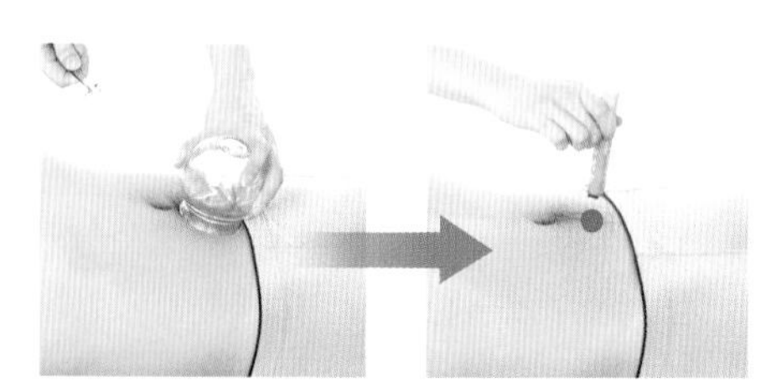

### 3. Qihai Point

**Location:** About 1.5 cun below the navel.

**Method:** Select and apply a cup of appropriate size to the point, retaining the cup for 10–15 minutes. With the cup removed, perform moxibustion with a moxa stick for 3–5 minutes until warmth is felt.

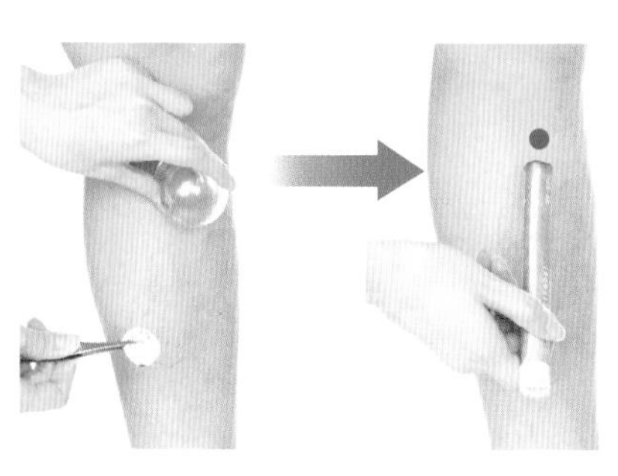

### 4. Yinlingquan Point

**Location:** In the depression on the inner edge of the shinbone below the knee.

**Method:** First knead Yinlingquan point with the thumb pulp for 2–3 minutes, and then cup this point, retaining the cup for 10–15 minutes. With the cup removed, perform moxibustion with a moxa stick for 3–5 minutes.

### 5. Pishu, Shenshu and Pangguangshu Points

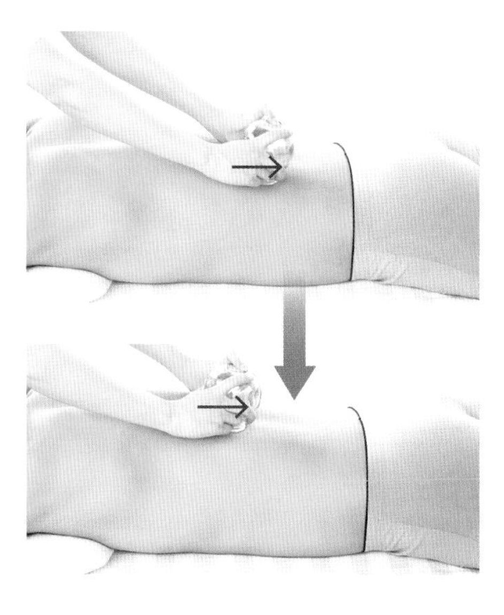

**Location:** Pishu point is 1.5 cun away horizontally from the eleventh thoracic vertebra; Shenshu point is 1.5 cun horizontally from the second lumbar spinal process; Pangguangshu point is in the sacral area, at the same level as the second posterior sacral foramen, 1.5 cun lateral to the median sacral crest.

**Method:** Use the moving cupping method. Move the cup on the bladder meridian on the back by segment along the meridian, and move it several times mainly on the Pishu, Shenshu, Pangguangshu points. Repeatedly push and pull on the points back and forth, until the skin becomes red. The cup may be retained on the abovementioned points for 10–15 minutes after the moving cupping.

### 6. Sanyinjiao Point

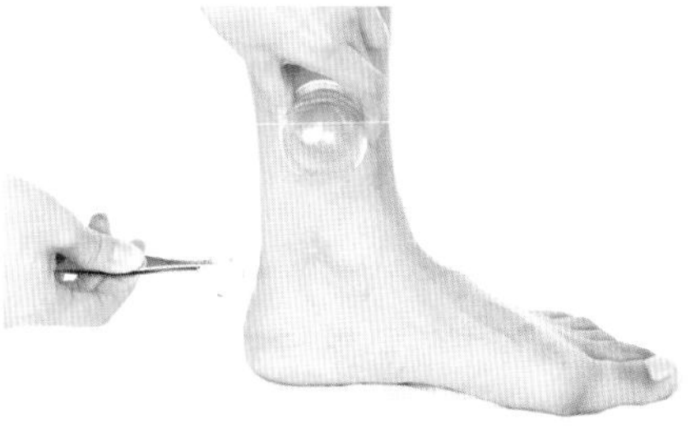

**Location:** At the rear edge of the shinbone, 3 cun above the ankle.

**Method:** First knead Sanyinjiao point with the thumb pulp for 2–3 minutes and then apply a cup to the point, retaining the cup for 10–15 minutes. With the cup removed, perform moxibustion with a moxa stick for 3–5 minutes, until warmth is felt.

### 7. Taixi Point

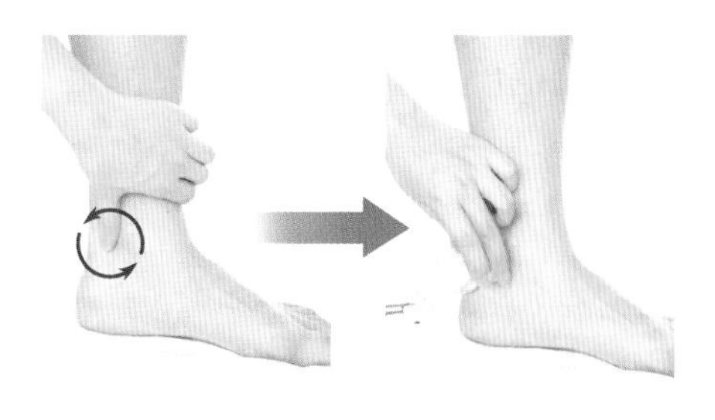

**Location:** In a cavity between the medial malleolus and Achilles tendon.

**Method:** First knead Taixi point with the thumb pulp for 2–3 minutes, and then select a cup of appropriate size and apply it to the point, retaining the cup for 10–15 minutes.

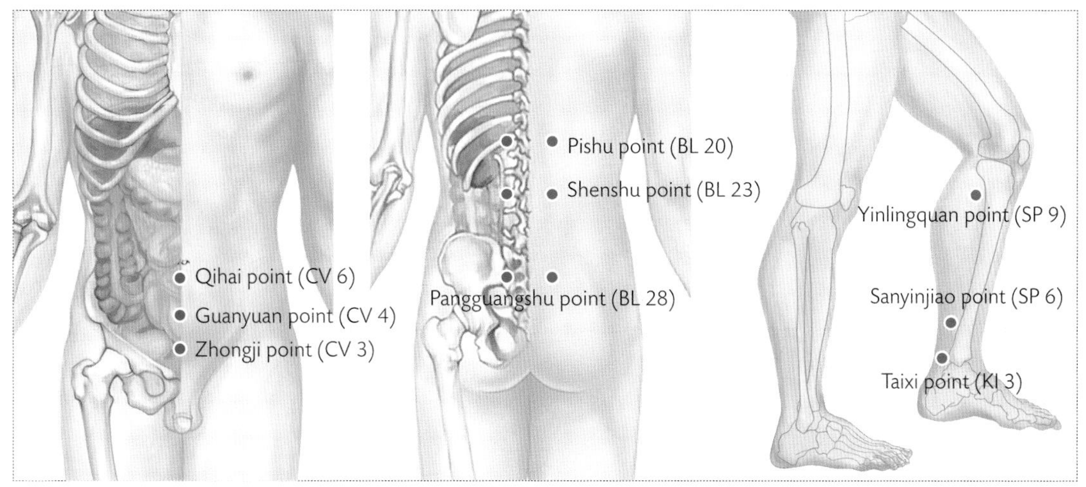

# 20 Constipation

As a complex symptom, constipation mainly means decrease in defecating frequency, reduced amount of stool, hard stool, difficulty in defecation, etc. In general, decrease in defecating frequency is the main symptom.

Patients should avoid abuse of laxatives which may lead to the body's dependence on some laxatives, thus resulting in constipation. They should make a reasonable arrangement of their life and work, and defecate regularly every day to form a conditioned reflex and develop good regular defecation. They should also eat more food rich in dietary fibers, such as apples, pears, bananas, red dates, grapes and a variety of vegetables, drink more water, actively participate in sports activities, and maintain an optimistic state of mind.

The cupping should be performed on Shenque, Tianshu, Shangjuxu, Zhigou, and Zusanli points.

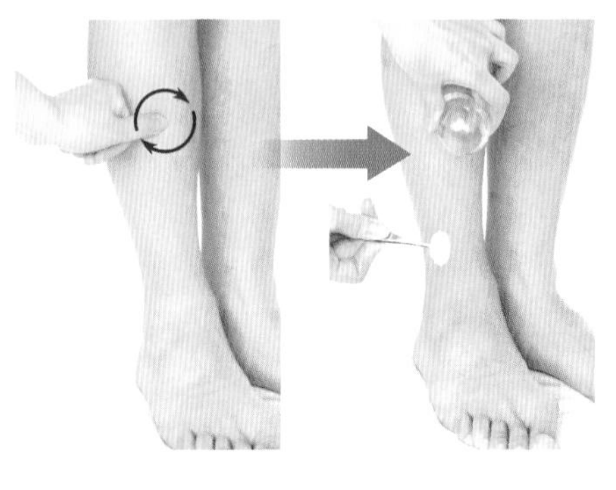

## Cupping Methods

### 1. Shangjuxu Point

**Location:** One middle finger cun (the length of the second section of the middle finger) on the outside of the tibial crest, 3 cun below the Zusanli point.

**Method:** First knead Shangjuxu point with the thumb pulp for 2–3 minutes, and then select a cup of appropriate size and apply it to the point, retaining the cup for 10–15 minutes. With the cup removed, perform moxibustion with a moxa stick for 3–5 minutes until warmth is felt.

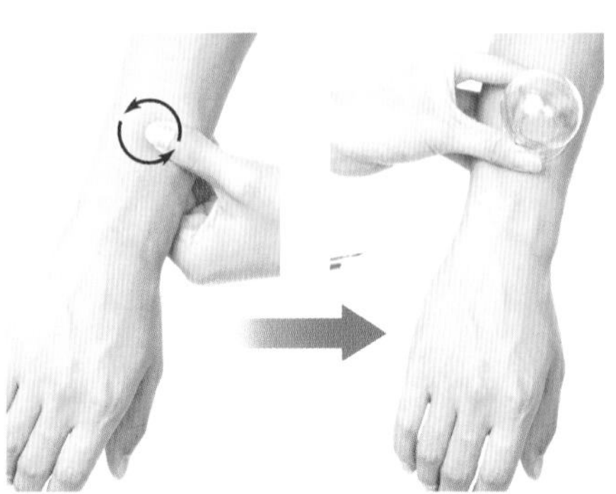

### 2. Zhigou Point

**Location:** In a cavity about 3 cun above the back of the wrist, between the two bones of the forearm.

**Method:** First knead Zhigou point with the thumb pulp for 2–3 minutes, and then select a cup of appropriate size and apply it to the point, retaining the cup for 10–15 minutes.

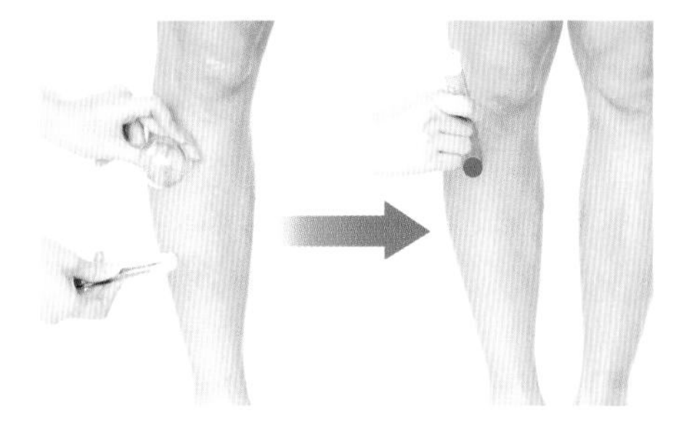

### 3. Zusanli Point

**Location:** About 3 cun below the knee on the outer side of the tibia.

**Method:** First knead Zusanli point with the thumb pulp for 2–3 minutes, and then select a cup of appropriate size and apply it to the point, retaining the cup for 10–15 minutes. With the cup removed, perform moxibustion with a moxa stick for 3–5 minutes until warmth is felt.

### 4. Shenque Point

**Location:** At the center of the navel.

**Method:** Centered on the umbilicus, massage the abdomen with the palm clockwise for around twenty circles, which should be performed gently, until the abdomen feels warm. Select and apply a cup of appropriate size to Shenque point, retaining the cup for 5–10 minutes. After the cup is removed, perform mild moxibustion with a moxa stick for 3–5 minutes until warmth is felt.

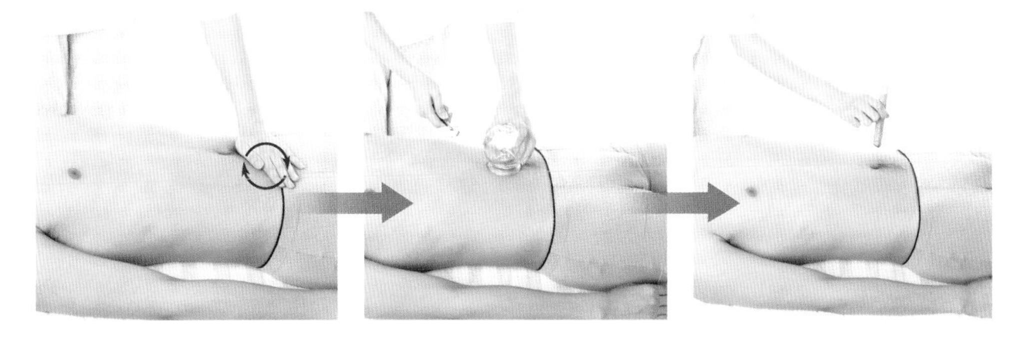

### 5. Tianshu Point

**Location:** About 2 cun horizontally away from the navel.

**Method:** First, press Tianshu point with the fingertip for 2–3 minutes, until a feeling of soreness and swelling is present. Then select a cup of appropriate size and apply it to the point, retaining the cup for 5–10 minutes.

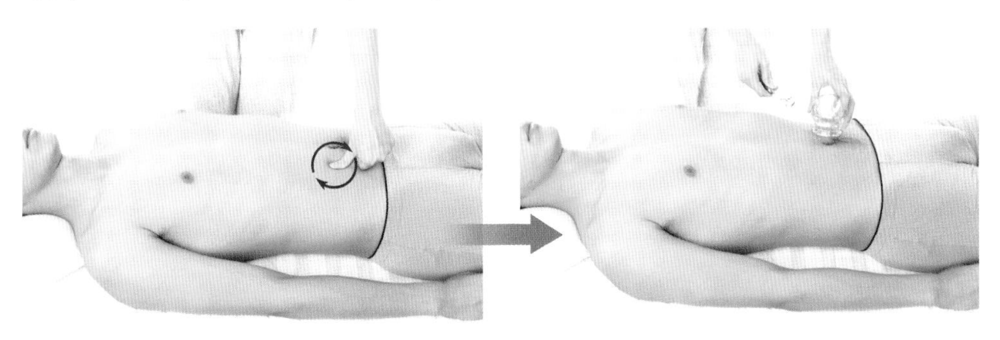

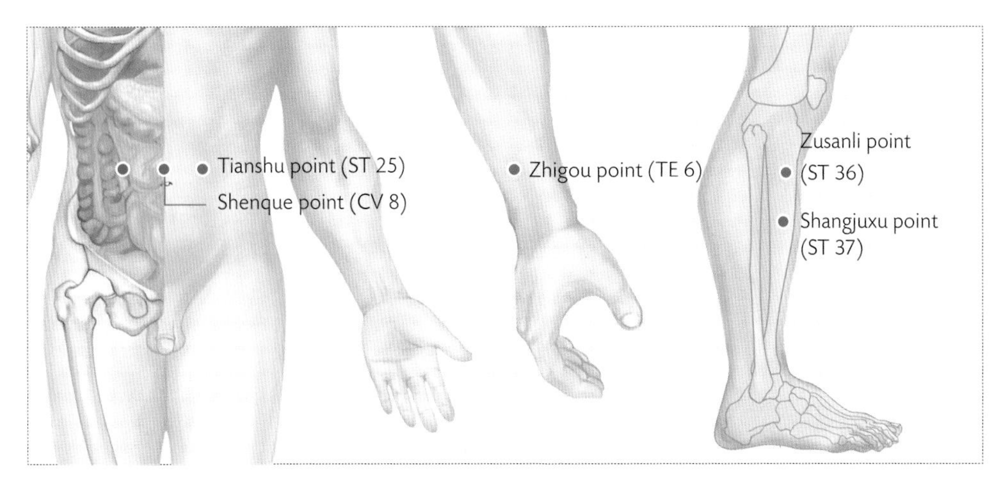

# 21 Hyperthyroidism

Patients with this disease are often characterized by excessive appetite, loss of weight, and exophthalmos, accompanied by palpitations, chest tightness, shortness of breath, prone to excitement, ect.

They should eat less iodine food like kelp, seaweed and other iodine-containing seafood. The cupping therapy has certain effects on alleviating hyperthyroidism. But those with thyroid crisis should be treated by combining appropriate Traditional Chinese Medicine and Western medicine.

The cupping can be applied to two groups of points, one group a day and two groups in turn, until the symptoms are alleviated or disappear. The first group includes Dazhui, Quchi, Taichong, and Taixi points, and the second group includes Xinshu, Pishu, Weishu, Shenshu, Ganshu, Shenmen, Jianshi, Neiguan, and Tongli points.

## Cupping Methods

### The First Group of Points

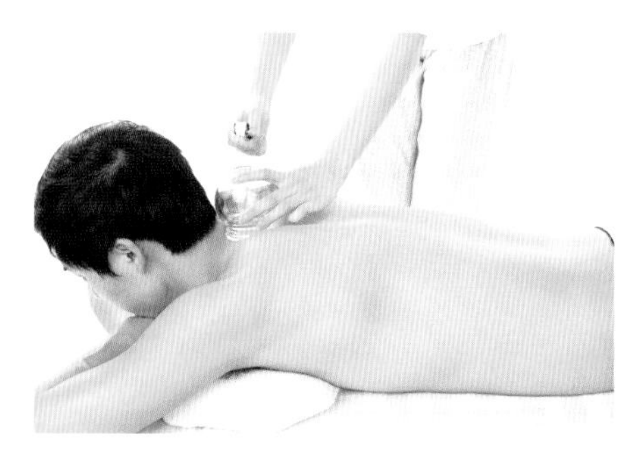

#### 1. Dazhui Point

**Location:** Under the spinous process of the seventh cervical vertebrae.

**Method:** Select a cup of appropriate size and apply it to Dazhui point. Retain the cup for 10–15 minutes.

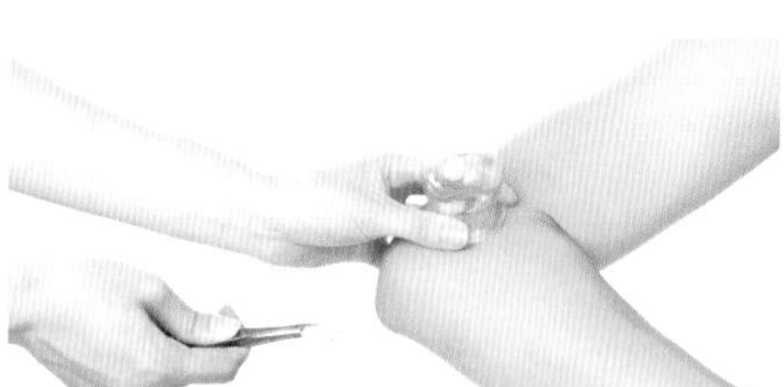

#### 2. Quchi Point

**Location:** With the elbow bent halfway, on the outer side of the cubital transverse crease.

**Method:** Select a cup of appropriate size and apply it to Quchi point. Retain the cup for 10–15 minutes.

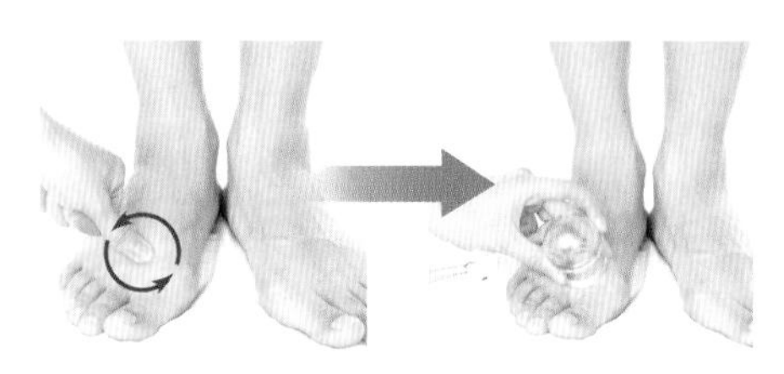

#### 3. Taichong Point

**Location:** On the foot in a notch between the first and second metatarsal bones.

**Method:** First knead Taichong point with the thumb pulp for 2–3 minutes, and then select and apply a cup of appropriate size to the point, retaining the cup for 10–15 minutes.

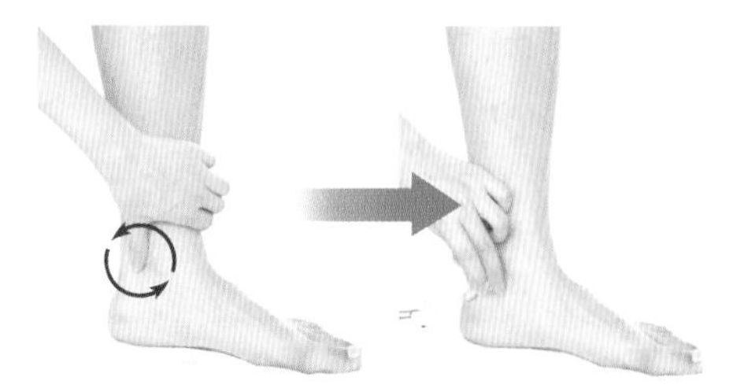

#### 4. Taixi Point

**Location:** In a cavity between the medial malleolus and Achilles tendon.

**Method:** First knead Taixi point with the thumb pulp for 2–3 minutes, and then select a cup of appropriate size and apply it to the point, retaining the cup for 10–15 minutes.

## The Second Group of Points

### 1. Xinshu, Pishu, and Weishu Points

**Location:** Xinshu point is under the fifth thoracic vertebra on the inner side of the scapula, 1.5 cun horizontally away; Pishu point is 1.5 cun away horizontally from the eleventh thoracic vertebra; Weishu point is about 1.5 cun below the spinous process of the twelfth thoracic vertebra.

**Method:** Use the moving cupping method, move the cup on the bladder meridian on the back by segment along the meridian. Move the cup several times focusing on Xinshu, Pishu, and Weishu points, and repeatedly push and pull on the points back and forth, until the skin becomes red. After the moving cupping is finished, retain the cup on Pishu and Weishu points for 10–15 minutes.

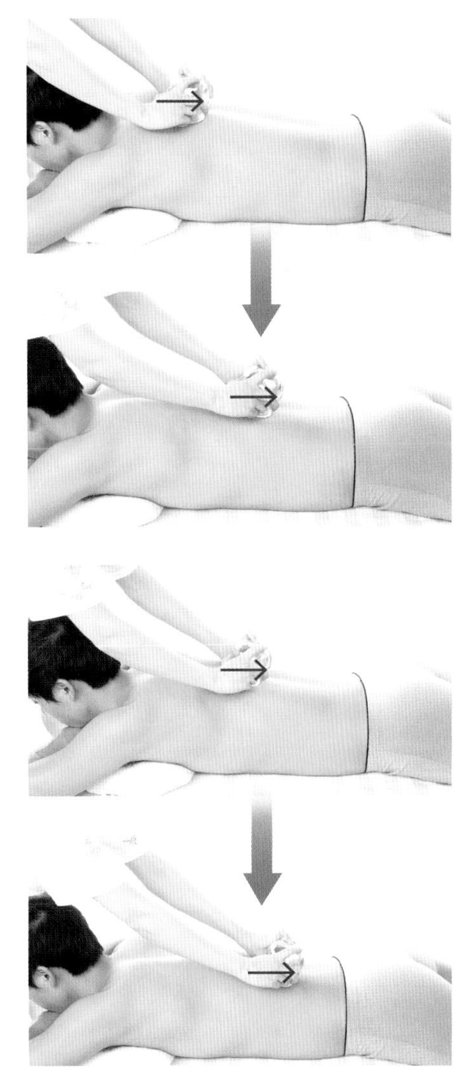

### 2. Shenshu and Ganshu Points

**Location:** Shenshu point is 1.5 cun horizontally from the second lumbar spinal process; Ganshu point is 1.5 cun away from the ninth thoracic spinal process on the inner side of the scapula.

**Method:** Use the moving cupping method. Move the cup on the bladder meridian on the back by segment along the meridian, and move it several times mainly on Shenshu and Ganshu points. Repeatedly push and pull on the points back and forth, until the skin becomes red. The cup may be retained on the abovementioned points for 10–15 minutes after the moving cupping.

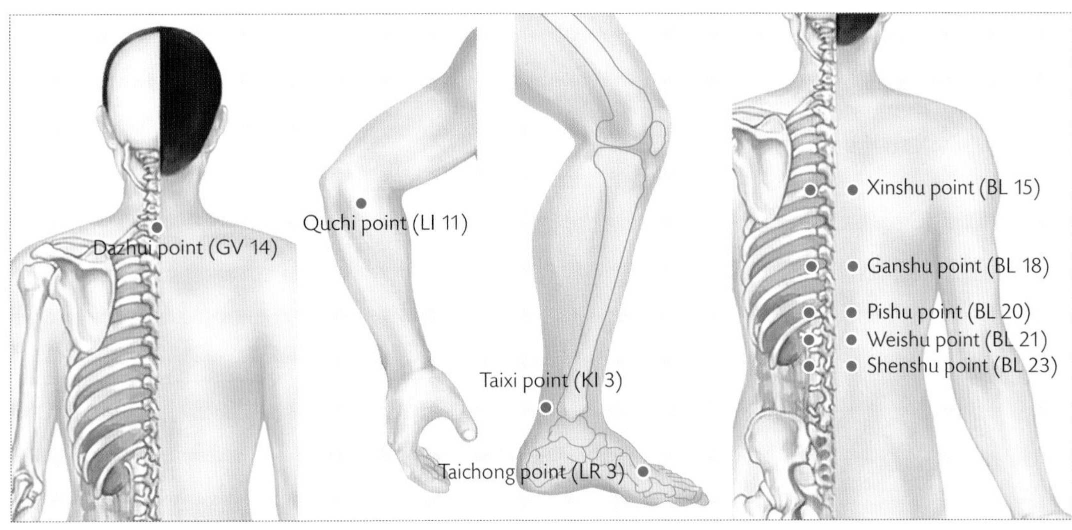

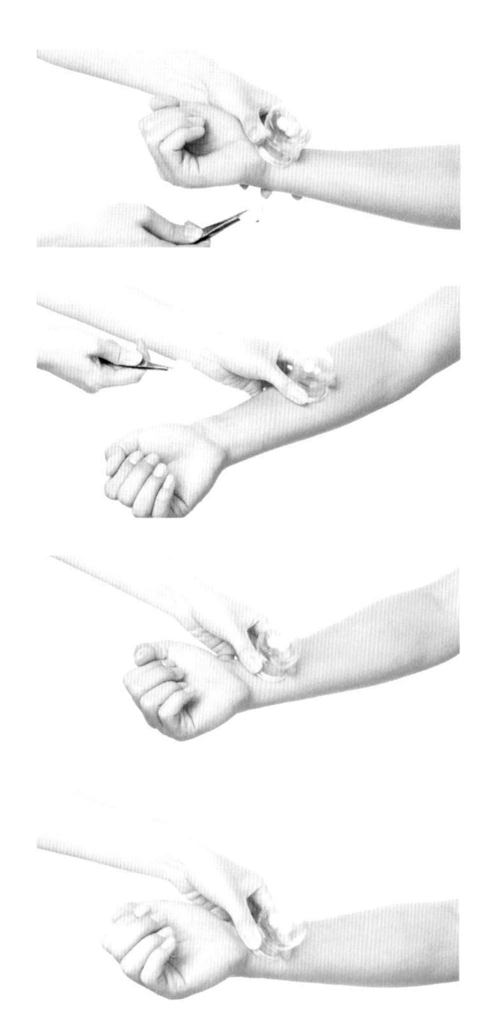

### 3. Shenmen Point

**Location:** On the inner wrist near the small finger when the palm is turned upward.

**Method:** First knead Shenmen point with the thumb pulp for 2–3 minutes, and then apply a cup to the point, retaining the cup for 5–10 minutes.

### 4. Jianshi Point

**Location:** On the anterior aspect of forearm, 3 cun above the palmar wrist crease, between the tendons of palmaris longus and flexor carpi radialis.

**Method:** First knead Jianshi point with the thumb pulp for 2–3 minutes, and then apply a cup to the point, retaining the cup for 5–10 minutes.

### 5. Neiguan Point

**Location:** Between the two tendons about 2 cun above the wrist joint.

**Method:** First knead Neiguan point with the thumb pulp for 2–3 minutes, and then apply a cup to the point, retaining the cup for 5–10 minutes.

### 6. Tongli Point

**Location:** In the anterior region of the forearm, on the radial side of the tendon of flexor carpi ulnaris, 1 cun proximal to the palmar wrist crease.

**Method:** First knead Tongli point with the thumb pulp for 2–3 minutes, and then apply a cup to the point, retaining the cup for 5–10 minutes.

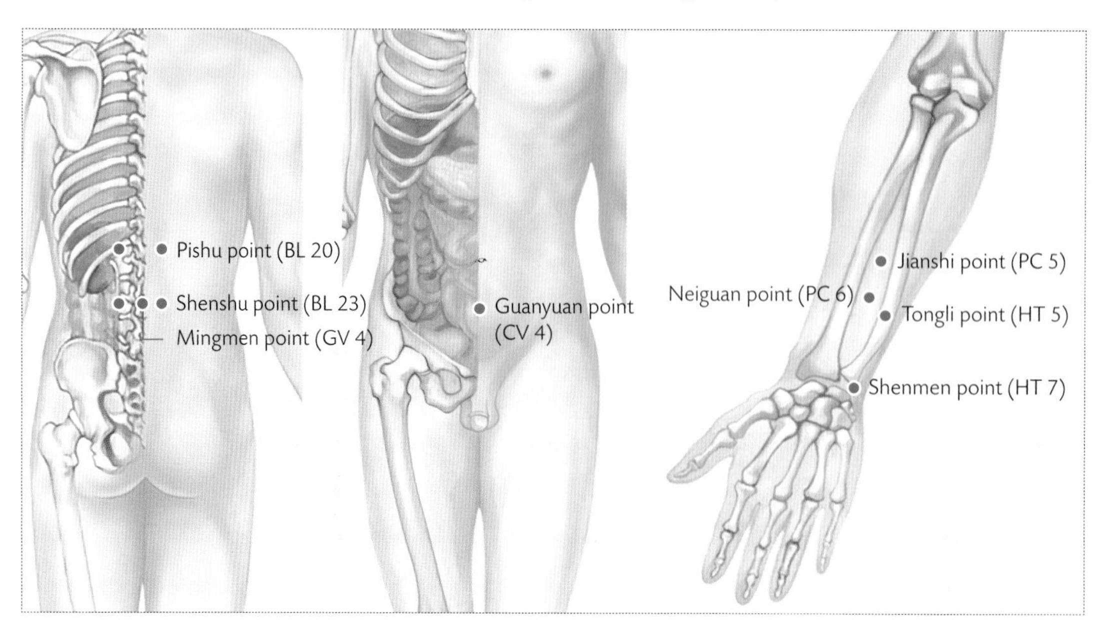

# 22 Hypothyroidism

Patients with this disease may feel myasthenia of limbs, decrease of endocrine function, low blood pressure, dizziness, muscle weakness, and have abnormal body shape, etc.

They should supplement iodized salt in their daily diet. Patients with hypothyroidism caused by iodine deficiency should eat appropriate amount of kelp, seaweed, etc., but should avoid eating any goitrogenic substance like oilseed rape, cassava, and walnut, and avoid eating food rich in cholesterol such as butter, animal brain and internal organs. Please know that the cupping therapy can only alleviate the hypothyroidism, but cannot completely replace other therapies.

The cupping should be performed on Pishu, Shenshu, Guanyuan, Mingmen, and Zusanli points, plus Taixi point for those with dizziness, Yanglingquan point for those with fatigue, and Shenmen and Zhaohai points for those with drowsiness.

## Cupping Methods

### 1. Pishu and Shenshu Points

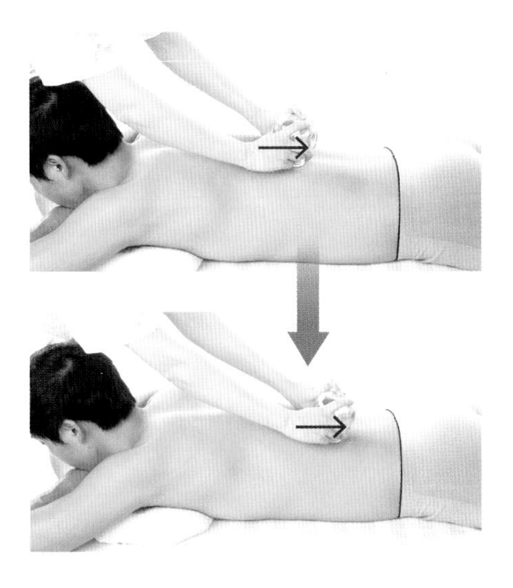

**Location:** Pishu point is 1.5 cun away horizontally from the eleventh thoracic vertebra; Shenshu point is 1.5 cun horizontally from the second lumbar spinal process.

**Method:** Use the moving cupping method by moving the cup on the bladder meridian on the back by segment along the meridian. Move the cup several times mainly on Pishu and Shenshu points, and repeatedly push and pull on the points back and forth, until the skin becomes red. The cup may be retained on the abovementioned points for 10–15 minutes after the moving cupping.

### 2. Guanyuan Point

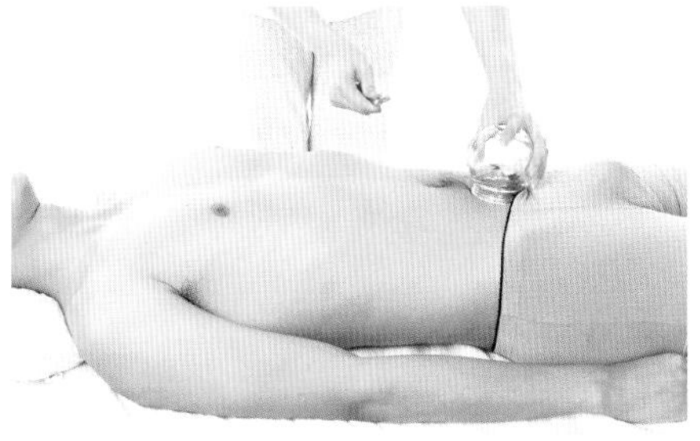

**Location:** About 3 cun below the navel.

**Method:** First knead Guanyuan point with the thumb pulp for 2–3 minutes, and then select and apply a cup of appropriate size to the point, retaining the cup for 10–15 minutes. With the cup removed, perform moxibustion with a moxa stick for 3–5 minutes until warmth is felt.

### 3. Mingmen Point

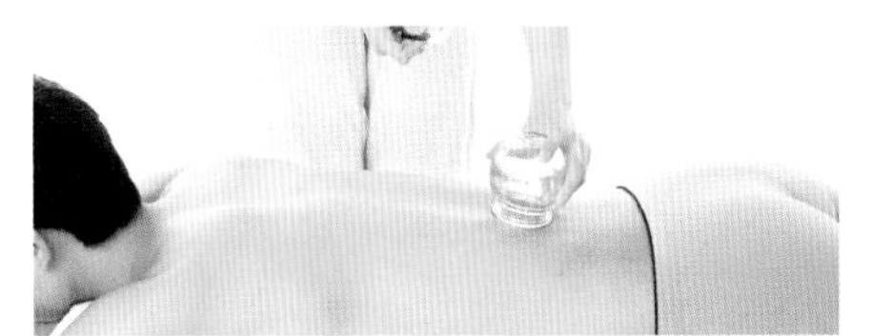

**Location:** In a cavity below the spinous process of the second cervical vertebra.

**Method:** Select and apply a cup of appropriate size to the point, retaining the cup for 5–10 minutes.

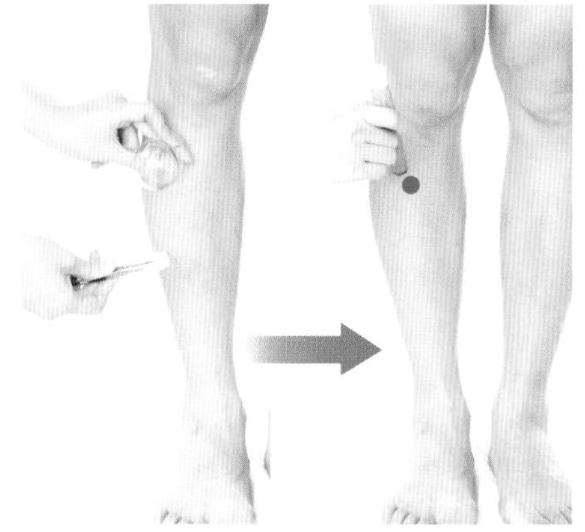

With the cup removed, perform moxibustion with a moxa stick for 3–5 minutes until warmth is felt.

### 4. Zusanli Point

**Location:** About 3 cun below the knee on the outer side of the tibia.

**Method:** First knead Zusanli point with the thumb pulp for 2–3 minutes, and then select a cup of appropriate size and apply it to the point, retaining the cup for 10–15 minutes. With the cup removed, perform moxibustion with a moxa stick for 3–5 minutes until warmth is felt.

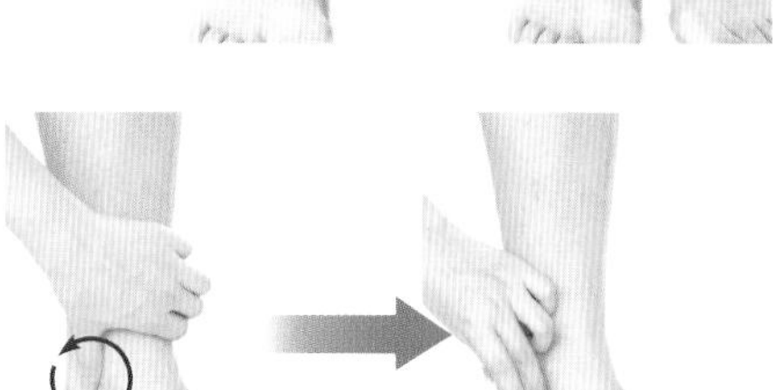

### 5. Taixi Point

**Location:** In a cavity between the medial malleolus and Achilles tendon.

**Method:** First knead Taixi point with the thumb pulp for 2–3 minutes, until soreness and swelling is felt. Then select a cup of appropriate size and apply it to the point, retaining the cup for 10–15 minutes.

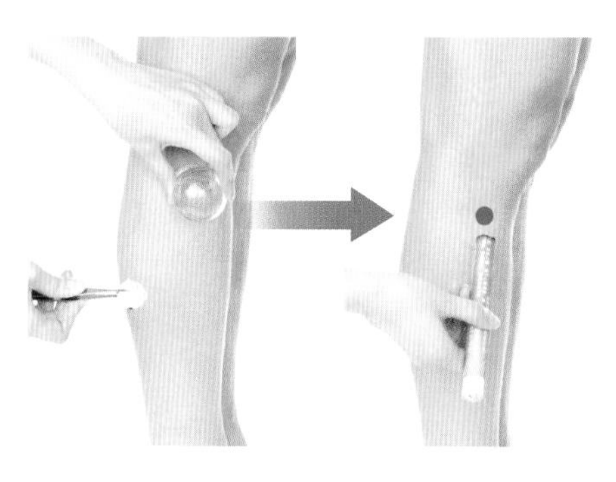

### 6. Yanglingquan Point

**Location:** On the outer side of the shin in a notch at the front lower part of the fibula.

**Method:** First knead Yanglingquan point with the thumb pulp for 2–3 minutes, and then select and apply a cup of appropriate size to the point, retaining the cup for 10–15 minutes. With the cup removed, perform moxibustion with a moxa stick for 3–5 minutes until warmth is felt.

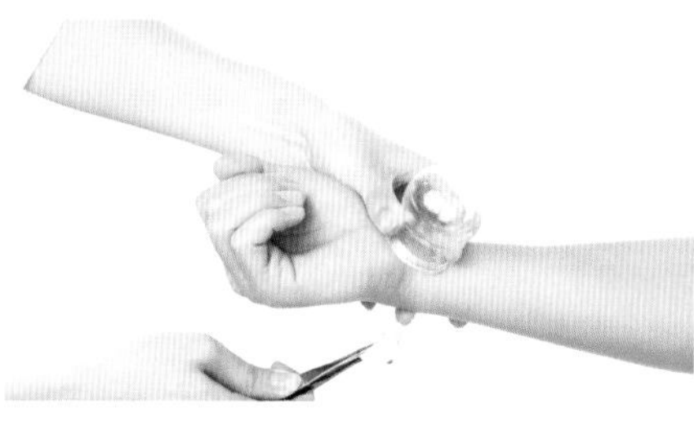

### 7. Shenmen Point

**Location:** On the inner wrist near the small finger when the palm is turned upward.

**Method:** First knead Shenmen point with the thumb pulp for 2–3 minutes, and then select and apply a small cup to the point, retaining the cup for 5–10 minutes.

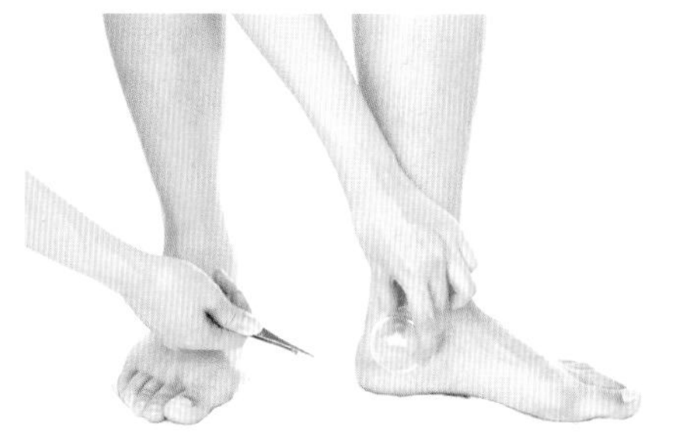

### 8. Zhaohai Point

**Location:** In a cavity below the protruding point in the interior of the ankle.

**Method:** First knead Zhaohai point with the thumb pulp for 2–3 minutes, until soreness and swelling is felt. Then apply a cup to the point, retaining the cup for 10–15 minutes.

# 23 Allergic Rhinitis

Patients with allergic rhinitis have paroxysmal itching of the nose, accompanied by eye itching, weeping, continuous sneezing, thin nasal discharge and stuffy nose, mostly on both sides, as well as hyposmia.

They should avoid contact with allergens, and put on more clothes during temperature changes and cold seasons to avoid catching a cold. In addition, they should strengthen physical exercise, try morning jogging and other sports, and may wash their faces or take baths with cold water to enhance the resistance of the body.

The cupping should be applied mainly to Yintang, Yingxiang, Hegu, Shousanli, and Quchi points.

## Cupping Methods

### 1. Yintang Point

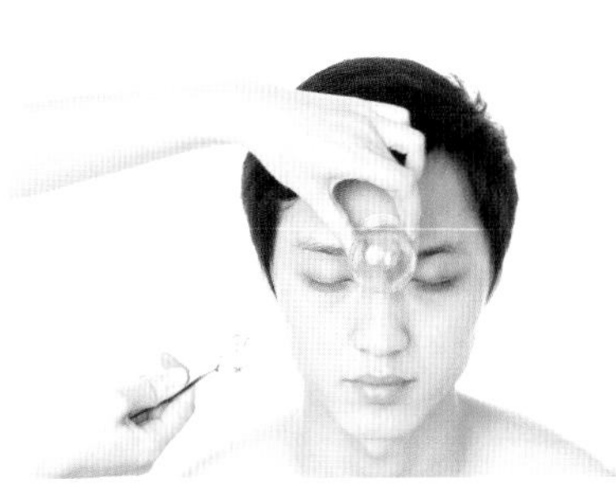

**Location:** At the central point right between the eyebrows.

**Method:** First, knead Yintang point with a finger pulp for 2–3 minutes, and then select and apply a small cup to the point, retaining the cup for 5–10 minutes.

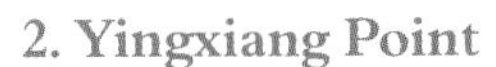

### 2. Yingxiang Point

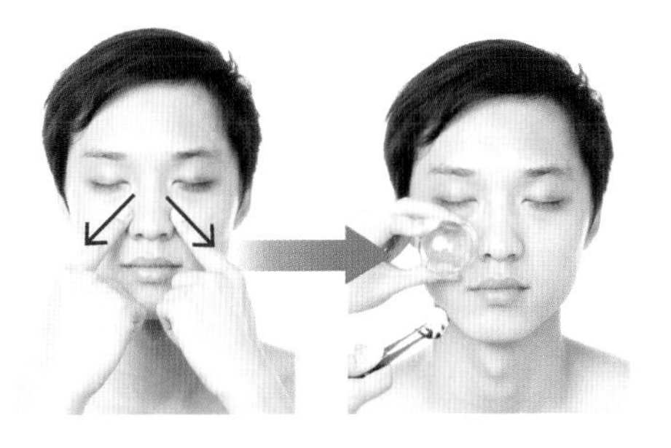

**Location:** Beside the wing of the nose, 0.5 cun away, in the nasolabial groove.

**Method:** First, rub Yinxiang point along both sides of the nosewing towards the nasion with the index finger for 2–3 minutes, and then select and apply a small cup to the point, retaining the cup for 5–10 minutes.

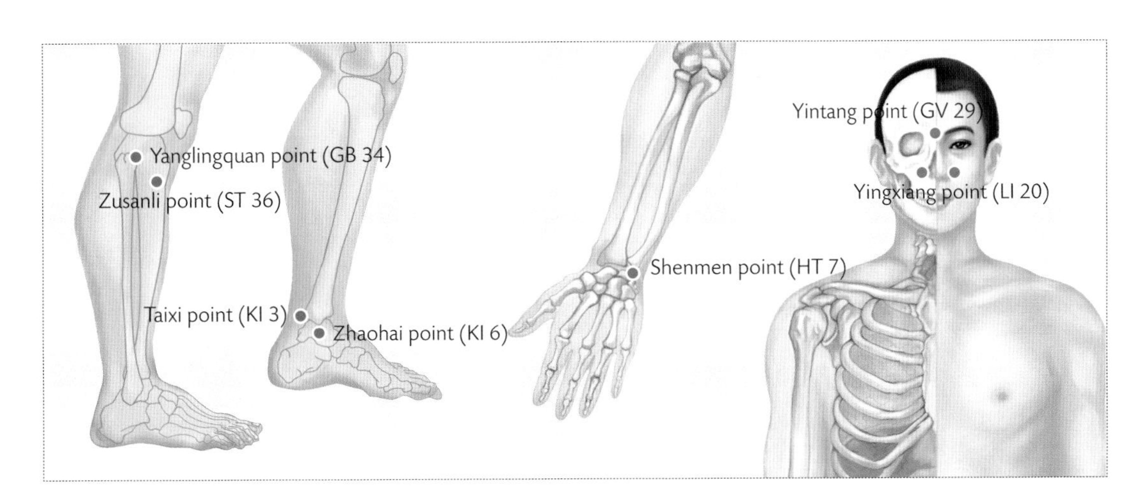

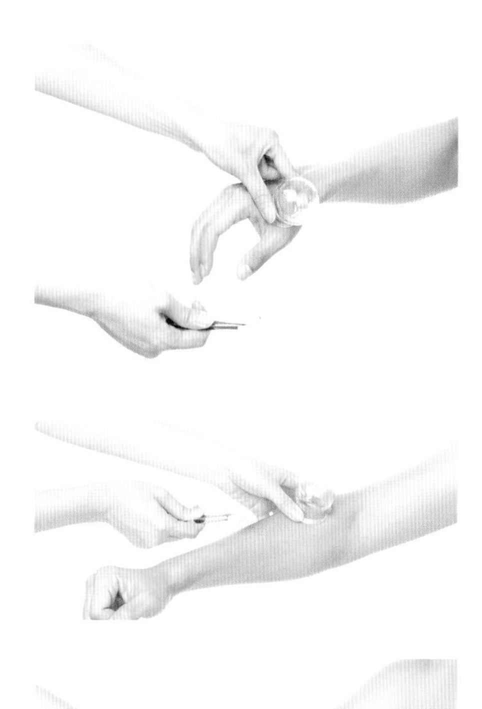

### 3. Hegu Point

**Location:** In the highest point on the back of the hand between the thumb base and the base of the index finger (in the webbing between these two fingers).

**Method:** First knead Hegu point with the thumb pulp for 2–3 minutes, until a feeling of soreness and swelling is present, and then select and apply a small cup to the point, retaining the cup for 5–10 minutes.

### 4. Shousanli Point

**Location:** 2 cun below the Quchi point.

**Method:** First knead Shousanli point with the thumb pulp for 2–3 minutes, and then select and apply a cup of appropriate size to the point, retaining the cup for 5–10 minutes.

### 5. Quchi Point

**Location:** With the elbow bent halfway, on the outer side of the cubital transverse crease.

**Method:** First knead Quchi point with the thumb pulp for 2–3 minutes, and then select and apply a cup of appropriate size to the point, retaining the cup for 5–10 minutes.

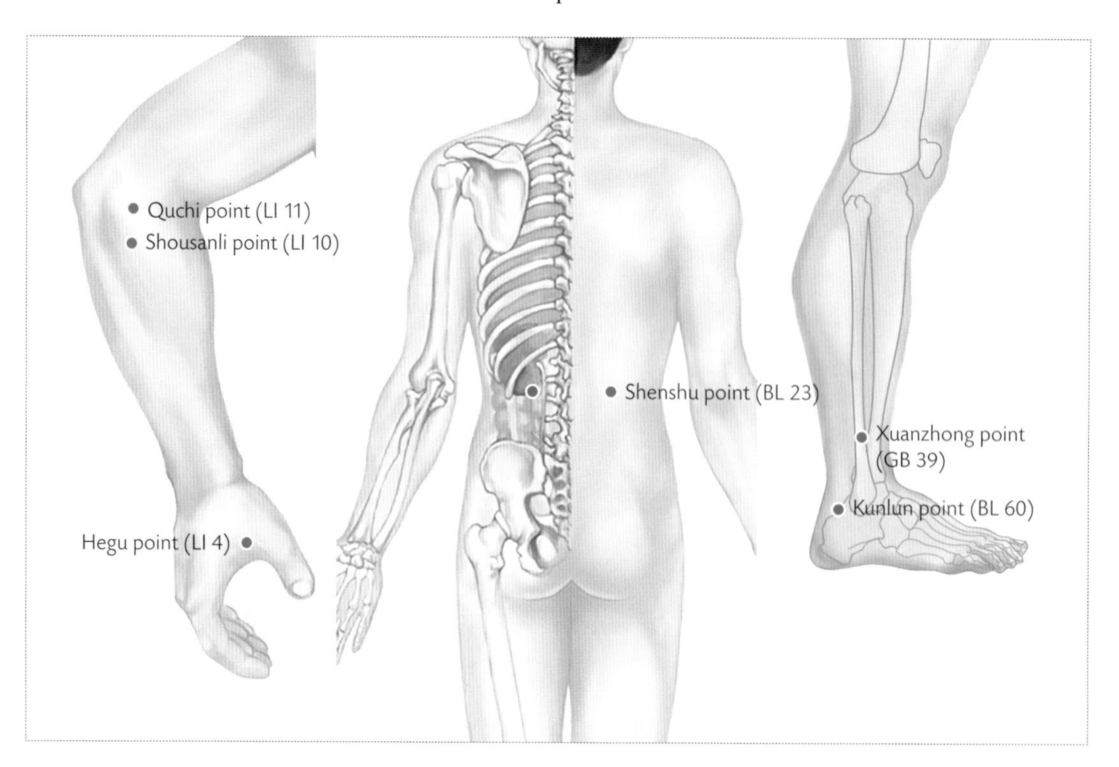

# 24 Gout

Gout often first occurs in the big toe, with the manifestations including redness and swelling of joints, feeling of burning and swelling, and severe pain when being touched gently or when the toe moves. Pain in fingers, toes, wrists, ankles and knee joints, or "chalk stone" may occur to prolonged patients.

The prevention and treatment of gout should be improved through diet and living habits. Control the daily intake of total calorie, eat less carbohydrate food, and food rich in fat, eat less sugar, honey, and tender lentils, green beans, soybeans, tofu, dried beans, and other high purine substances, avoid or abstain from eating animal offal, shrimps and crabs, concentrated broth, edible fungi, seaweed, anchovies, sardines, clams, beans, beers, and other high purine food, and limit the intake of salt, avoid drinking alcohol, and avoid eating hotpot. Drinking more water and eating more vegetables (e.g. potatoes) and fruits (e.g. green plums, lemon) can reduce blood and urine acidity. Watermelon and white gourd are alkaline foods that are beneficial to patients with gout. Pasta and alkali porridge can promote uric acid excretion and protect the kidneys as they have alkaline substances. It is advisable to eat these food.

The cupping should focus on around the affected areas. With the cup removed, perform moxibustion with a moxa stick for 3–5 minutes until warmth is felt. Cupping may also be applied to Shenshu, Xuanzhong and Kunlun points.

## Cupping Methods

### 1. Shenshu Point

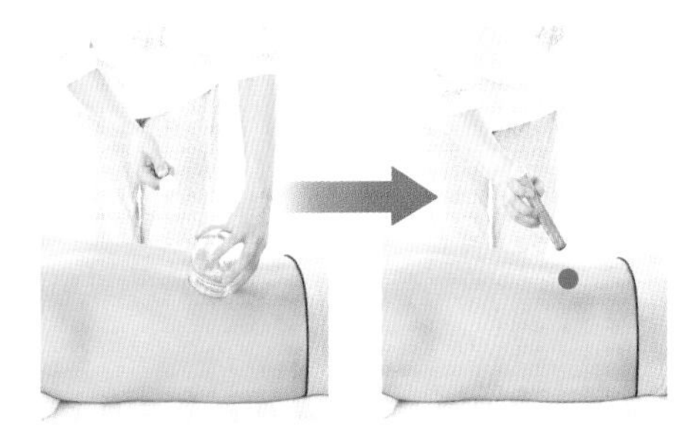

**Location:** 1.5 cun horizontally from the second lumbar spinal process.

**Method:** Select and apply a cup of appropriate size to Shenshu point, retaining the cup for 10–15 minutes. With the cup removed, perform moxibustion with a moxa stick for 3–5 minutes until warmth is felt.

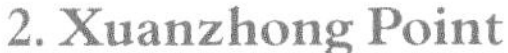

### 2. Xuanzhong Point

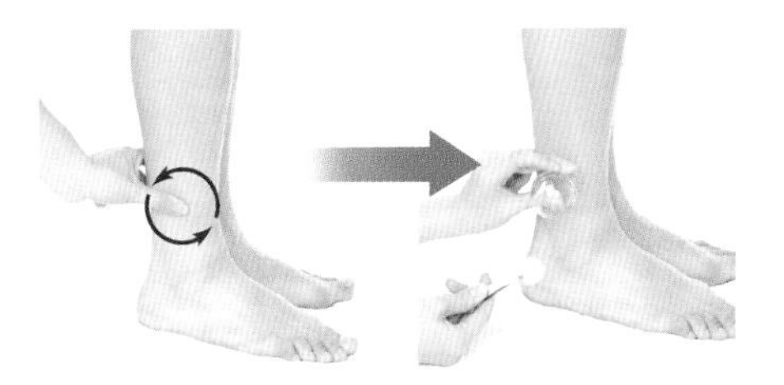

**Location:** In a cavity 3 cun above the outer ankle tip.

**Method:** First knead Xuanzhong point with the thumb pulp for 2–3 minutes until one feels sore and swelling at the point, and then select an appropriate cup and apply it to the point, retaining the cup for 10–15 minutes.

### 3. Kunlun Point

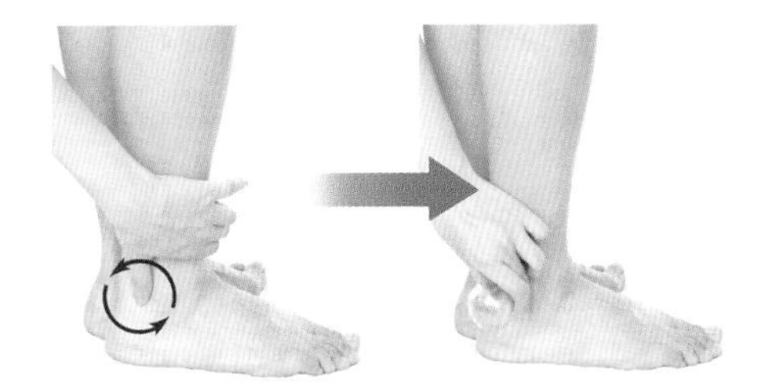

**Location:** In a cavity directly in the rear of the lateral malleolus.

**Method:** First knead Kunlun point with the thumb pulp for 2–3 minutes until one feels sore and swelling at the point, and then select an appropriate cup and apply it to the point, retaining the cup for 10–15 minutes.

# 25 Indigestion

Indigestion is characterized by intermittent feelings of discomfort or pain, fullness, heartburn (acid reflux), and belching in the upper abdomen. Patients with this disease are unwilling to eat or eat little due to such discomforts as chest tightness, premature satiety (which means feeling of "fullness" after eating less than normal food intake), and abdominal distention.

The patients should not eat too sour, too spicy, irritating, raw, cold, or indigestible food, but can eat porridge cooked with hawthorn, malt, sweet ferment rice, and dried tangerine peel, which is conducive to the restoration of gastric motility, and promote digestion.

The cupping should be performed on Zhongwan, Liangmen, Neiguan, and Zusanli points.

## Cupping Methods

### 1. Zhongwan Point

**Location:** On the upper abdomen, 4 cun above the center of the umbilicus, on the anterior midline.

**Method:** First massage the abdomen above the bellybutton for about ten circles with the palm or corporately the index finger, the middle finger, and the ring finger. Then select a cup of appropriate size, and apply it to Zhongwan point, retaining the cup for 10–15 minutes. With the cup removed, perform moxibustion with a moxa box for 3–5 minutes until warmth is felt.

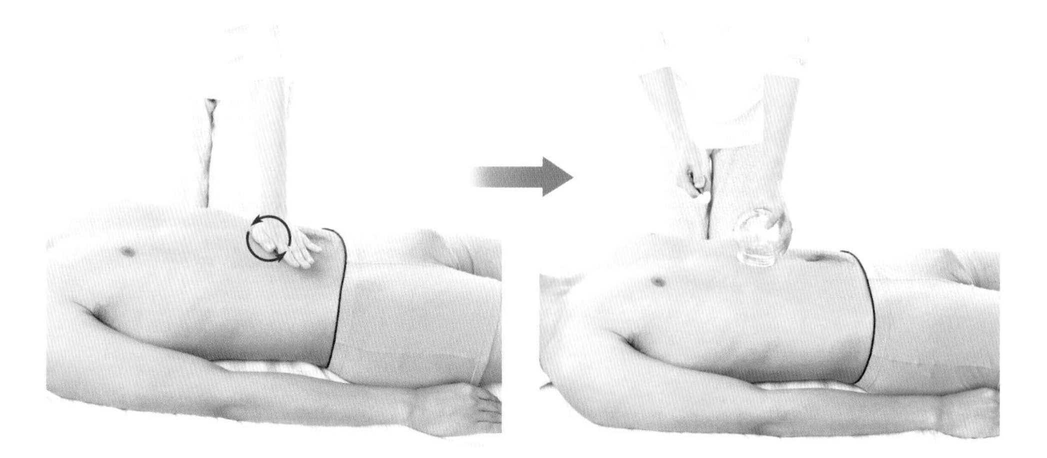

### 2. Liangmen Point

**Location:** On the upper abdomen, 4 cun above the umbilicus, 2 cun lateral to the anterior midline.

**Method:** First knead Liangmen point with the thumb pulp for 2–3 minutes and then apply a cup to the point, retaining the cup for 10–15 minutes.

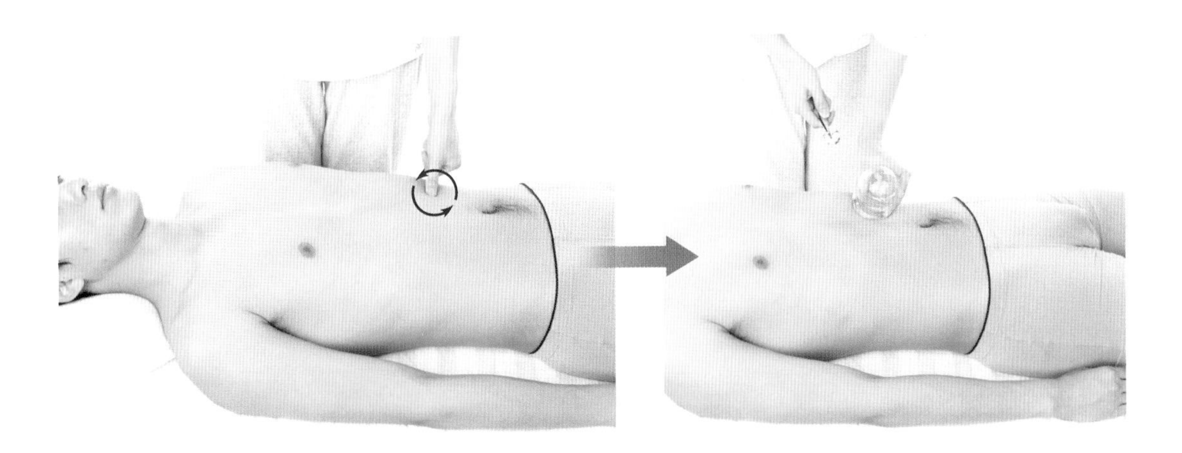

### 3. Neiguan Point

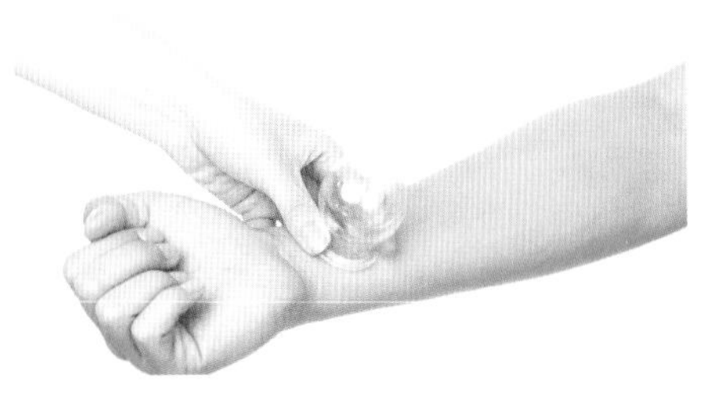

**Location:** Between the two tendons about 2 cun above the wrist joint bend.

**Method:** First knead Neiguan point with the thumb pulp for 2–3 minutes, and then select and apply a cup of appropriate size to the point, retaining the cup for 10–15 minutes.

### 4. Zusanli Point

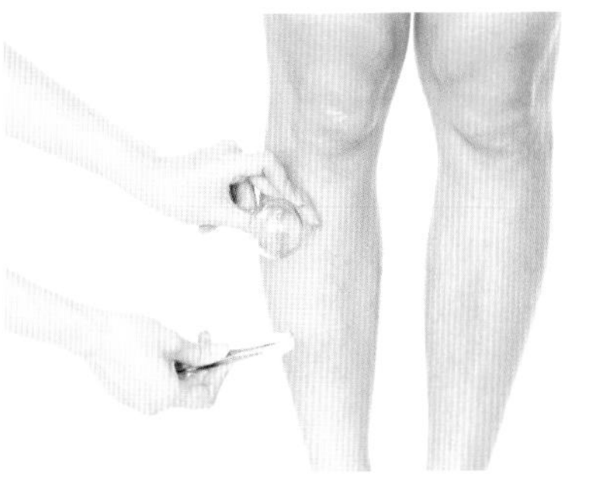

**Location:** About 3 cun below the knee on the outer side of the tibia.

**Method:** First knead Zusanli point with the thumb pulp for 2–3 minutes, and then select a cup of appropriate size and apply it to the point, retaining the cup for 10–15 minutes. With the cup removed, perform moxibustion with a moxa stick for 3–5 minutes until warmth is felt.

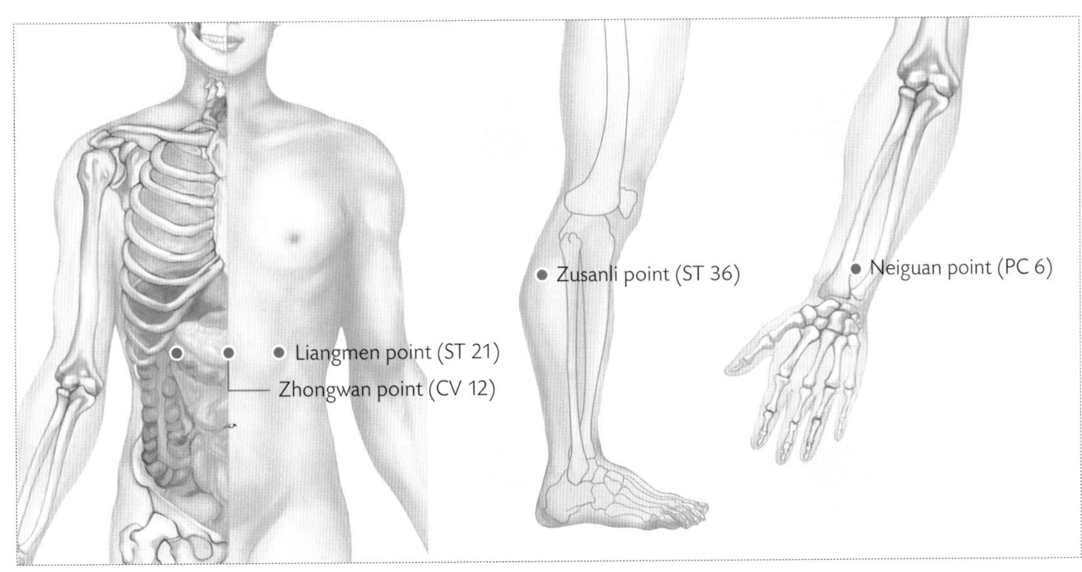

# 26 Cholecystitis

Acute cholecystitis often occurs after eating greasy supper, with symptoms including persistent pain and paroxysmal exacerbations in the right upper abdomen, which can radiate to the right shoulder, often accompanied by nausea, vomiting, and fever, as well as yellow skin and eyes in severe cases.

See a doctor immediately in case of continued attack of cholecystitis so as not to delay the treatment. Operative therapy may be considered for those with repeated attack of cholecystitis. The patients should avoid eating fatty pork, lamb, chicken, pepper, etc., and should not eat greasy food.

The cupping should be applied to Ganshu, Danshu, Qimen, Yanglingquan, and Dannang points.

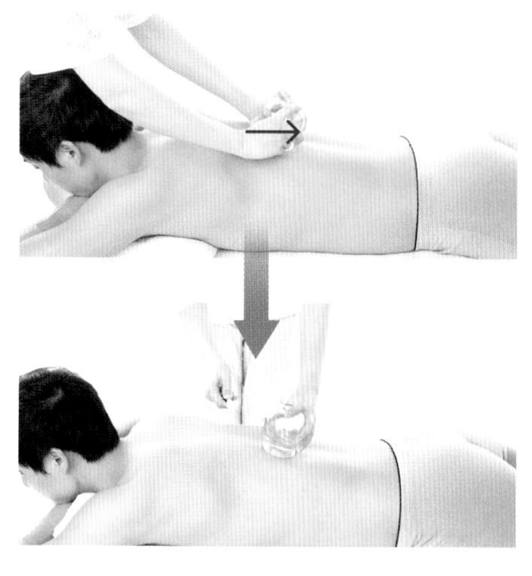

## Cupping Methods

### 1. Ganshu and Danshu Points

**Location:** Ganshu point is 1.5 cun away from the ninth thoracic spinal process on the inner side of the scapula; Danshu point is in the spine area, 1.5 cun lateral to the posterior midline of the lower border of the spinous process of the tenth thoracic vertebra.

**Method:** Use the moving cupping method. Select a cup of appropriate size and move it on the bladder meridian on the back by segment along the meridian, until the skin becomes red. Cup on Ganshu and Danshu points after the moving cupping, and retain the cup for 10–15 minutes.

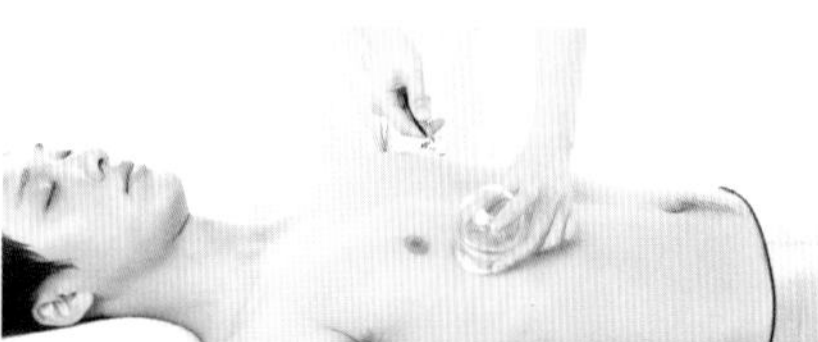

### 2. Qimen Point

**Location:** In the sixth intercostal space directly below the nipple.

**Method:** Select and apply a cup of appropriate size to the point, retaining the cup for 10–15 minutes.

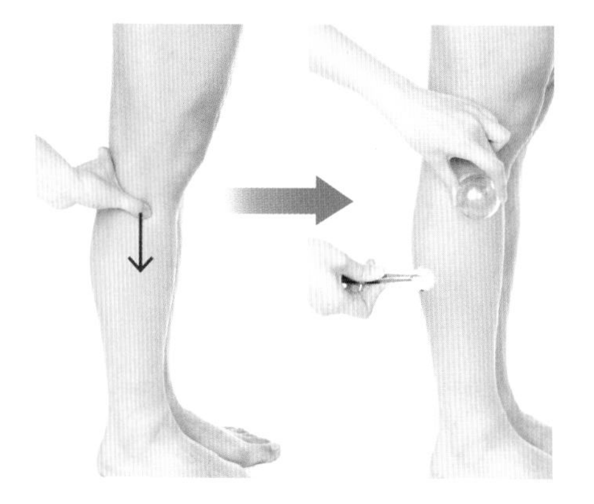

### 3. Yanglingquan and Dannang Points

**Location:** Yanglingquan point is on the outer side of the shin in a notch at the front lower part of the fibula; Dannang point is on the lateral side of the calf, 2 cun directly below the head of the fibula.

**Method:** First, knead with the thumb pulp from Yanglingquan point to Dannang point for 2–3 minutes, and then select and apply a cup of appropriate size to these two points, retaining the cup for 10–15 minutes. After the cup is removed, perform moxibustion with a moxa stick for 3–5 minutes until warmth is felt.

# 27 Anemia

Patients with anemia often have a pale complexion, abnormal heartbeat, dizziness, fatigue, shortness of breath, palpitations, and other symptoms, which may be aggravated after activities. The main causes of anemia include deficiency of iron, bleeding, hemolysis, and hematopoietic dysfunction.

The patients with anemia should pay attention to their diets, and eat porridge cooked with coix seeds, red dates, corns, black sesame seeds often, and eat other foods that tonify qi and blood. They should have balanced meals, and eat more fresh vegetables and fruits to supplement various elements required by the human body, especially iron. In addition, they should strike a proper balance between work and rest, and engage in appropriate sports activities.

The cupping should be performed on Baihui, Guanyuan, Mingmen, Shenshu, and Zusanli points. Choose 2–3 points each time.

## Cupping Methods

### 1. Baihui Point

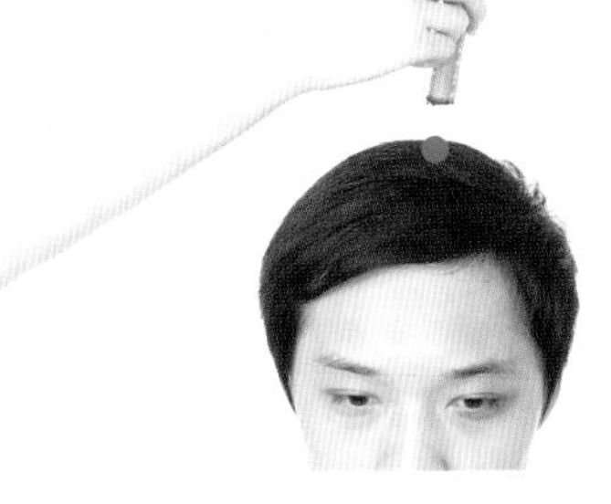

**Location:** On the head, 5 cun superior to the anterior hairline, on the anterior midline.

**Method:** Cup on Baihui point for 10–15 times by using the flash cupping method. Do not retain the cup. Then perform moxibustion with a moxa stick for 3–5 minutes until warmth is felt.

### 2. Guanyuan Point

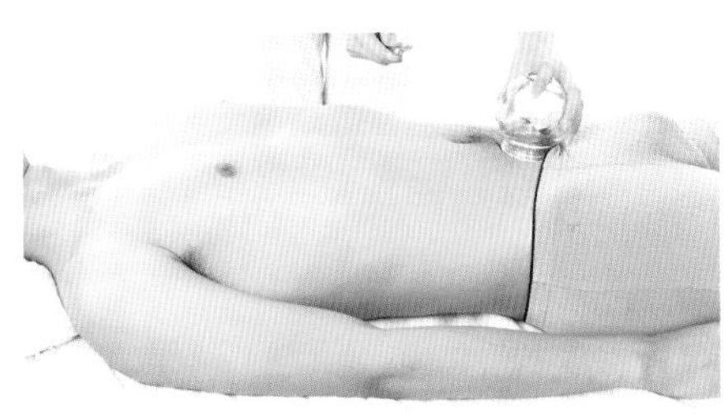

**Location:** About 3 cun below the navel.

**Method:** First knead Guanyuan point with the thumb pulp for 2–3 minutes, and then apply a cup to the point, retaining the cup for 10–15 minutes. With the cup removed, perform moxibustion with a moxa stick for 3–5 minutes warmth is felt.

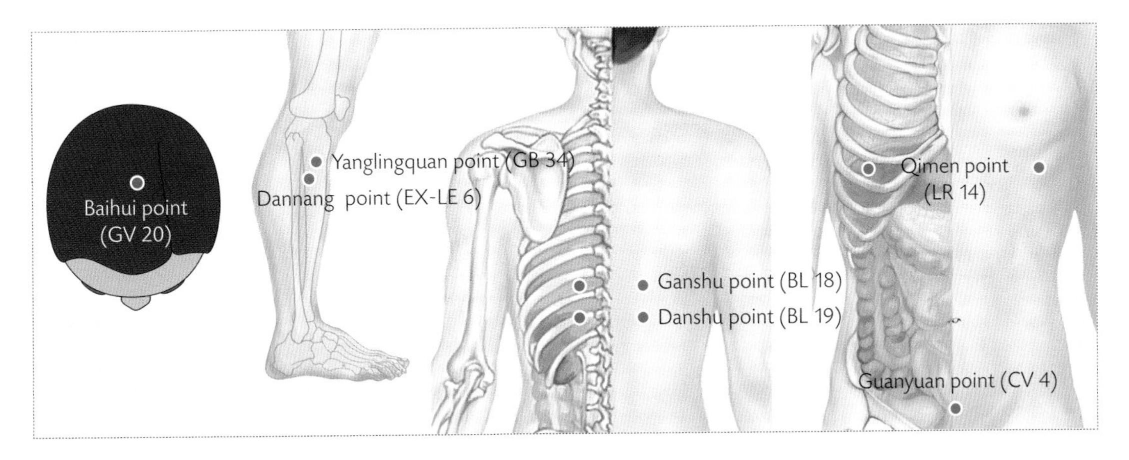

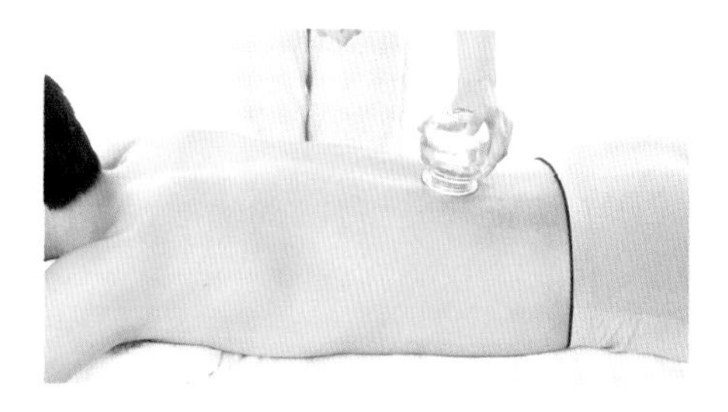

### 3. Mingmen Point

**Location:** In a cavity below the spinous process of the second cervical vertebra.

**Method:** Select and apply a cup of appropriate size to the point, retaining the cup for 5–10 minutes. After the cup is removed, perform moxibustion with a moxa stick for 3–5 minutes until warmth is felt.

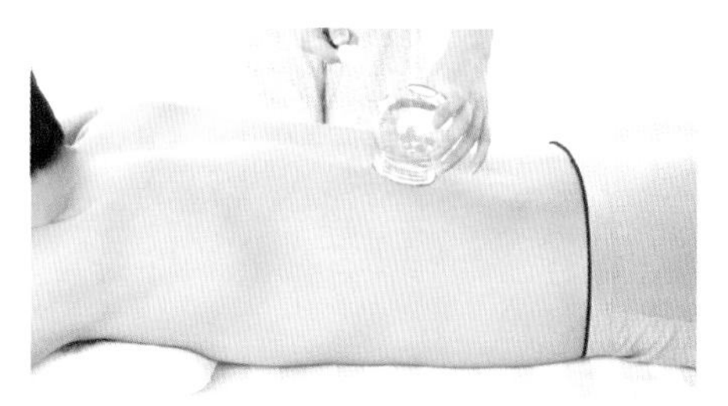

### 4. Shenshu Point

**Location:** 1.5 cun horizontally from the second lumbar spinal process.

**Method:** Select and apply a cup of appropriate size to the point, retaining the cup for 5–10 minutes. After the cup is removed, perform moxibustion with a moxa stick for 3–5 minutes until warmth is felt.

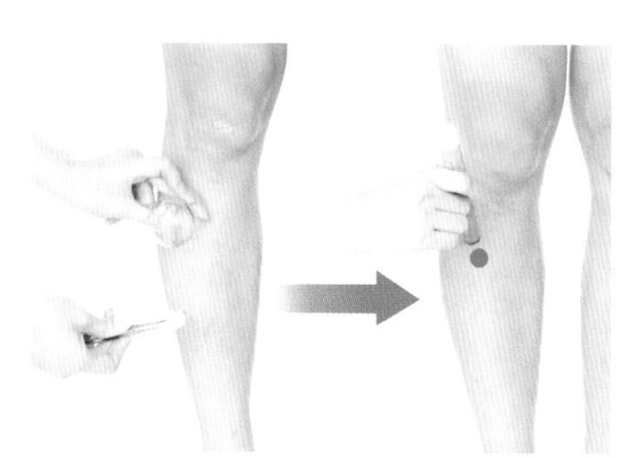

### 5. Zusanli Point

**Location:** About 3 cun below the knee on the outer side of the tibia.

**Method:** First knead Zusanli point with the thumb pulp for 2–3 minutes, and then select a cup of appropriate size and apply it to the point, retaining the cup for 10–15 minutes. With the cup removed, perform moxibustion with a moxa stick for 3–5 minutes until warmth is felt.

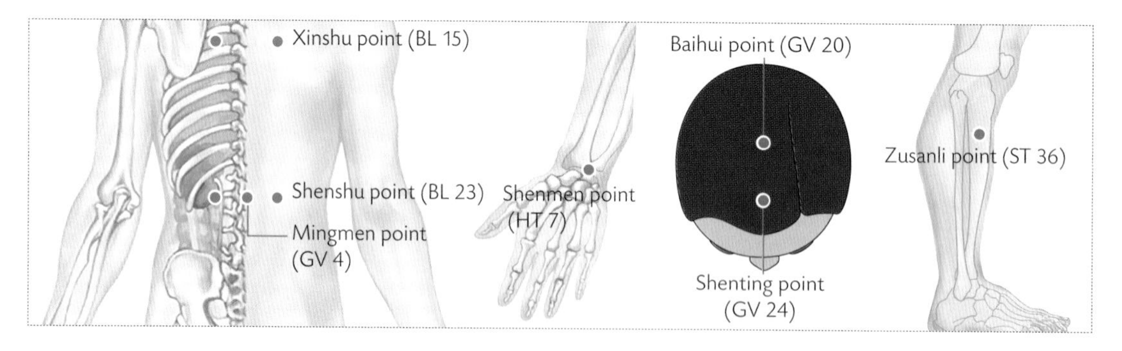


# 28 Alzheimer's Disease

The signs of Alzheimer's disease in the early stages are suspicious personality and changes in sleep circadian rhythm, developing into speaking unclearly, and being muddleheaded in the later stages, and complete mental retardation, lying in bed with the inability to take care of oneself in the advanced stage.

To avoid Alzheimer's disease, old people should use the brain frequently, for example, read more books and learn new things to stimulate the vitality of nerve cells. They should also eat walnuts, carrots, kelp, fish often, as they are conducive to improving memory. Strengthen the care for old patients with Alzheimer's disease, and observe and communicate with them frequently. Old people often have other organ dysfunction or some diseases. Serious consequences could be caused as the patients are blunted in sensibility and poor in responsiveness if they are not carefully observed, frequently asked, or treated in time.

The cupping should focus on Baihui, Shenting, Xinshu, Shenshu, and Shenmen points.

## Cupping Methods

### 1. Baihui Point

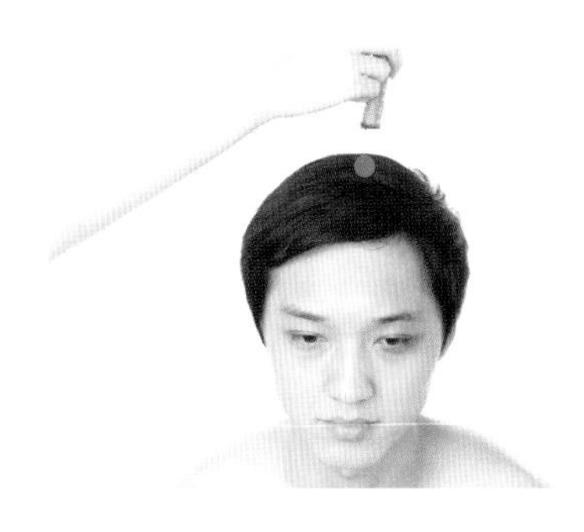

**Location:** On the head, 5 cun superior to the anterior hairline, on the anterior midline.

**Method:** Cup on Baihui point for 10–15 times by using the flash cupping method. Do not retain the cup. Then perform moxibustion with a moxa stick for 3–5 minutes until warmth is felt.

### 2. Shenting Point

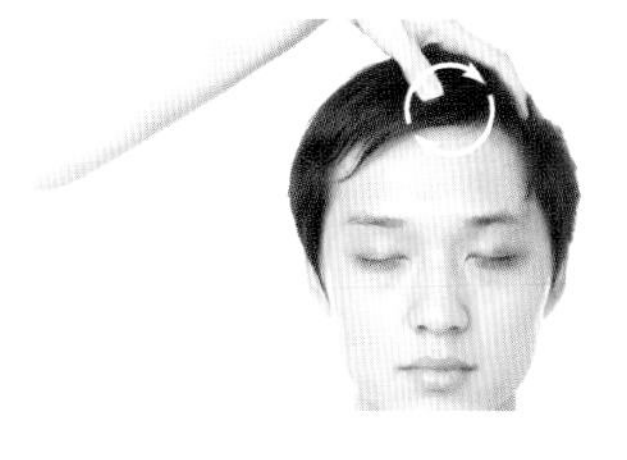

**Location:** On the head on the midline, 0.5 cun superior to the anterior hairline.

**Method:** Cup on Shenting point for 10–15 times by using the flash cupping method. Do not retain the cup. Knead the point for 2–3 minutes after the cup is removed.

### 3. Xinshu and Shenshu Points

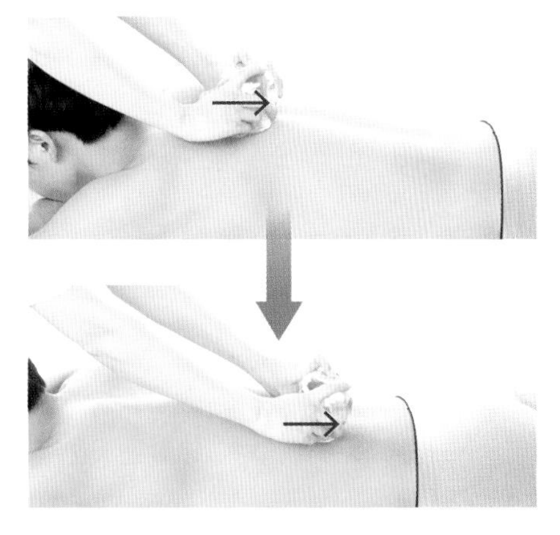

**Location:** Xinshu point is under the fifth thoracic vertebra on the inner side of the scapula, 1.5 cun horizontally away; Shenshu point is 1.5 cun horizontally from the second lumbar spinal process.

**Method:** Use the moving cupping method. Move the cup on the bladder meridian on the back by segment along the meridian, and move the cup several times mainly on Xinshu and Shenshu points. Repeatedly push and pull on the points back and forth, until the skin becomes red. The cup may be retained on the abovementioned points for 10–15 minutes after the moving cupping.

### 4. Shenmen Point

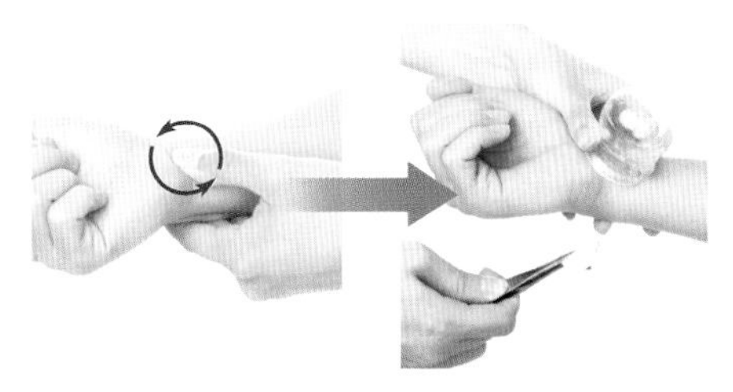

**Location:** On the inner wrist near the small finger when the palm is turned upward.

**Method:** First knead Shenmen point with the thumb pulp for 2–3 minutes, and then select and apply a small cup to the point, retaining the cup for 5–10 minutes.

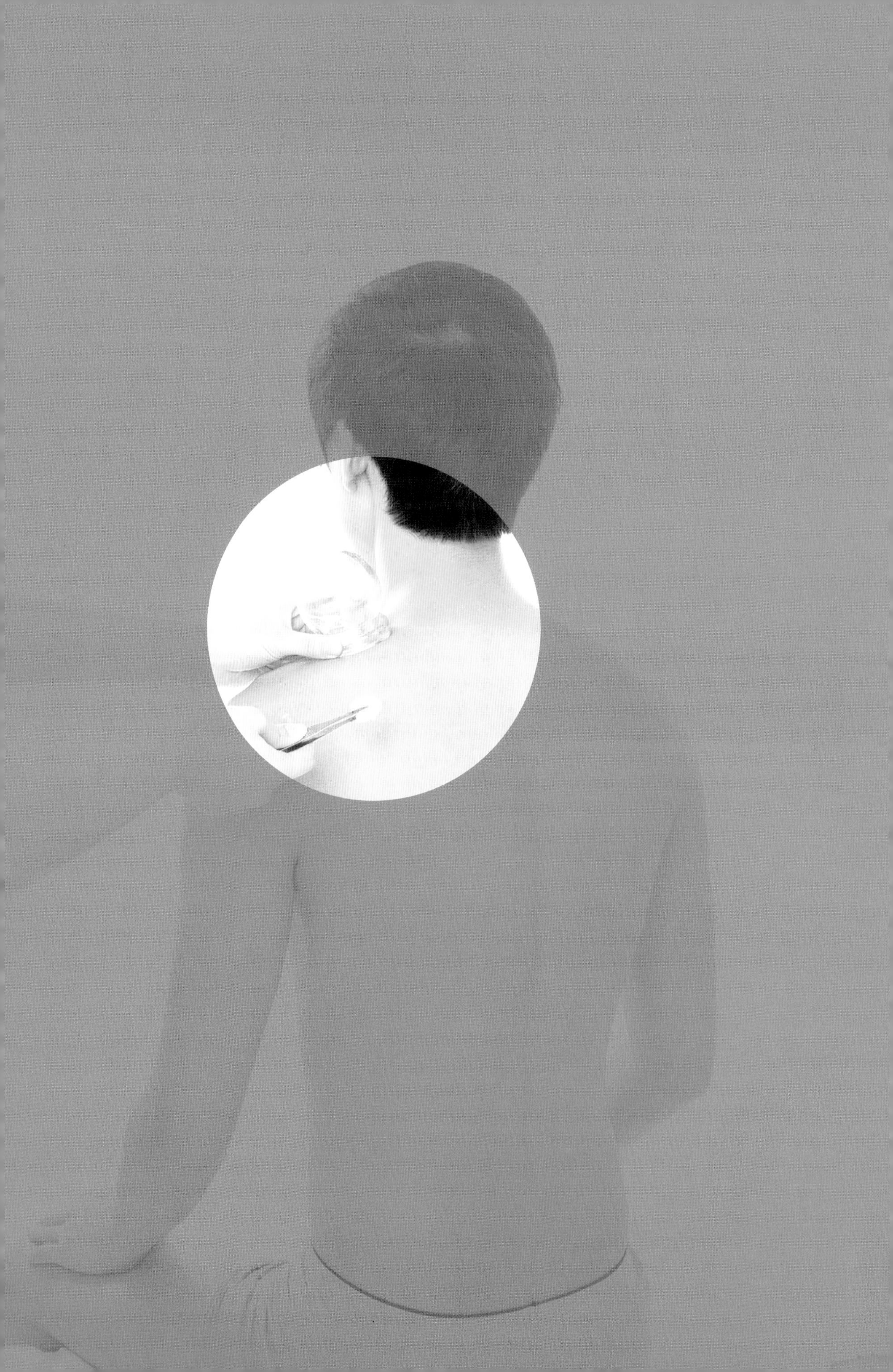

# Chapter Six
## Surgical Diseases

Surgical diseases are generally caused by a long period of overwork, improper sleep or sitting gesture, etc., though not life-threatening, they are always accompanied by unbearable pain. Once they attack, it could be difficult to stand and walk, let alone work. Cupping can not only be effectively but also quickly alleviate the pain caused by surgical diseases.

## 1 Cervical Spondylosis

The patients feel soreness in their heads, necks, shoulders, backs and arms. They suffer neck stiffness and limited movement, which may radiate to their heads and upper limbs. Some are accompanied by giddiness, and the severe ones are accompanied by nausea and vomiting, and dizziness and cataplexy in a few cases.

To prevent cervical spondylosis, one should correct bad posture and habits, avoid working with the neck held at a single posture for a long time. One should rest for about ten minutes after working for about one hour to alleviate the tension and spasm of neck muscles. One should try to use low pillow during sleep to prevent neck fatigue. In addition, one should keep neck warm. Cupping, massage, and acupuncture can be used jointly, which can achieve better effects on early cervical disease.

The cupping should be performed on Fengchi, Jianjing, Dazhui, and Tianzong points, plus Jianliao, Jianzhen, Shousanli, and Quchi points for those with poor movement of upper limbs.

### Cupping Methods

#### 1. Fengchi Point

**Location:** In the depression on both sides of the large tendon behind the nape of the neck, next to the lower edge of the skull.

**Method:** First knead Fengchi point with the thumb pulp for 1–3 minutes. Then apply a cup to the point, retaining the cup for 15–20 minutes. With the cup removed, perform moxibustion with a moxa stick for 3–5 minutes until warmth is felt.

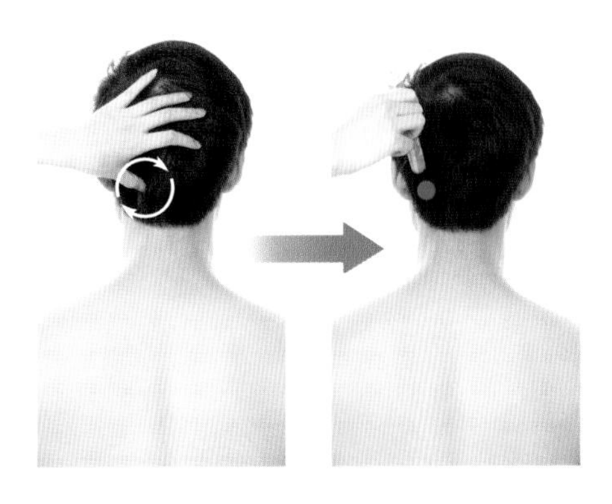

### 2. Jianjing Point

**Location:** At the midpoint of the top on the shoulder.

**Method:** Knead Jianjing point with the palm heel for 1–3 minutes, retaining the cup for 15–20 minutes. With the cup removed, perform moxibustion with a moxa stick for 3–5 minutes until warmth is felt.

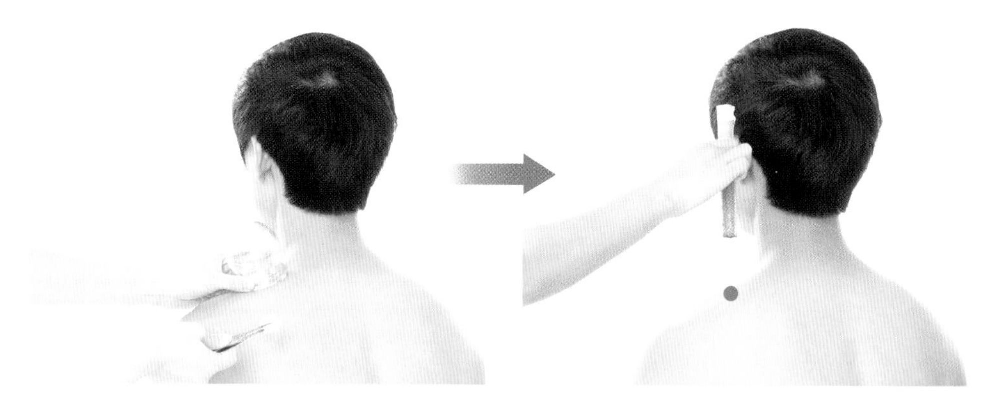

### 3. Dazhui Point

**Location:** Under the spinous process of the seventh cervical vertebrae.

**Method:** Knead Dazhui point with the palm heel for 1–3 minutes, retaining the cup for 15–20 minutes. With the cup removed, perform moxibustion with a moxa stick for 3–5 minutes until warmth is felt.

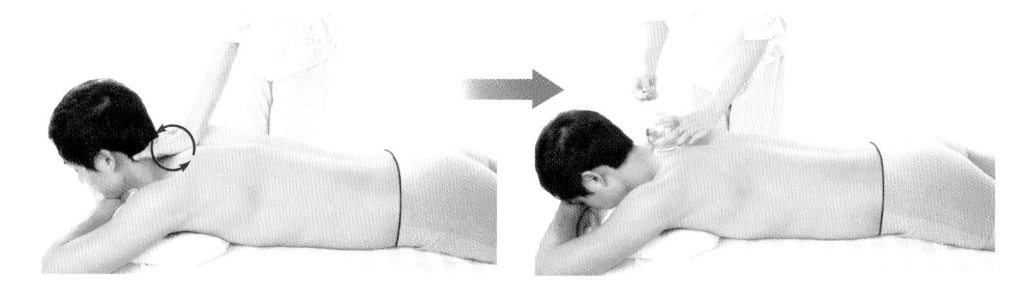

### 4. Tianzong Point

**Location:** In the depression at the center of the scapula.

**Method:** Knead Tianzong point with the palm heel for 1–3 minutes, retaining the cup for 15–20 minutes. With the cup removed, perform moxibustion with a moxa stick for 3–5 minutes until warmth is felt.

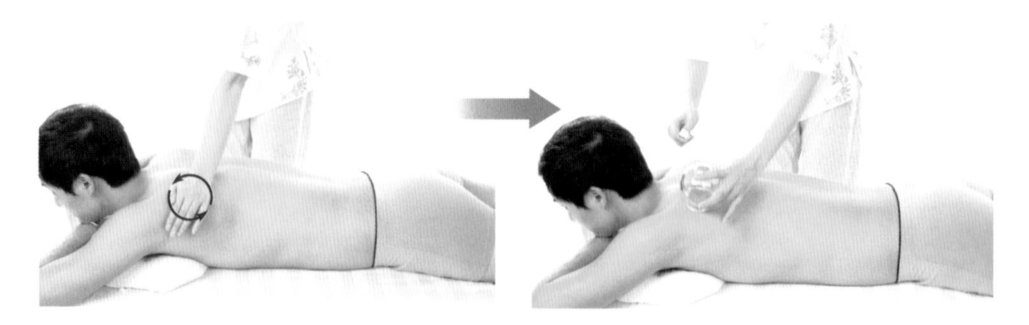

### 5. Jianliao Point

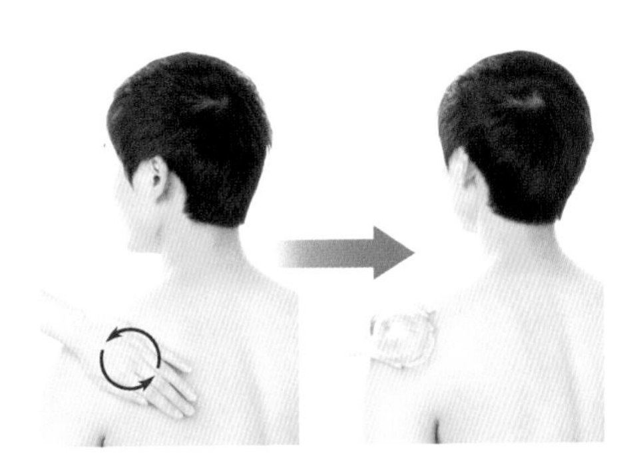

**Location:** In the deltoid muscle area, in the depression between acromial angle and the greater tubercle of humerus.

**Method:** Knead Tianzong point with the palm heel for 1–3 minutes, retaining the cup for 15–20 minutes. With the cup removed, perform moxibustion with a moxa stick for 3–5 minutes until warmth is felt.

### 6. Jianzhen Point

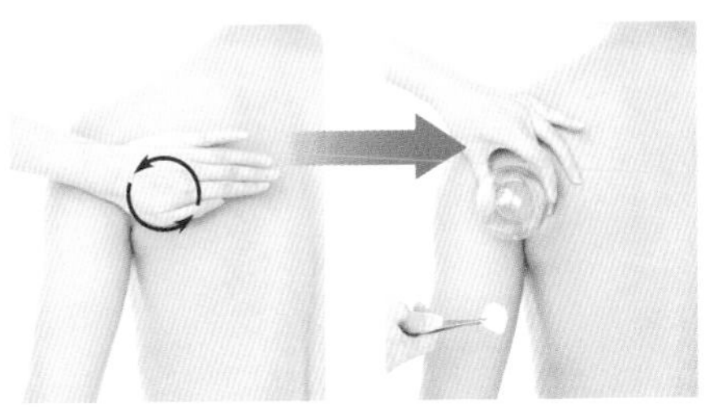

**Location:** At the lower back of the shoulder joint.

**Method:** Knead Jianzhen point with the palm heel for 1–3 minutes, retaining the cup for 15–20 minutes. With the cup removed, perform moxibustion with a moxa stick for 3–5 minutes until warmth is felt.

### 7. Shousanli Point

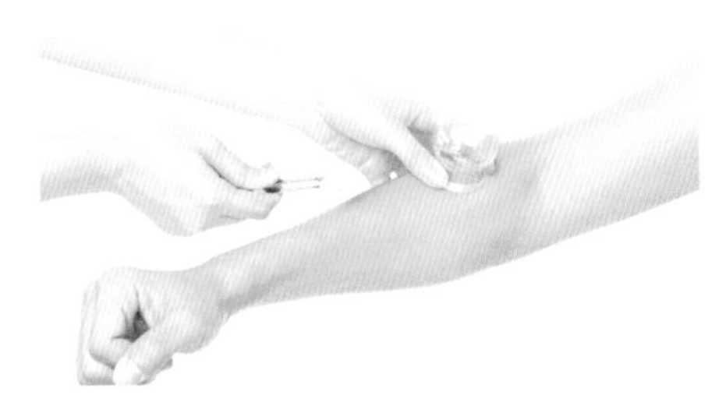

**Location:** 2 cun below the Quchi point.

**Method:** Knead Shousanli point with the palm heel for 1–3 minutes, retaining the cup for 15–20 minutes. With the cup removed, perform moxibustion with a moxa stick for 3–5 minutes until warmth is felt.

### 8. Quchi Point

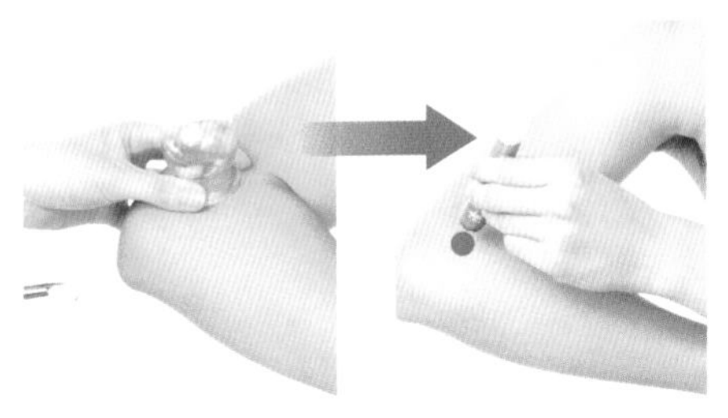

**Location:** With the elbow bent halfway, on the outer side of the cubital transverse crease.

**Method:** Knead Quchi point with the palm heel for 1–3 minutes, retaining the cup for 15–20 minutes. With the cup removed, perform moxibustion with a moxa stick for 3–5 minutes until warmth is felt.

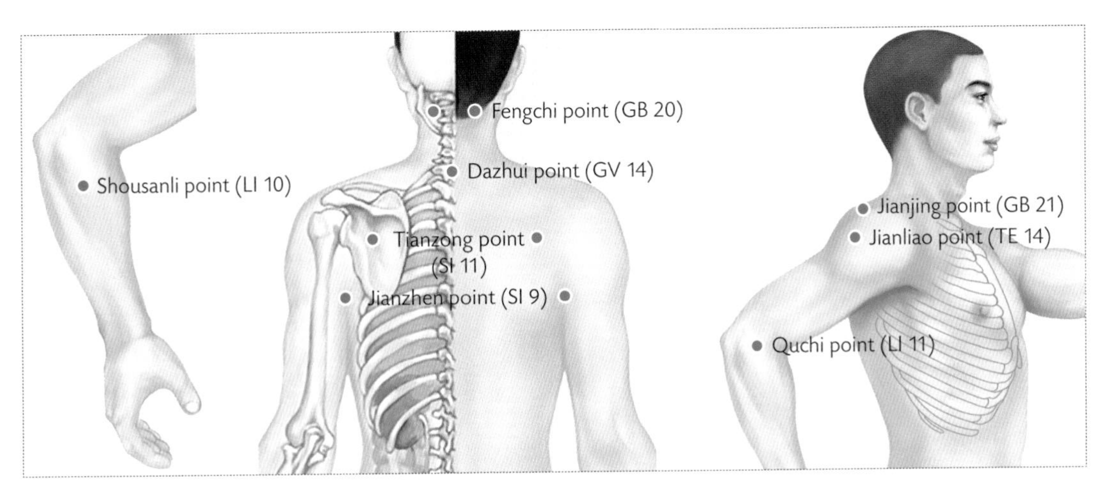

# 2 Periarthritis of Shoulder

Shoulder pain will manifest in the early stage, with a knife-cut feeling in severe cases, and may often radiate to arms and aggravate at night. Joint stiffness, loss of movement ability, muscle atrophy, and so on may appear in the later stage.

During treatment, patients should actively do shoulder joint exercise, and keep the shoulders warm to avoid coldness, so as to avoid aggravation of symptoms or recurrence. Cupping, massage, and acupuncture should be used jointly, which can achieve better effects on periarthritis of the shoulder.

The cupping can be applied to two groups of points, one group a day and two groups in turn, until the symptoms are alleviated or disappear. The first group includes Jianzhen, Jianliao, Jianyu, and Jianjing points, and the second group mainly includes Quchi, Waiguan, Tiaokou, Yanglingquan, and Chengshan points.

## Cupping Methods

### The First Group of Points

#### 1. Jianzhen Point

**Location:** At the lower back of the shoulder joint.

**Method:** Knead Jianzhen point with the palm heel for 1–3 minutes, retaining the cup for 15–20 minutes. With the cup removed, perform moxibustion with a moxa stick for 3–5 minutes until warmth is felt.

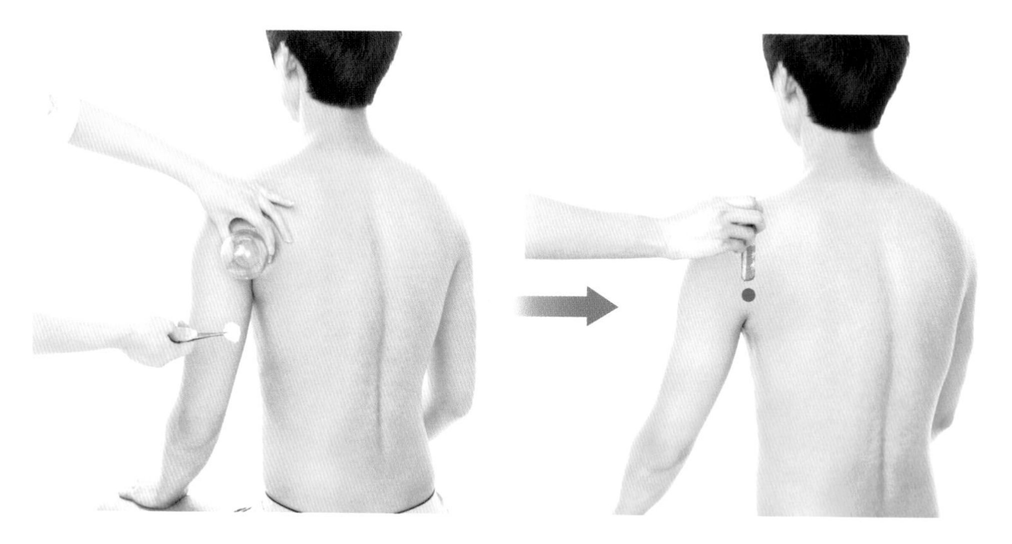

#### 2. Jianliao Point

**Location:** In the deltoid muscle area, in the depression between acromial angle and the greater tubercle of humerus.

**Method:** Knead Jianliao point with the palm heel for 1–3 minutes, retaining the cup for 15–20 minutes. With the cup removed, perform moxibustion with a moxa stick for 3–5 minutes until warmth is felt.

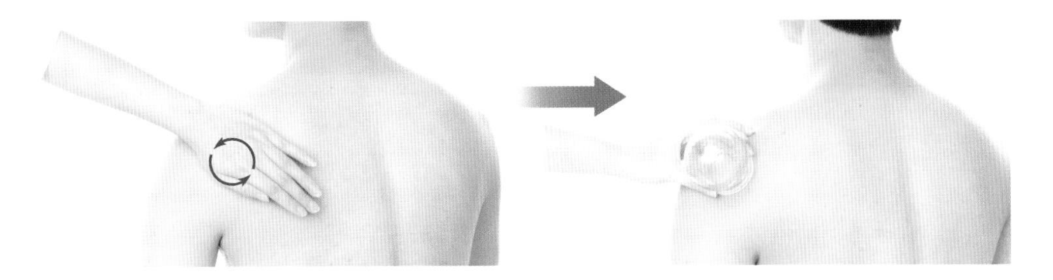

### 3. Jianyu Point

**Location:** In a cavity just before the shoulder peak when one raises the upper arm horizontally.

**Method:** Knead Jianyu point with the palm heel for 1–3 minutes, retaining the cup for 15–20 minutes. With the cup removed, perform moxibustion with a moxa stick for 3–5 minutes until warmth is felt.

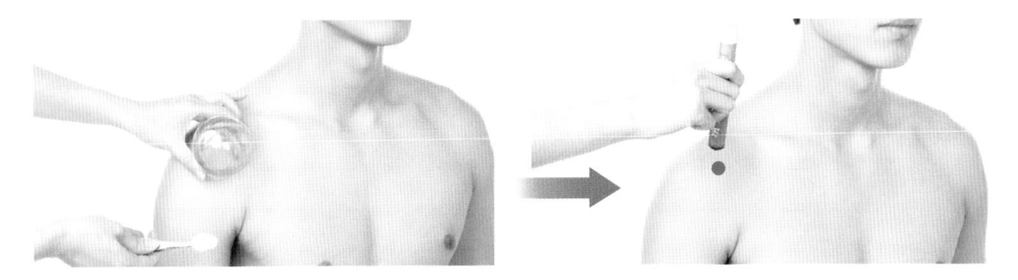

### 4. Jianjing Point

**Location:** At the midpoint of the top on the shoulder.

**Method:** Knead Jianjing point with the palm heel for 1–3 minutes, retaining the cup for 15–20 minutes. With the cup removed, perform moxibustion with a moxa stick for 3–5 minutes until warmth is felt.

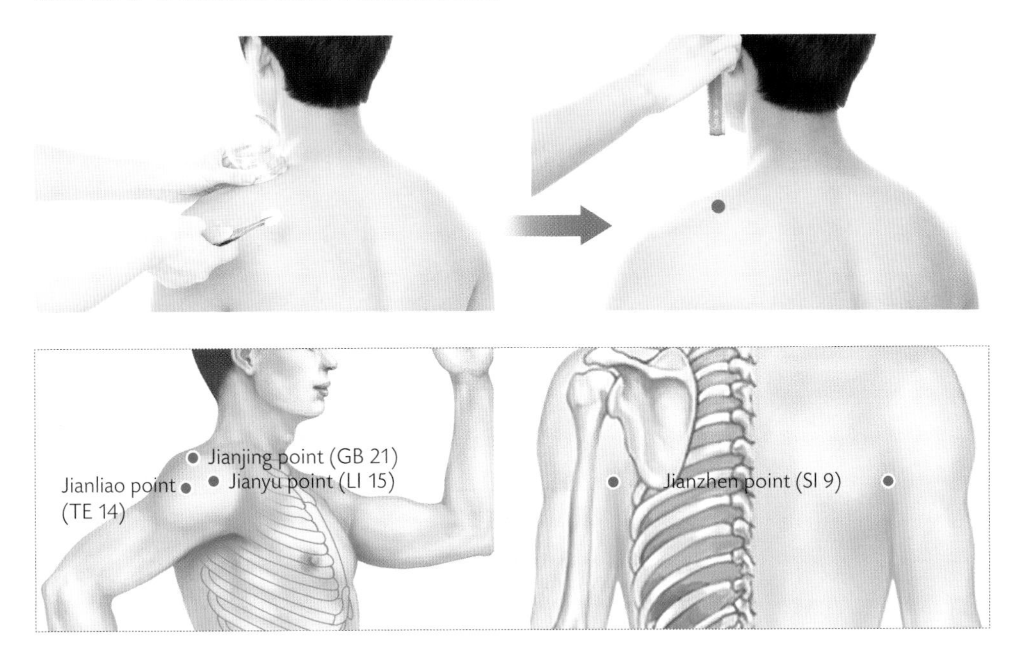

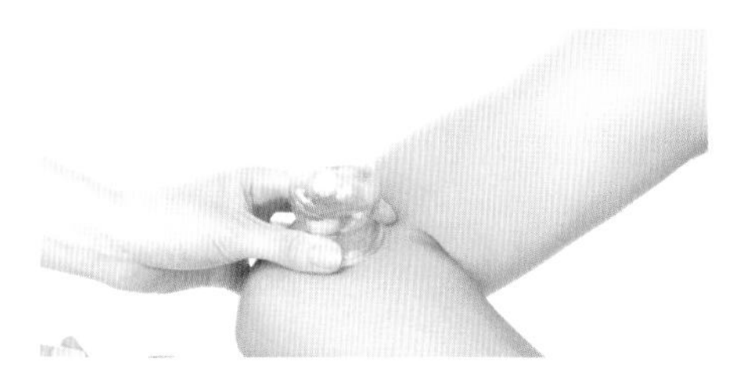

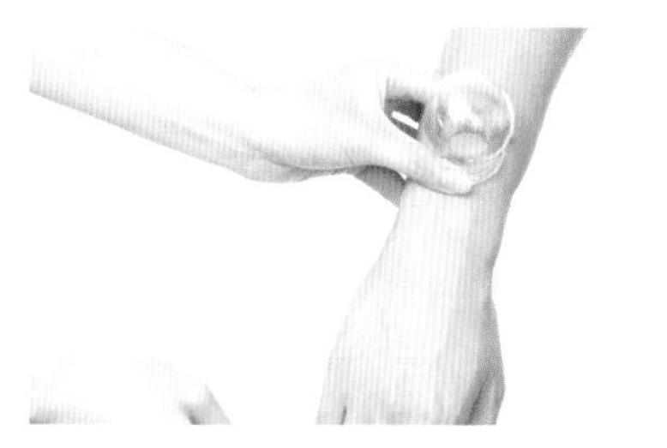

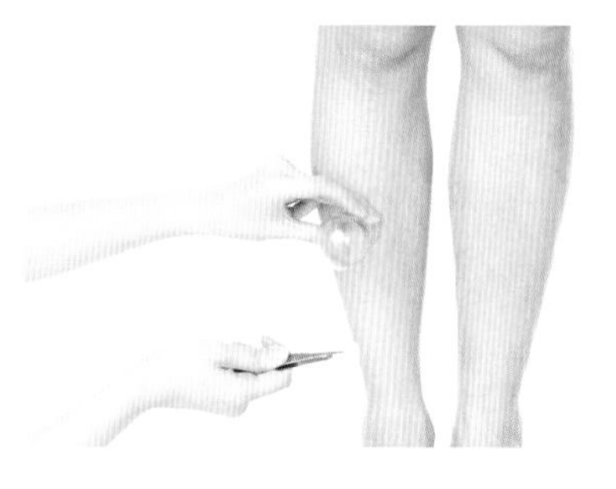

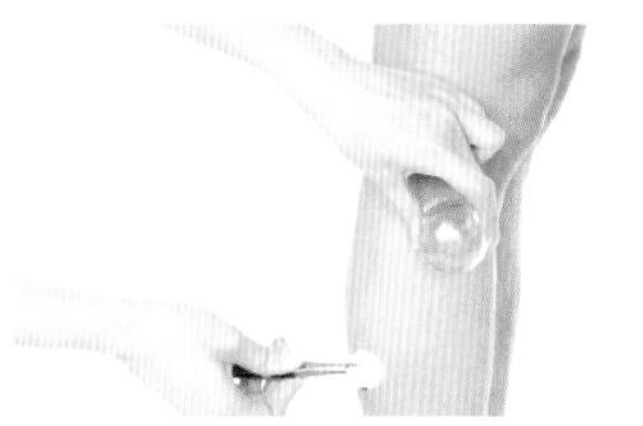

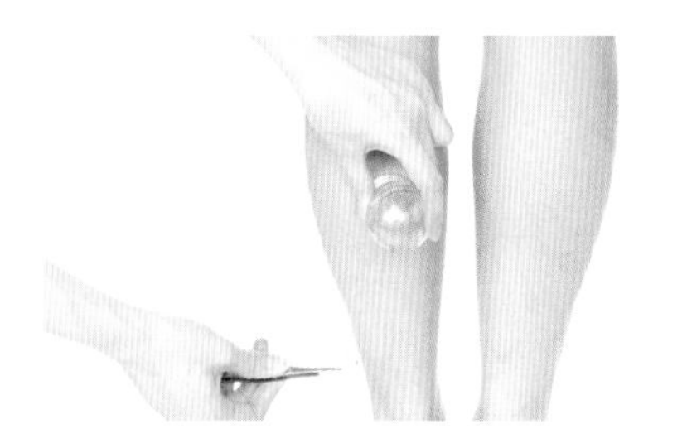

### The Second Group of Points

#### 1. Quchi Point

**Location:** With the elbow bent halfway, on the outer side of the cubital transverse crease.

**Method:** Select an appropriate cup and apply it to Quchi point, retaining the cup for 10–15 minutes.

#### 2. Waiguan Point

**Location:** The Waiguan point is in the middle on the outside of the arm, between the ulna and radius about 2 cun away from the horizontal line of the wrist joint.

**Method:** Select an appropriate cup and apply it to Waiguan point, retaining the cup for 10–15 minutes.

#### 3. Tiaokou Point

**Location:** At the posterior shank, two centimeters outside the tibial crest, on the midpoint of the line connecting the small bone protruding under the knee and the outer ankle.

**Method:** Select an appropriate cup and apply it to Tiaokou point, retaining the cup for 10–15 minutes.

#### 4. Yanglingquan Point

**Location:** On the outer side of the shin in a notch at the front lower part of the fibula.

**Method:** Select an appropriate cup and apply it to Yanglingquan point, retaining the cup for 10–15 minutes.

#### 5. Chengshan Point

**Location:** In a cavity in the middle of the rear of the lower leg, at the top of the depression between the two muscles of the calf.

**Method:** Select an appropriate cup and apply it to Chengshan point, retaining the cup for 10–15 minutes.

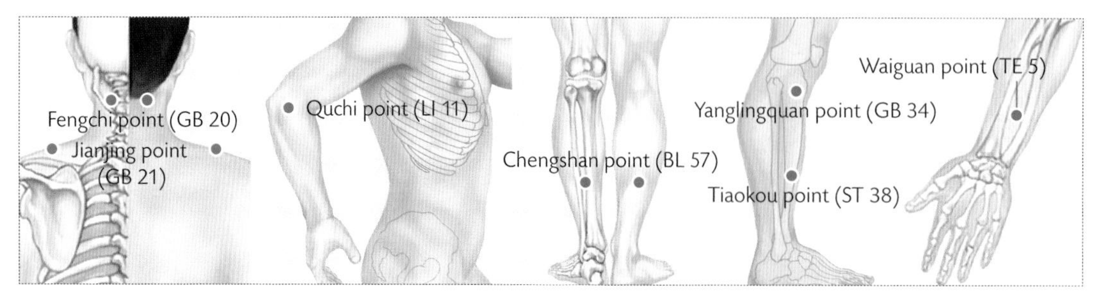

# 3 Stiff Neck

One with stiff neck suddenly feels pain and discomfort on the back of the neck or upper back, and cannot rotate the neck freely. Those with severe symptoms also have difficulty in bending or lifting the head, even with their heads at an abnormal position, deviating towards the affected side.

To avoid stiff neck, one should pay attention to his sleeping posture in daily life, do not make pillows too high, and maintain the cervical spine in the normal physiological curve during sleep. After the cupping, patients should move their necks appropriately, and meanwhile, pay attention to the warmth of the neck. They should consider the possibility of cervical spondylosis in case of recurrence of stiff neck, and are suggested to seek medical advice in time.

The cupping can be applied to three groups of points, one group a day and three groups in turn, until the symptoms disappear. The first group includes Ashi, Fengchi, and Jianjing points. The second group includes Neiguan and Chengshan points. The third group includes Xuanzhong point and foot trapezius muscle reflex zone.

## Cupping Methods

### The First Group of Points

#### 1. Ashi Point

**Location:** Painful point.

**Method:** First, knead Ashi point with the palm heel for 3–5 minutes, and then cup the point before retaining the cup for 15–20 minutes.

#### 2. Fengchi Point

**Location:** In the depression on both sides of the large tendon behind the nape of the neck, next to the lower edge of the skull.

**Method:** First knead Fengchi point with the thumb pulp for 1–3 minutes, until a feeling of soreness and swelling is present. Then cup the point, retaining the cup for 15–20 minutes. With the cup removed, perform moxibustion with a moxa stick for 3–5 minutes until warmth is felt.

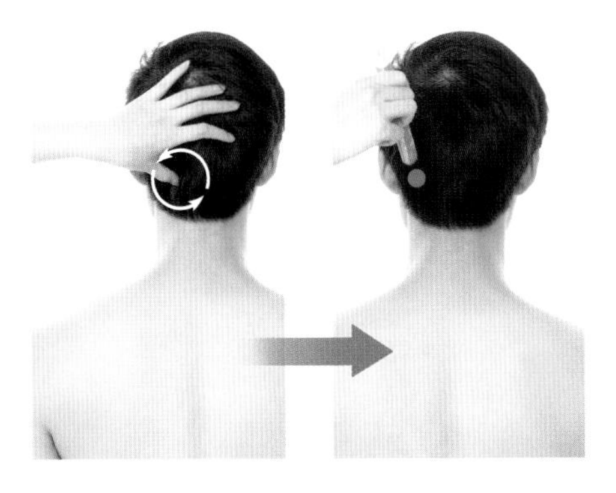

#### 3. Jianjing Point

**Location:** At the midpoint of the top on the shoulder.

**Method:** Knead Jianjing point with the palm heel for 1–3 minutes, retaining the cup for 15–20 minutes. With the cup removed, perform moxibustion with a moxa stick for 3–5 minutes until warmth is felt.

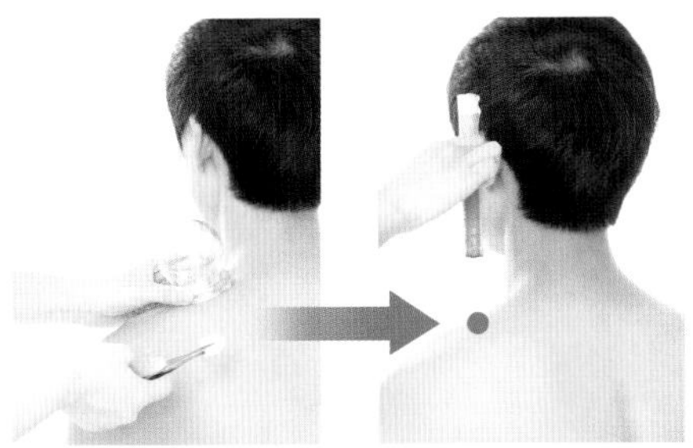

## The Second Group of Points

### 1. Neiguan Point

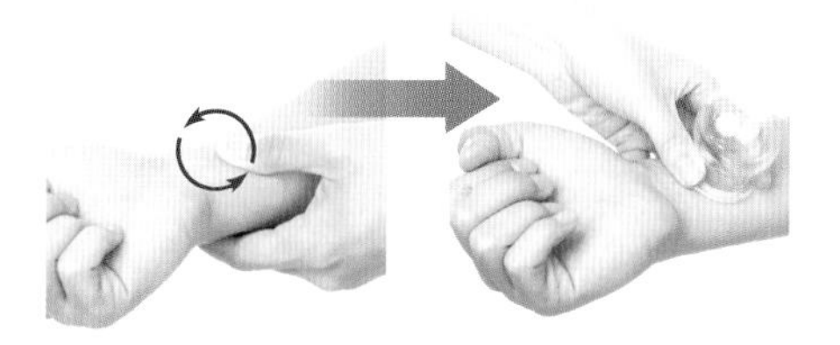

**Location:** Between the two tendons about 2 cun above the wrist joint bend.

**Method:** First, press Neiguan point with the thumb, until one feels soreness on the shoulders and the neck. Then cup Neiguan point, retaining the cup for 15 minutes. With the cup removed, turn the head around, until it can move freely.

### 2. Chengshan Point

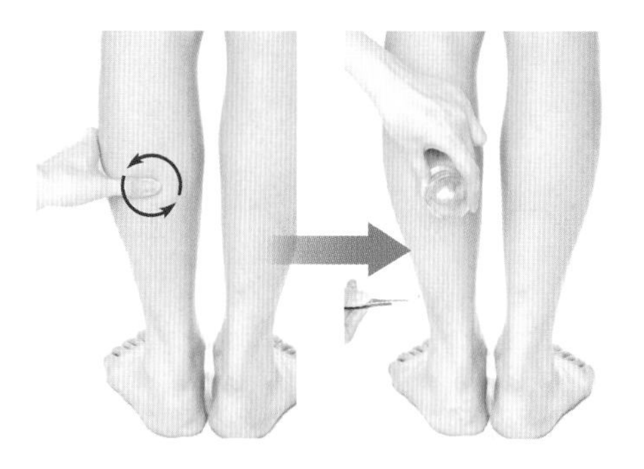

**Location:** In a cavity in the middle of the rear of the lower leg, at the top of the depression between the two muscles of the calf.

**Method:** First knead Chengshan point with the thumb pulp for 2–3 minutes until a feeling of soreness and swelling is present. Then select and apply a cup of appropriate size to the point, retaining the cup for 10–15 minutes.

## The Third Group of Points

### 1. Xuanzhong Point

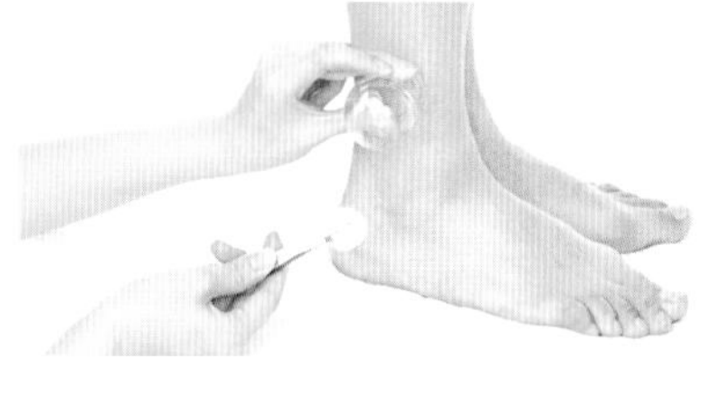

**Location:** In a cavity 3 cun above the outer ankle tip.

**Method:** Select a cup of appropriate size and apply it to Xuanzhong point, retaining the cup for 15–20 minutes.

### 2. Foot Trapezius Muscle Reflex Zone

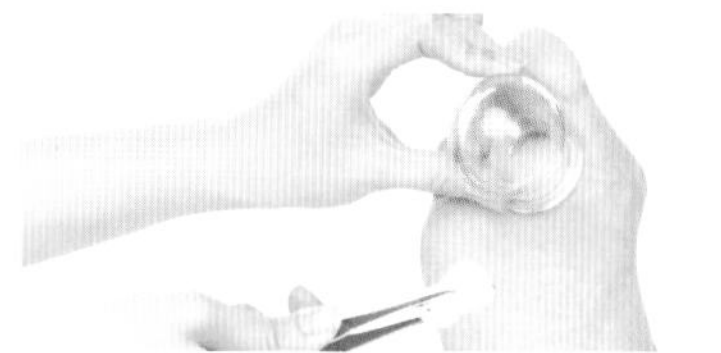

**Location:** See the picture as follows.

**Method:** Select a cup of appropriate size and apply it to foot trapezius muscle reflex zone. Retain the cup for 15–20 minutes.

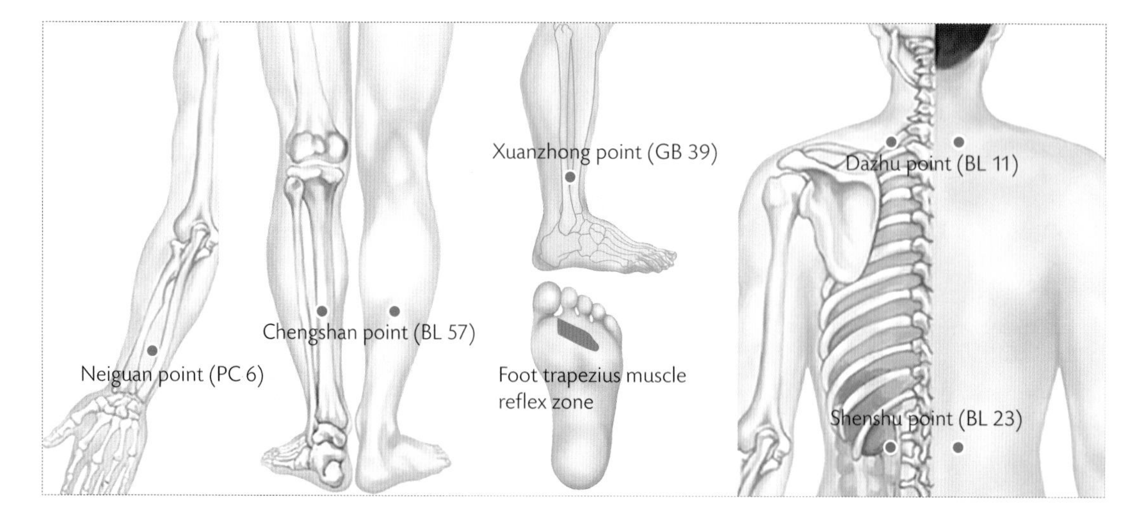

**Ashi Point**
Ashi point is also known as the indefinite point, that is to say this kind of points has no fixed location or name, but is determined depending on the location of the disease, mostly located in the vicinity of the disease. The point is identified at the region where the pain is.

# 4 Rheumatoid Arthritis

The main symptoms are chronic and symmetric pain, swelling, and deformity in multiple joints, mostly on the hands, wrists, feet, and other small joints.

One should actively receive treatment to prevent complications once he is found having rheumatoid arthritis. Patients should not smoke and should avoid passive smoking, so as to prevent aggravation of arthritis. In terms of diet, they should eat less dairy products, fat meat, high animal fat, high cholesterol food or sweets, and drink less alcohol, coffee, tea, or other related beverages. They may eat appropriate amount of animal blood, eggs, fish, shrimps, bean products, potatoes, beef, chicken, beef tendon meat, and other food rich in histidine, arginine, nucleic acid, and collagen.

During cupping, select local Ashi points on the wrist, ankle, knee joints, and elbow joints. You can also add Dazhu and Shenshu points. Do not cup small joints.

## Cupping Methods

### 1. Ashi Point

**Location:** Painful point.

**Method:** First, knead Ashi point with the thumb pulp for 2–3 minutes, and then cup the point before retaining the cup for 15–20 minutes.

### 2. Dazhu Point

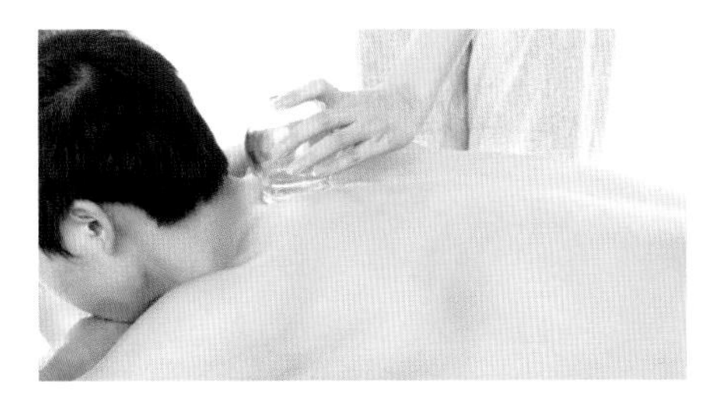

**Location:** In the spine area, 1.5 cun lateral to the posterior midline of the lower border of the spinous process of the first thoracic vertebra.

**Method:** Select a cup of appropriate size and apply it to the point, retaining the cup for 15–20 minutes.

### 3. Shenshu Point

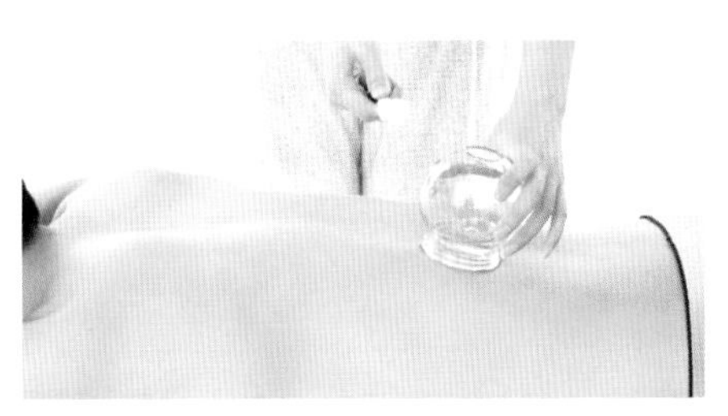

**Location:** 1.5 cun horizontally from the second lumbar spinal process.

**Method:** Select a cup of appropriate size and apply it to the point, retaining the cup for 15–20 minutes.

# 5 Lumbar Disc Herniation

This type of patient will feel low back pain, accompanied by radiating pain, numbness or cold on the lower limb, which may radiate to the outer part of the leg, heal, or toe.

Patients in the early stages should take enough rest, avoid catching a cold or being tired. They should correct their bad postures, and do appropriate functional exercise to enhance the strength of lower back muscles and maintain the stability of the spine. The cupping should be used jointly with appropriate massage, acupuncture, and drug therapy, which can achieve good effects.

Cup Yaoyangguan, Mingmen, Shenshu, and Dachangshu points for those with waist symptoms, and Huantiao, Fengshi, Weizhong, Chengshan, Yanglingquan, and Kunlun points for those with lower limb symptoms.

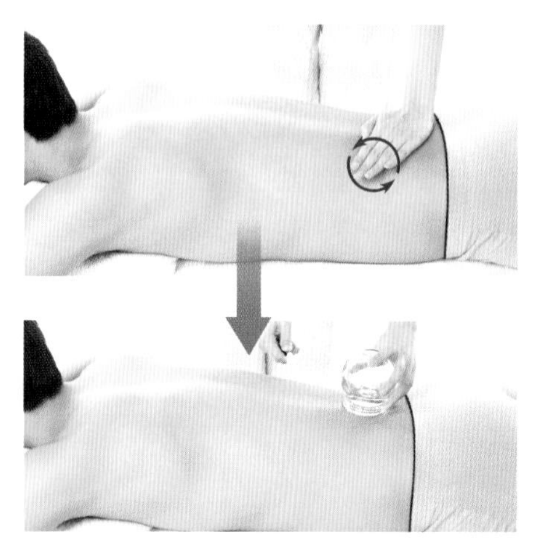

## Cupping Methods

### Cup the Following Points for Those with Waist Symptoms

**1. Yaoyangguan Point**

**Location:** In a cavity below the fourth lumbar vertebra.

**Method:** First knead Yaoyangguan point with the palm for 2–3 minutes, and then select and apply a cup of appropriate size to the point, retaining the cup for 10–15 minutes. With the cup removed, perform moxibustion with a moxa box for 3–5 minutes until warmth is felt.

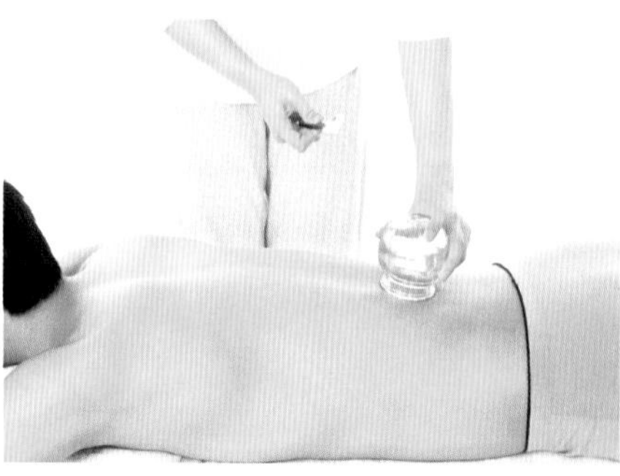

**2. Mingmen Point**

**Location:** In a cavity below the spinous process of the second cervical vertebra.

**Method:** First knead Mingmen point with the palm for 2–3 minutes, and then select and apply a cup of appropriate size to the point, retaining the cup for 10–15 minutes. With the cup removed, perform moxibustion with a moxa box for 3–5 minutes until warmth is felt.

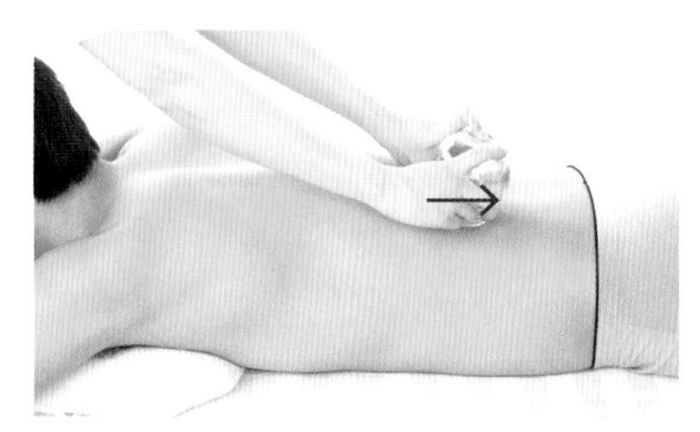

**3. Shenshu and Dachangshu Points**

**Location:** Shenshu point is 1.5 cun horizontally from the second lumbar spinal process; Dachangshu point is about 1.5 cun away from the fourth lumbar vertebra on two sides.

**Method:** First, knead Shenshu and Dachangshu points with the palm for 2–3 minutes, and then apply a cup of appropriate size to the points, continuously moving the cup on these two points, retaining the cup on each point for 10–15 minutes. With the cup removed, perform moxibustion with a moxa box for 3–5 minutes until warmth is felt.

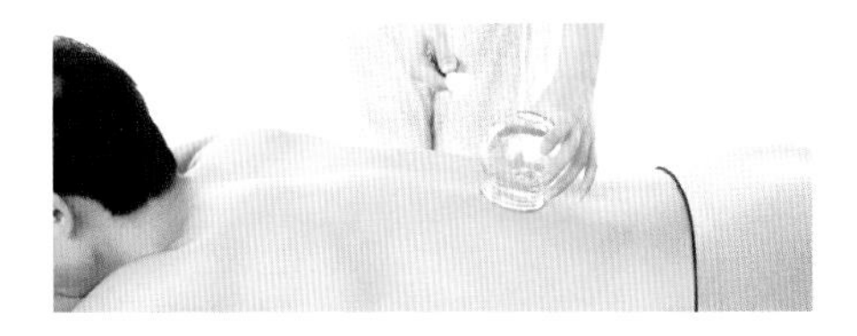

### Cup the Following Points for Those with Lower Limb Symptoms

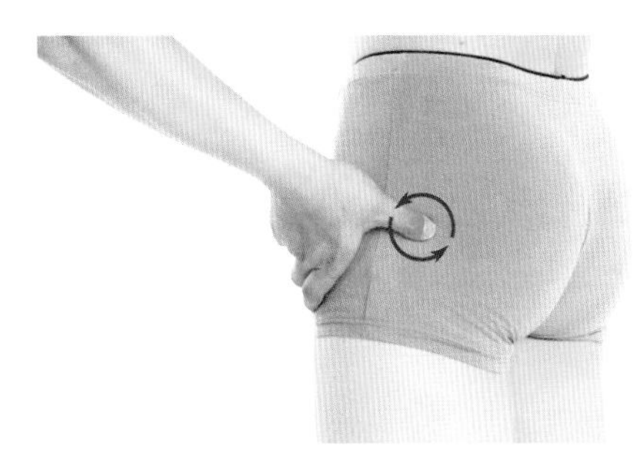

#### 1. Huantiao Point

**Location:** In the depression on the outer side of the gluteus maximus, on both sides when standing.

**Method:** First, massage Huantiao point with the thumb before cupping. Retain the cup for 15–20 minutes.

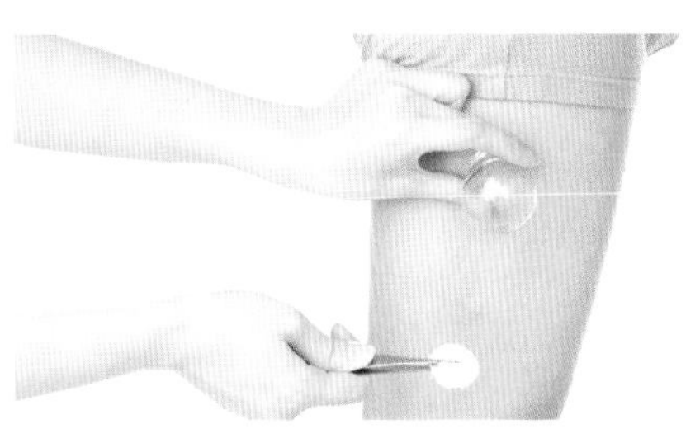

#### 2. Fengshi Point

**Location:** With the arm lying naturally at the side, the point where the tip of the middle finger touches the leg.

**Method:** First, massage Huantiao point with the thumb before cupping. Retain the cup for 15–20 minutes.

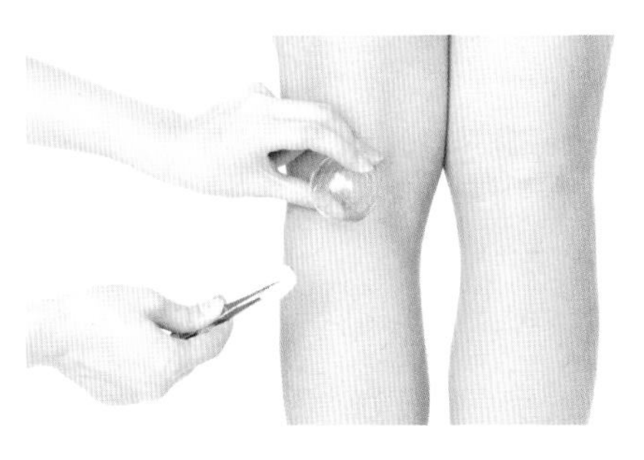

#### 3. Weizhong Point

**Location:** Right in the middle of popliteal crease (at the back of the knee).

**Method:** First knead Weizhong point with the thumb tip for 2–3 minutes, preferably with a heavy force, until one feels sore and swelling at the point. Then apply a cup of appropriate size to the point, and retain the cup for 10–15 minutes.

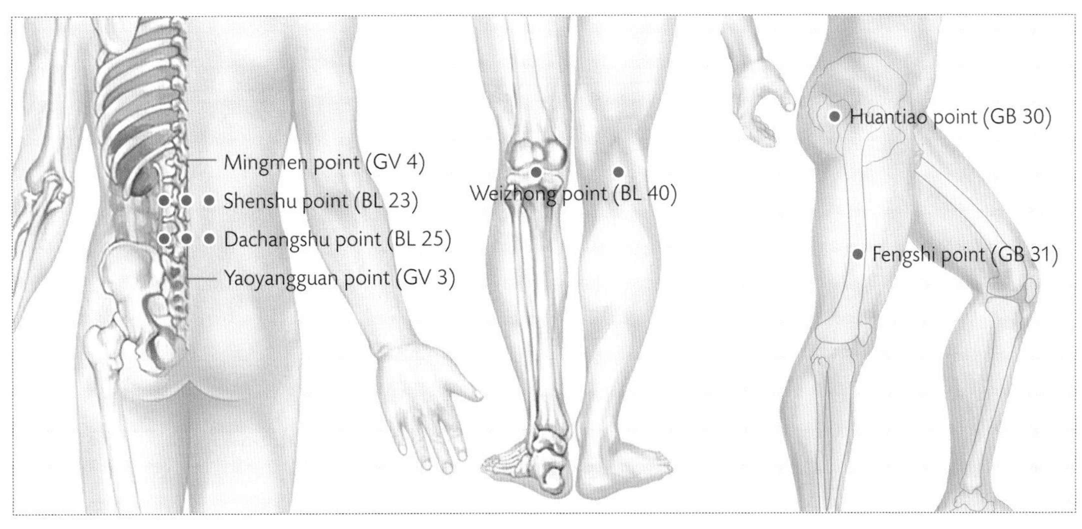

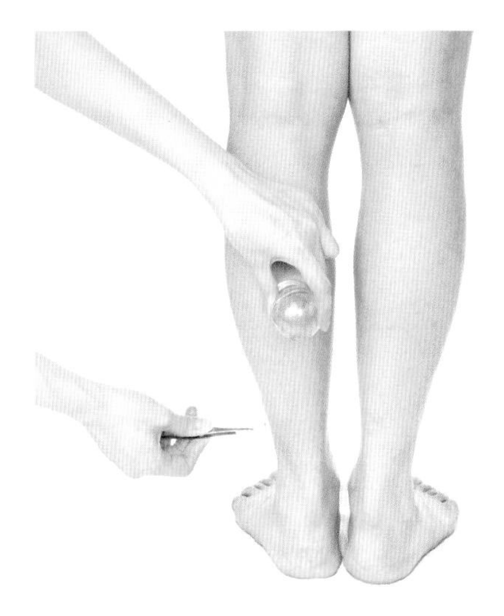

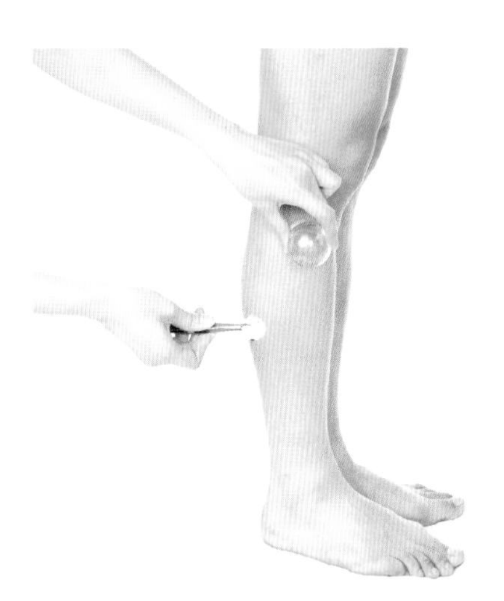

### 4. Chengshan Point

**Location:** In a cavity in the middle of the rear of the lower leg, at the top of the depression between the two muscles of the calf.

**Method:** First knead Chengshan point with the thumb tip for 2–3 minutes, preferably with a heavy force, until one feels sore and swelling at the point. Then apply a cup of appropriate size to the point, and retain the cup for 10–15 minutes.

### 5. Yanglingquan Point

**Location:** On the outer side of the shin in a notch at the front lower part of the fibula.

**Method:** Select a cup with appropriate size and apply it to the point, retaining the cup for 15–20 minutes.

### 6. Kunlun Point

**Location:** In a cavity directly in the rear of the lateral malleolus.

**Method:** Select a cup with appropriate size and apply it to the point, retaining the cup for 15–20 minutes.

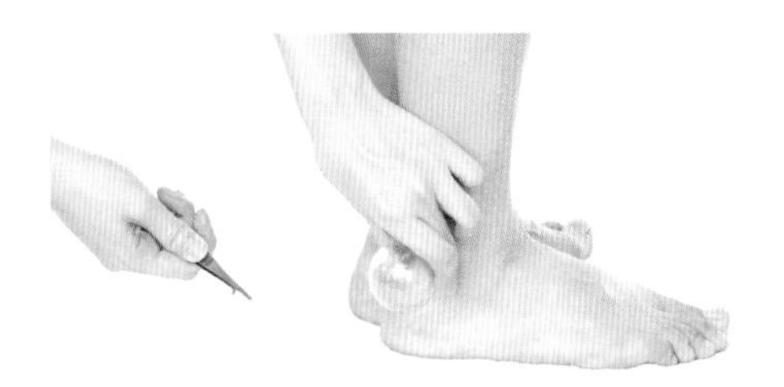

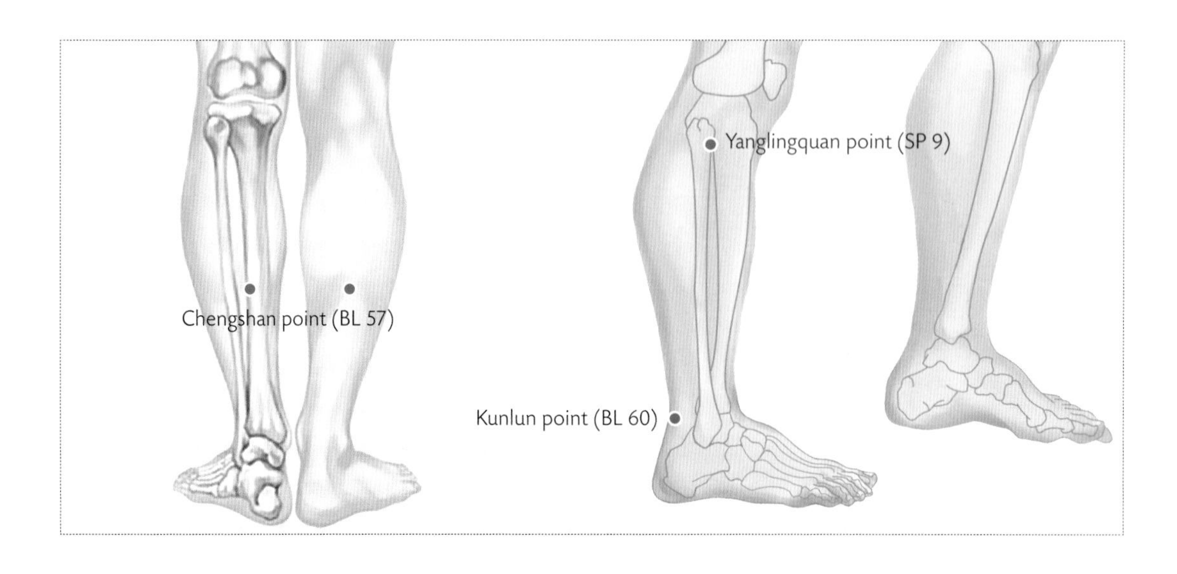

# 6 Chronic Lumbar Muscle Strain

Chronic lumbar muscle strain has manifestations including long-term recurrence of pain, soreness, and discomfort in the lower back. The symptoms may be alleviated after rest or appropriate activities, but may be aggravated after fatigue, in rainy days, and after being exposed to wind, cold, and dampness.

Patients may sleep on hard beds, and have enough rest in the early stages of pain and strengthen functional exercise in the alleviation period. Those who have sat in the office for a long time should change their positions frequently and correct their bad postures. Cupping may be applied together with massage, acupuncture and external application of medicines invigorating the kidney and supporting yang.

The cupping should be performed on Ashi, Chengshan and Weizhong points.

## Cupping Methods

### 1. Ashi Point

**Location:** Painful point.

**Method:** Use the moving cupping method. Move the cup on the bladder meridian on the back by segment along the meridian, and move it several times mainly on the Ashi point. Repeatedly push and pull on the point back and forth, until the skin becomes red. The cup may be retained on the abovementioned point for 10–15 minutes after the moving cupping. With the cup removed, perform moxibustion with a moxa stick for 3–5 minutes until warmth is felt.

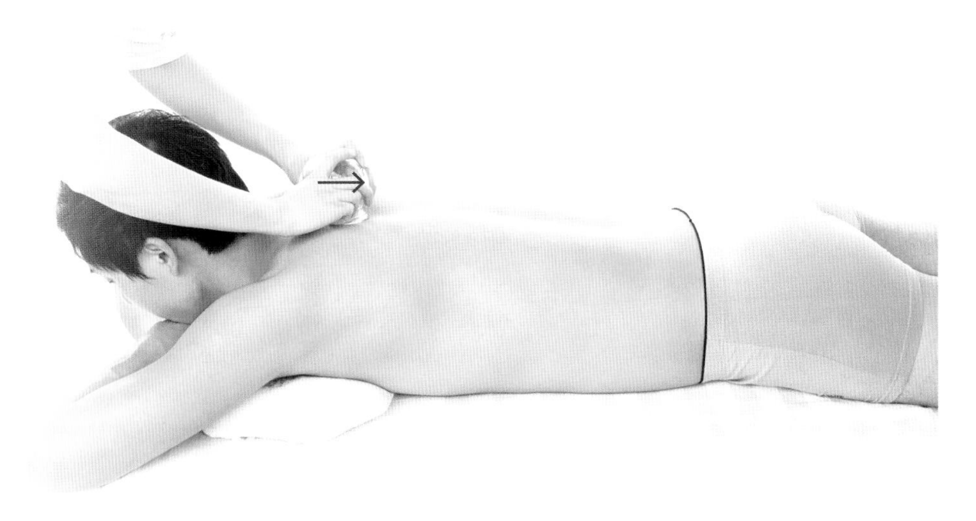

### 2. Chengshan Point

**Location:** In a cavity in the middle of the rear of the lower leg, at the top of the depression between the two muscles of the calf.

**Method:** First knead Chengshan point with the thumb tip for 2–3 minutes, preferably with a heavy force, until one feels sore and swelling at the point. Then apply a cup of appropriate size to the point, and retain the cup for 10–15 minutes.

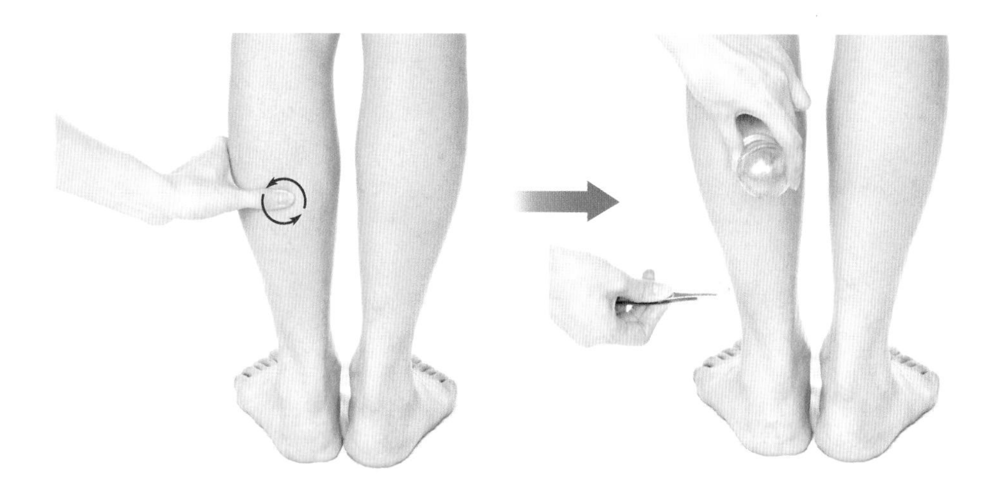

### 3. Weizhong Point

**Location:** Right in the middle of popliteal crease (at the back of the knee).

**Method:** First knead Weizhong point with the thumb tip for 2–3 minutes, preferably with a heavy force, until one feels sore and swelling at the point. Then apply a cup of appropriate size to the point, and retain the cup for 10–15 minutes.

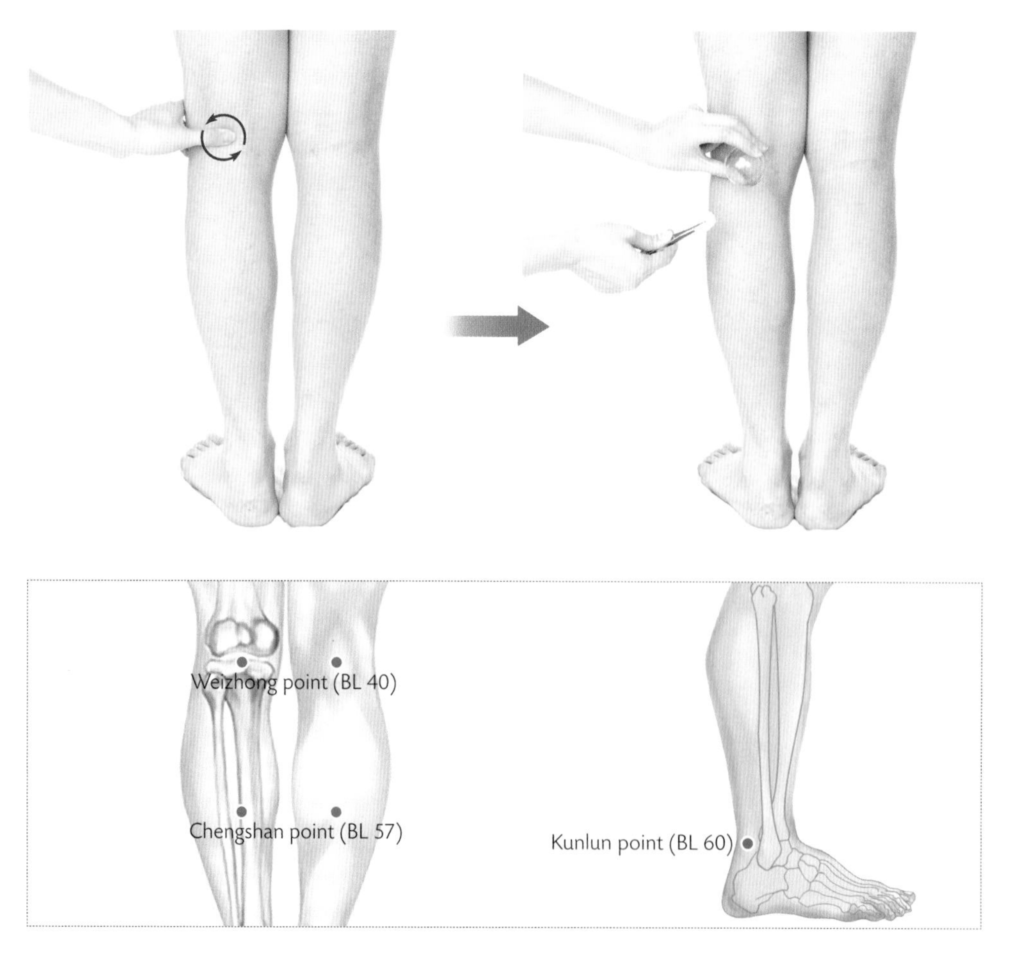

# 7 Heel Pain

The symptom of patients with this disease is pain or local tenderness on the heels when walking or standing. Pain will increase when walking after rest, but may alleviate after walking for a short period, and aggravate again after walking for a long time, and then alleviate again after rest, with probable local swelling.

Patients should walk less so that the feet may have sufficient rest, and should wear soft soles or place a sponge pad under the affected foot. Hot compress can be applied to local parts with some blood stasis medicine or soak feet in warm water every day.

The cupping should be applied to Ashi, Taixi, Chengshan, and Kunlun points.

## Cupping Methods

### 1. Ashi Point

**Location:** Painful point.

**Method:** First, knead Ashi point with the thumb pulp for 2–3 minutes, and then cup the point before retaining the cup for 15–20 minutes.

### 2. Chengshan Point

**Location:** In a cavity in the middle of the rear of the lower leg, at the top of the depression between the two muscles of the calf.

**Method:** Select a cup of appropriate size and apply it to the point, retaining the cup for 15–20 minutes.

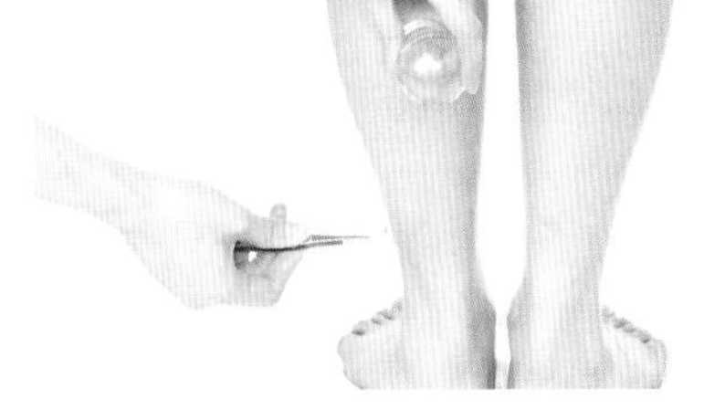

### 3. Kunlun Point

**Location:** In a cavity directly in the rear of the lateral malleolus.

**Method:** Select a cup of appropriate size and apply it to the point, retaining the cup for 15–20 minutes.

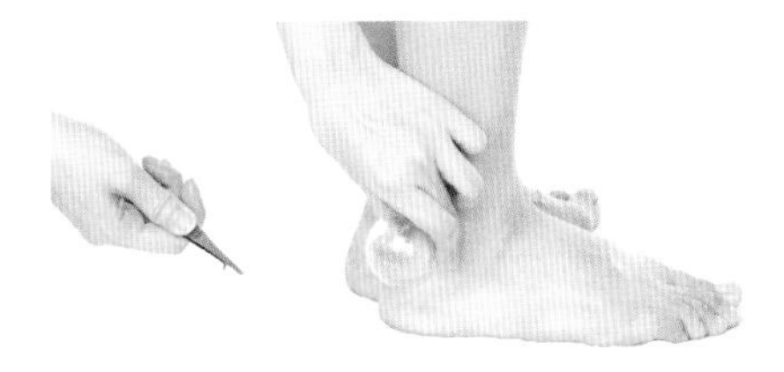

### 4. Taixi Point

**Location:** In a cavity between the medial malleolus and Achilles tendon.

**Method:** Select a cup of appropriate size and apply it to the point, retaining the cup for 15–20 minutes.

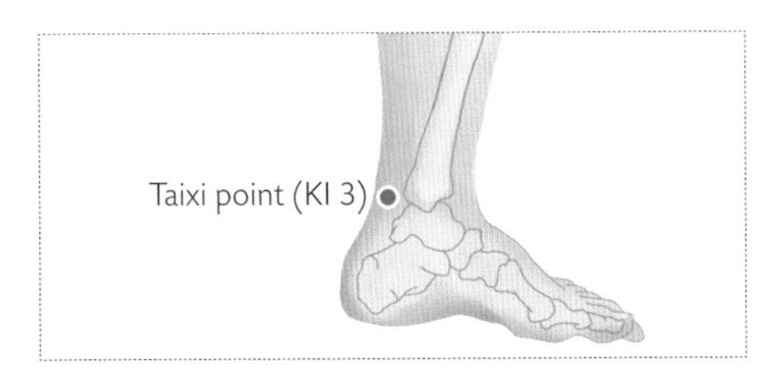


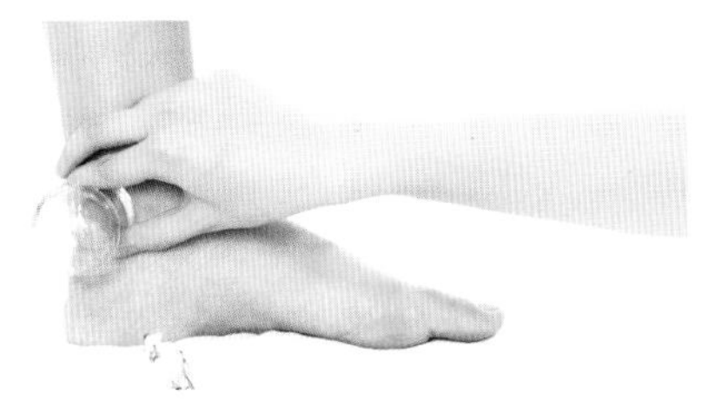

# 8 Thromboangiitis Obliterans

During the attack of the disease, patients feel cold in the skin of the affected limb, have fear of cold and feel pain, with pale and dry skin with desquamation, and muscular atrophy.

Patients should pay attention to the warmth of the limbs in the early stage, and should not soak their feet if there are diabrotic spots.

The cupping should be performed on Weizhong, Xuehai, Geshu, Futu, and Taiyuan points.

## Cupping Methods

### 1. Futu Point

**Location:** 6 cun above the outer upper margin of the patella.

**Method:** Select and apply a cup of appropriate size to Futu point, retaining the cup for 5–10 minutes. With the cup removed, perform moxibustion with a moxa box for 3–5 minutes until warmth is felt.

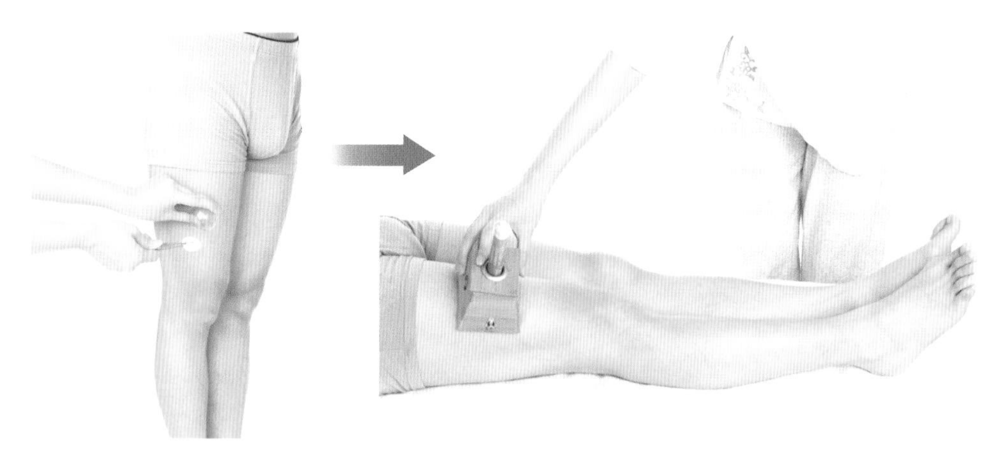

### 2. Geshu Point

**Location:** 1.5 cun away from the spinous process of the seventh thoracic vertebra.

**Method:** Select and apply a cup of appropriate size to Geshu point, retaining the cup for 5–10 minutes. With the cup removed, perform moxibustion with a moxa box for 3–5 minutes until warmth is felt.

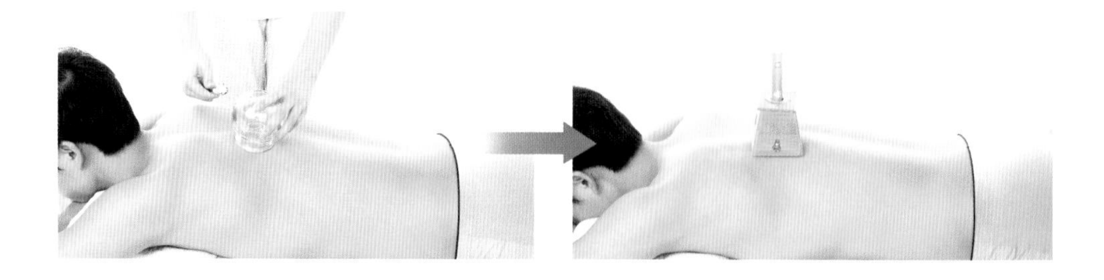

### 3. Weizhong Point

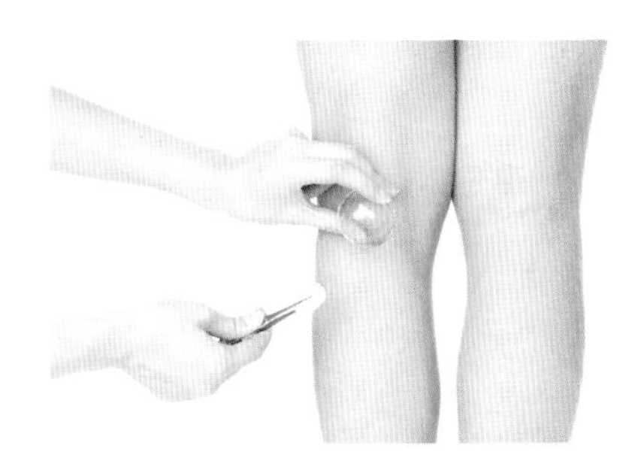

**Location:** Right in the middle of popliteal crease (at the back of the knee).

**Method:** Select and apply a cup of appropriate size to Weizhong point, retaining the cup for 5–10 minutes. With the cup removed, perform moxibustion with a moxa box for 3–5 minutes until warmth is felt.

### 4. Xuehai Point

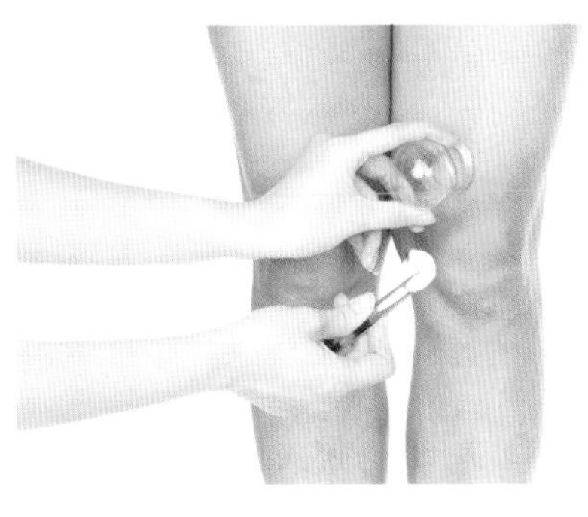

**Location:** In a cavity about 2 cun away from the inner upper corner of the patella, when the knee is bent.

**Method:** Select and apply a cup of appropriate size to Xuehai point, retaining the cup for 5–10 minutes. With the cup removed, perform moxibustion with a moxa box for 3–5 minutes until warmth is felt.

### 5. Taiyuan Point

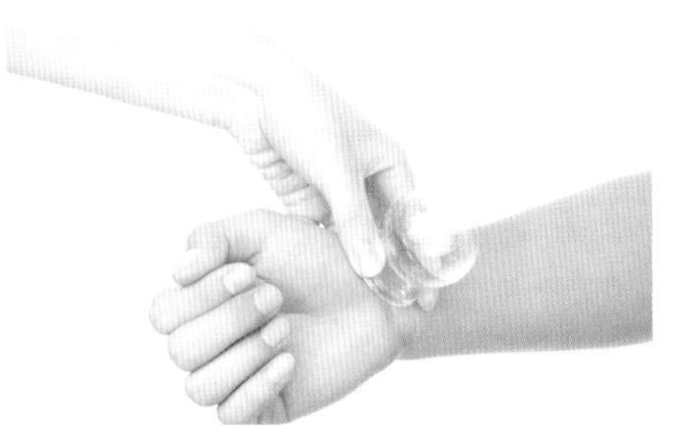

**Location:** In the anterior region of the wrist, between the radial styloid process and the scaphoid bone, in the depression at the ulnar side of abductor pollicis longus tendon.

**Method:** Select and apply a cup of appropriate size to Taiyuan point, retaining the cup for 15–20 minutes.

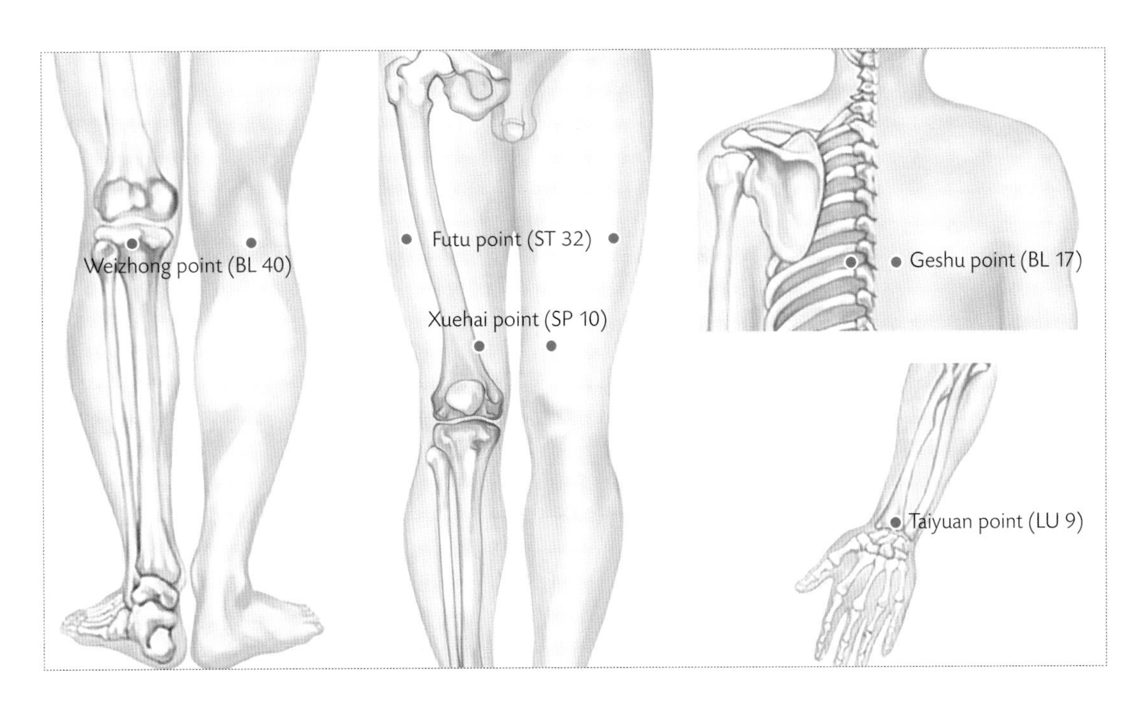

# 9 Varicosity

Patients with varicosity are characterized by swelling and heaviness of affected limbs, and proneness to fatigue, swell, and curve or even clump of leg veins. They may also suffer mild edema on ankle, skin atrophy, pigmentation on the lower legs and ankles and chronic ulcers.

Patients should have appropriate rest and should not stand for a long time. When they are sleeping, they should raise their lower limbs, use elastic cloth to tighten the varicose parts, and see a doctor in the event of serious complications.

The cupping should be applied to Sanyinjiao, Geshu, and Xuehai points.

## Cupping Methods

### 1. Sanyinjiao Point

**Location:** At the rear edge of the shinbone, 3 cun above the ankle.

**Method:** First knead Sanyinjiao point with the thumb pulp for 2–3 minutes, and then select and apply a cup of appropriate size to the point, retaining the cup for 10–15 minutes. With the cup removed, perform moxibustion with a moxa stick for 3–5 minutes.

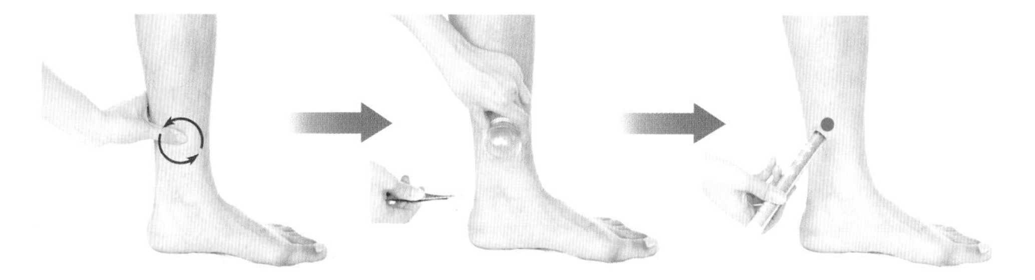

### 2. Geshu Point

**Location:** At the point 1.5 cun away from the spinous process of the seventh thoracic vertebra.

**Method:** Select a cup of appropriate size and apply it to Geshu point. Retain the cup for 5–10 minutes. With the cup removed, perform moxibustion with a moxa box for 3–5 minutes.

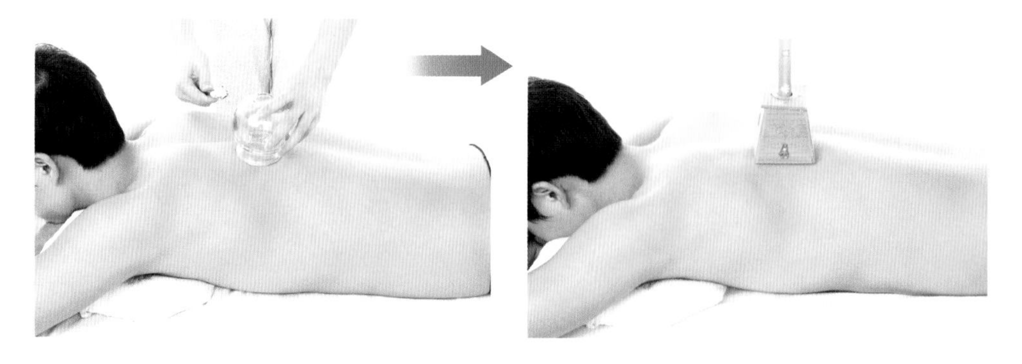

### 3. Xuehai Point

**Location:** In a cavity about 2 cun away from the inner upper corner of the patella, when the knee is bent.

**Method:** First knead Xuehai point with the thumb pulp for 2–3 minutes, and then select and apply a cup of appropriate size to the point, retaining the cup for 5–10 minutes. With the cup removed, perform moxibustion with a moxa box for 3–5 minutes until warmth is felt.

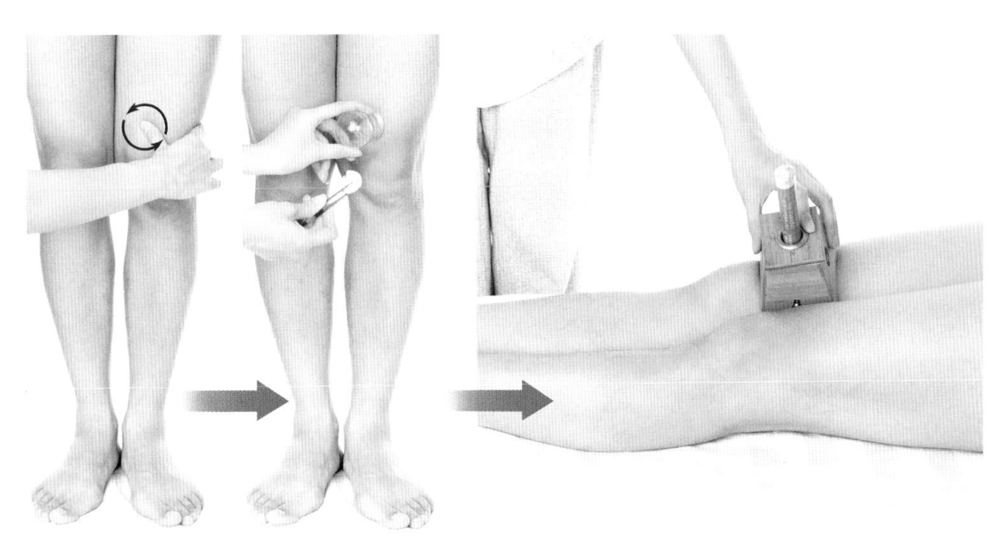

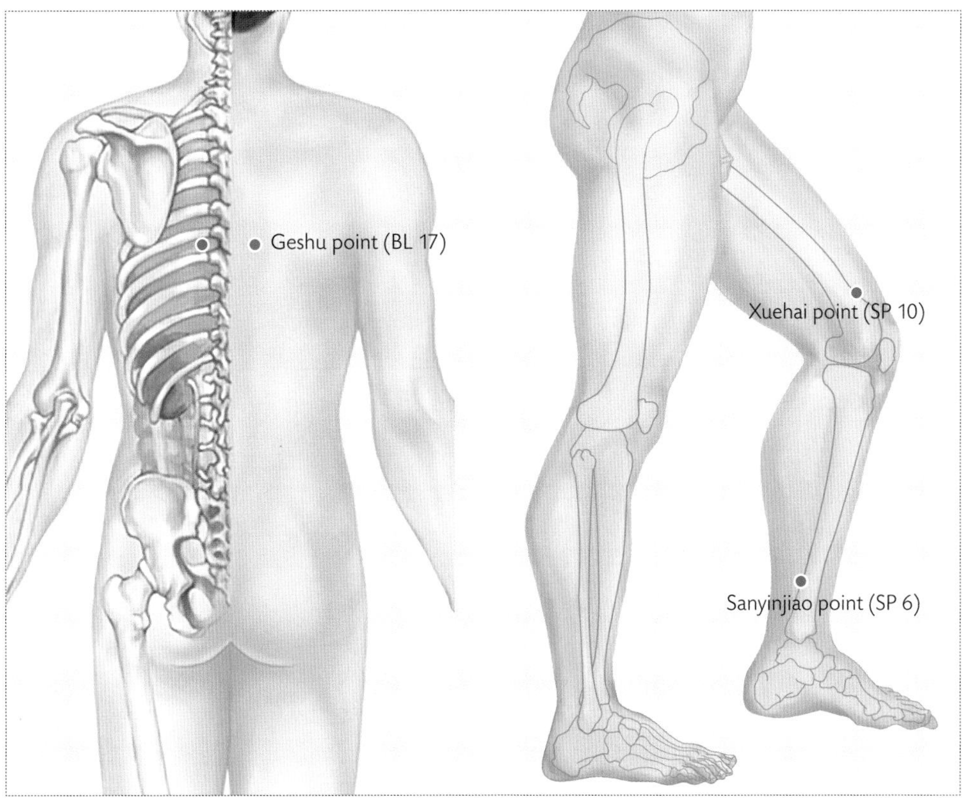

# 10 Hemorrhoids

Patients with hemorrhoids have rectal bleeding, mostly in the early stages of defecation, probably associated with pain. Some may have anal prolapse, which could restore automatically, but needs the help of hands when the case is serious. Hemorrhoids is the most common proctologic disease.

To prevent hemorrhoids, patients should develop good defecation habits, and eat more fresh vegetables, bananas, and other food that help relax the bowel to relieve constipation in daily life, avoid eating spicy food, strengthen the exercise of the anus, and develop the habit of regular defecation to keep the bowls open and prevent constipation. In the event of long-term sustained blood in the stool, they should consider the possibility of other diseases and see a doctor.

The cupping should be performed on Dachangshu, Xuehai, Ciliao, and Geshu points.

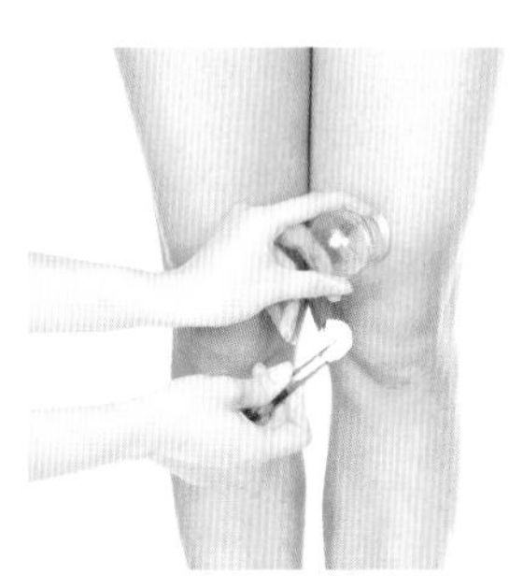

## Cupping Methods

### 1. Xuehai Point

**Location:** In a cavity about 2 cun away from the inner upper corner of the patella, when the knee is bent.

**Method:** Select and apply a cup of appropriate size to Xuehai point, retaining the cup for 10–15 minutes.

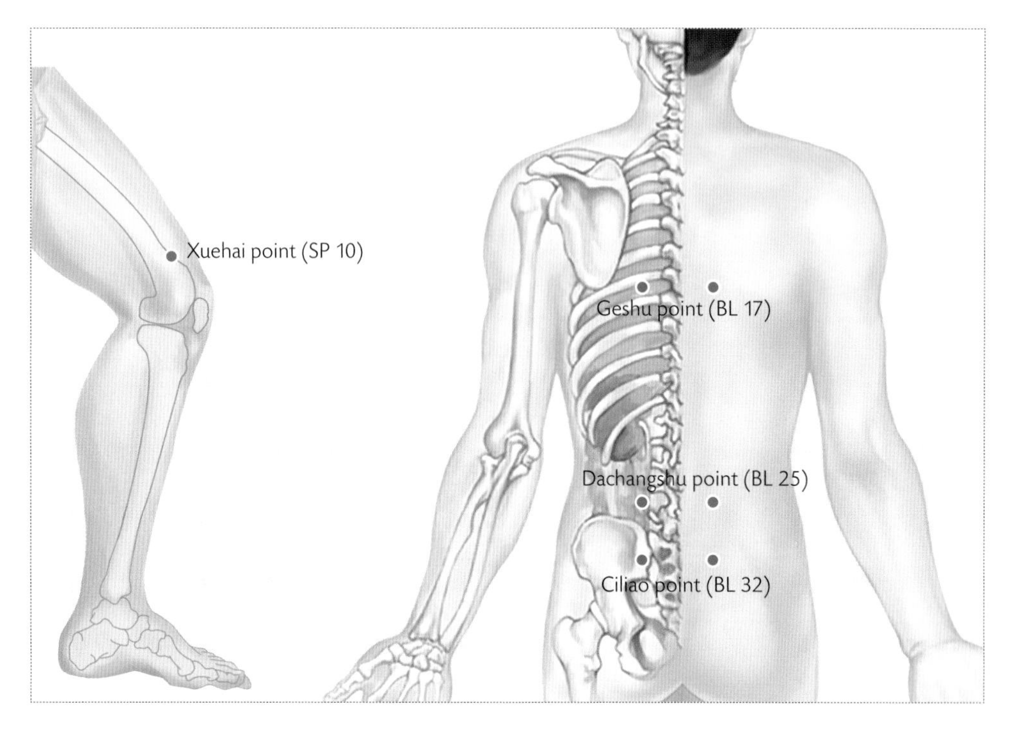

### 2. Dachangshu Point

**Location:** About 1.5 cun away from the fourth lumbar vertebra on two sides.

**Method:** Select a cup of appropriate size and apply it to Dachangshu point and move continuously on the lumbosacral region, until the skin becomes red. Retain the cup on the point for 10–15 minutes.

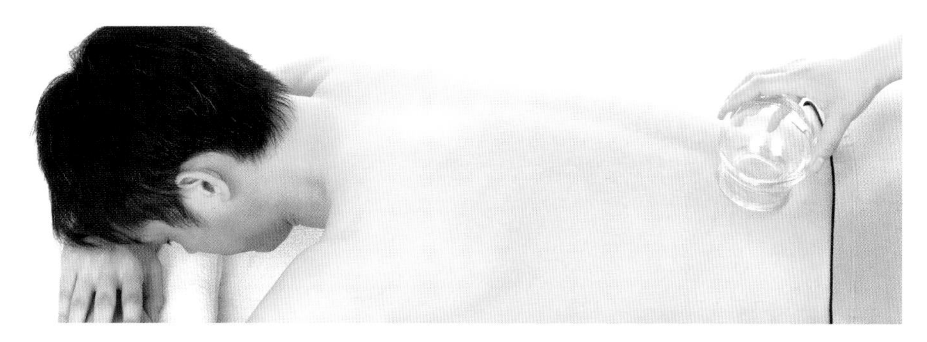

### 3. Ciliao Point

**Location:** In the sacral region, in the second posterior sacral foramen.

**Method:** Select a cup of appropriate size and apply it to Ciliao point, until the skin becomes red. Retain the cup for 10–15 minutes.

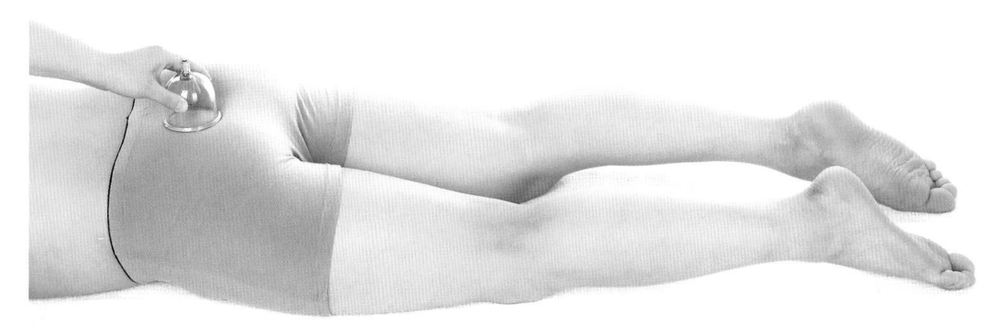

### 4. Geshu Point

**Location:** 1.5 cun away from the spinous process of the seventh thoracic vertebra.

**Method:** Select a cup of appropriate size and apply it to Geshu point. Retain the cup for 10–15 minutes.

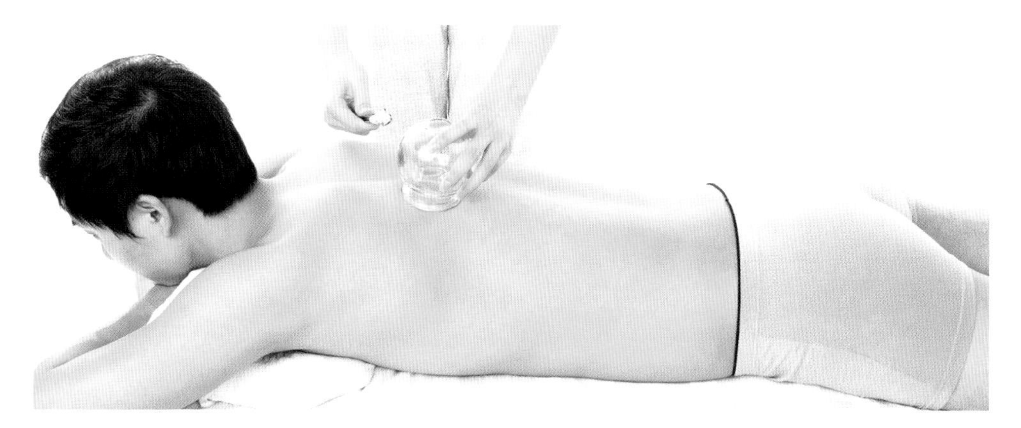

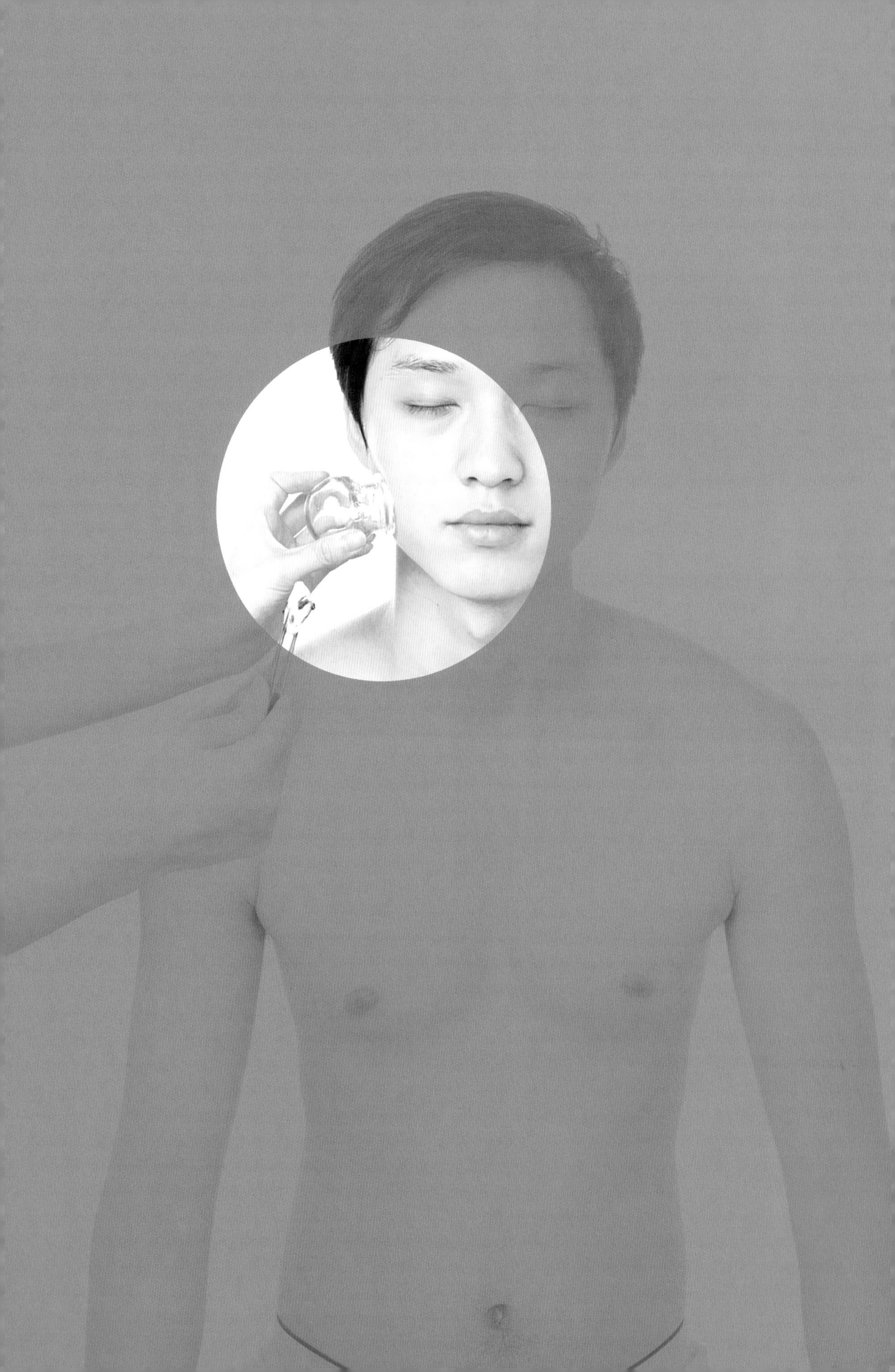

# Chapter Seven
# Diseases of the Five Sense Organs

There is an old Chinese saying that "a toothache is not an illness, yet the pain hurts so badly." People who have experienced toothache know how seriously toothache may affect their daily life and work. As the mouth, nose, eyes, ears, and throat are on the head and face, the attack of this disease may also directly damage the beauty of the face, and the five organs are particularly susceptible to this. These five-sense-organ diseases often make people very uncomfortable. Therefore, it is very important to receive cupping timely to alleviate related symptoms.

## 1 Toothache

At the time of an attack, toothache can be severe, and can break out or aggravate when the teeth are exposed to coldness, heat, sourness, sweetness, and other stimuli, with gum swelling or discharge of pus, bleeding, gingival atrophy, looseness of tooth, inability to bite, etc.

In daily life, one should pay attention to oral hygiene, develope a good habit of brushing their teeth in the morning and evening, and rinse mouth after a meal. See a dentist immediately when tooth decay is found. Do not eat sugar, biscuits, and starchy food before going to bed. Patients should eat more food which can clear stomach heat and liver heat, such as pumpkin, watermelon, water chestnuts, celery, radish, etc., and should not eat food that is too hard, and eat less food that are too acid, too cold, or overheated. Do not take in hot and heat-inducing drinks and food.

The cupping should be applied to Dazhui, Jiache, and Waiguan points, in conjunction with Weishu point for those with excessive stomach heat, as well as Taixi and Shenshu points for those with kidney deficiency.

### Cupping Methods

**1. Dazhui Point**

**Location:** Under the spinous process of the seventh cervical vertebrae.

**Method:** Select a cup of appropriate size and apply it to Dazhui point. Retain the cup for 10–15 minutes.

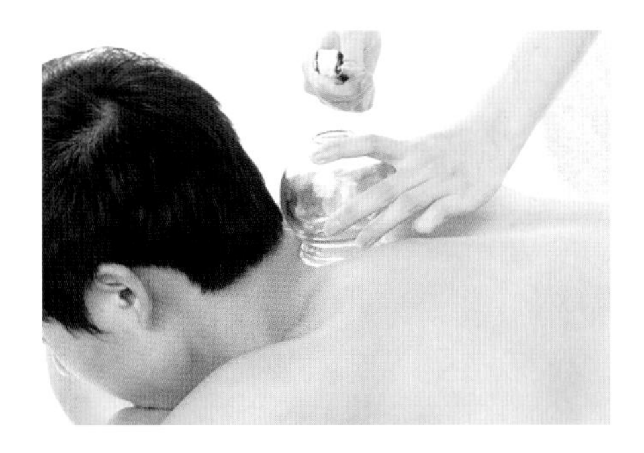

### 2. Jiache Point

**Location:** In a cavity about 1 cun in the upper part of the lower jaw corner, i.e. the highest point of the zygomaxillary muscle when one chews.

**Method:** Select a cup of appropriate size and cup on Jiache point using the flash cupping method for 10–15 times. Do not retain the cup. Then perform moxibustion with a moxa stick for 3–5 minutes until warmth is felt.

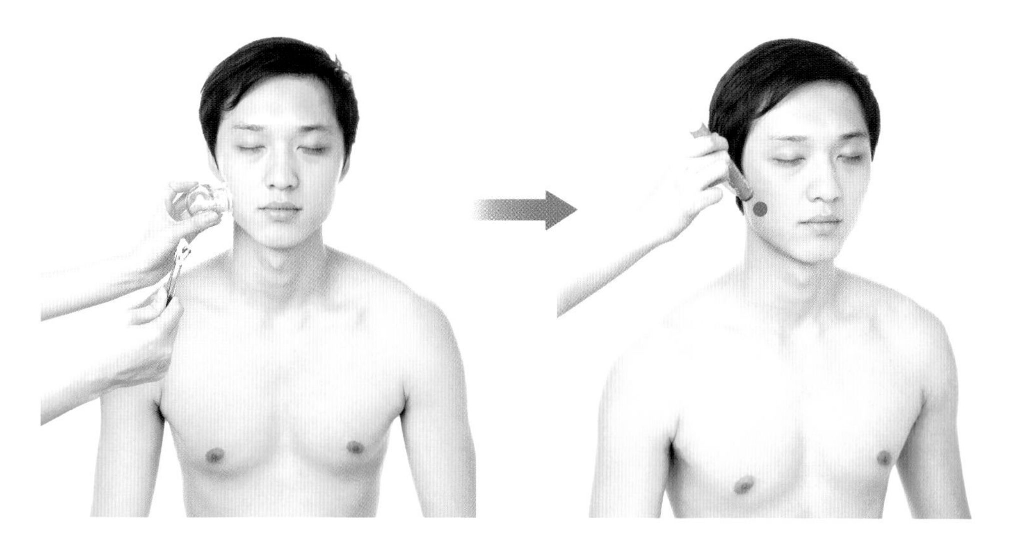

### 3. Waiguan Point

**Location:** The Waiguan point is in the middle on the outside of the arm, between the ulna and radius about 2 cun away from the horizontal line of the wrist joint.

**Method:** First knead Waiguan point with the thumb pulp for 2–3 minutes, until a feeling of soreness and swelling is present, and then select and apply a cup of appropriate size to the point, retaining the cup for 10–15 minutes.

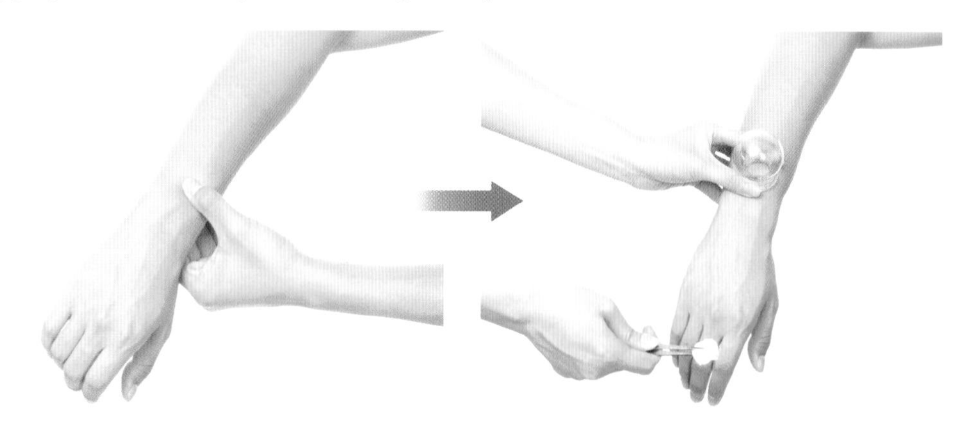

### 4. Taixi Point

**Location:** In a cavity between the medial malleolus and Achilles tendon.

**Method:** First knead Taixi point with the thumb pulp for 2–3 minutes until a feeling of soreness and swelling is present, and then select a cup of appropriate size and apply it to the point, retaining the cup for 10–15 minutes.

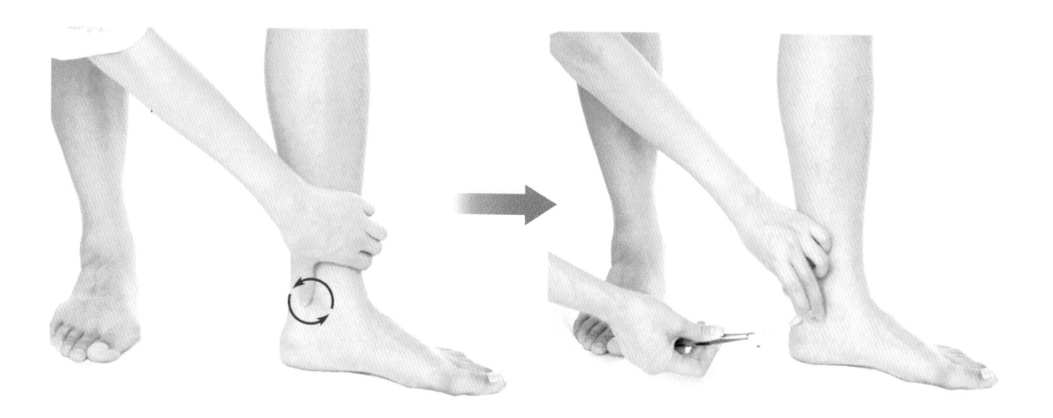

### 5. Weishu Point

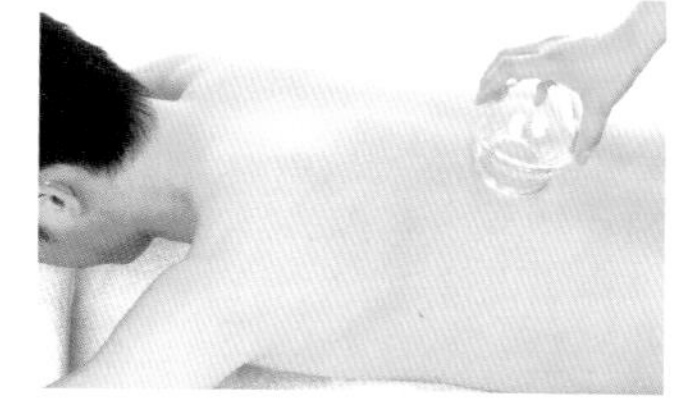

**Location:** About 1.5 cun below the spinous process of the twelfth thoracic vertebra.

**Method:** Select a cup of appropriate size and apply it to the point, retaining the cup for 10–15 minutes.

### 6. Shenshu Point

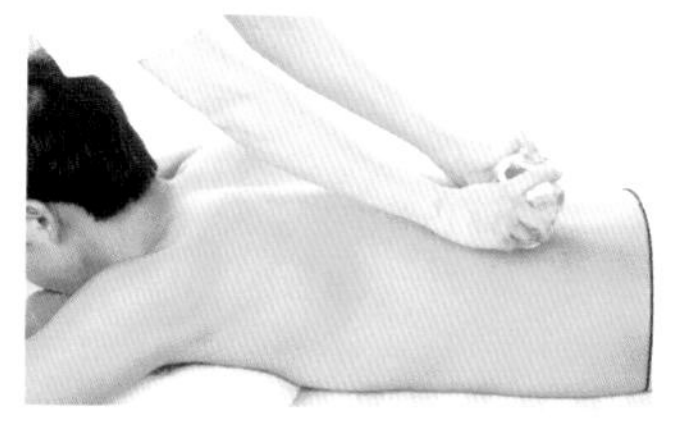

**Location:** 1.5 cun horizontally from the second lumbar spinal process.

**Method:** Select a cup of appropriate size and apply it to the point, retaining the cup for 10–15 minutes.

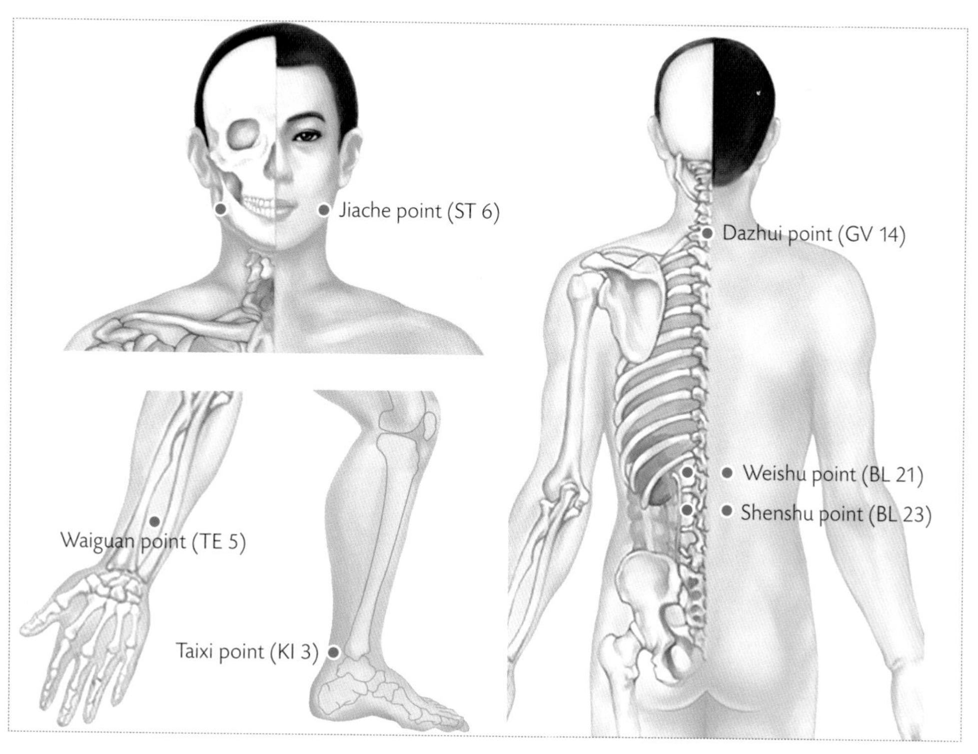

# 2 Deafness and Tinnitus

Deafness is a general term for various symptoms of hearing loss. Patients consciously feel ringing in the ears or head, but without corresponding external sound source in the surrounding environment. The ringing can occur on one side or both sides.

Patients should cautiously use or prohibit from using drugs that damage the hearing nerves. To restore hearing, they should maintain a good mental state, develop scientific habits of diet, and eat more food rich in zinc, iron, and calcium.

The cupping should be applied to Waiguan, Baihui, and Tinggong points, plus Ganshu, Danshu, and Taichong points for excess syndromes, and Taixi, Shenshu, and Sanyinjiao points for deficiency syndromes.

## Cupping Methods

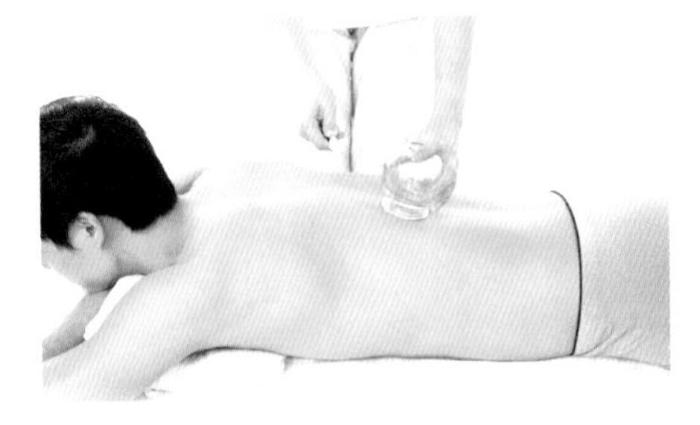

### 1. Ganshu and Danshu Points

**Location:** Ganshu point is 1.5 cun away from the ninth thoracic spinal process on the inner side of the scapula; Danshu point is in the spine area, 1.5 cun lateral to the posterior midline of the lower border of the spinous process of the tenth thoracic vertebra.

**Method:** Select and apply a cup of appropriate size to Ganshu and Danshu points, retaining the cup for 10–15 minutes.

### 2. Shenshu Point

**Location:** 1.5 cun horizontally from the second lumbar spinal process.

**Method:** Select a cup of appropriate size and apply it to the point, retaining the cup for 10–15 minutes. Then perform moxibustion with a moxa stick for 3–5 minutes until warmth is felt.

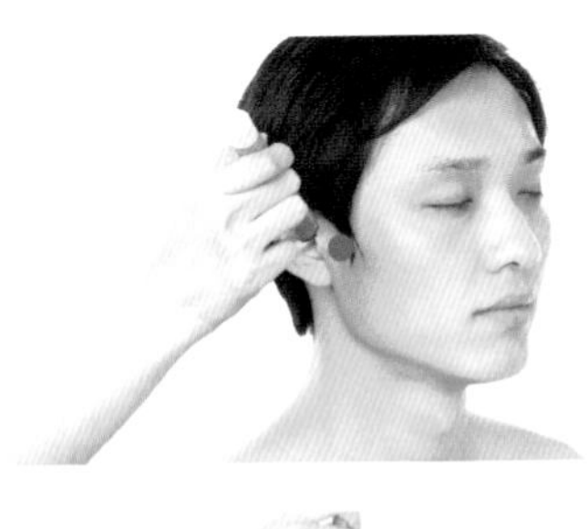

### 3. Tinggong Point

**Location:** With the mouth open, in a cavity before the tragus on a line with the earlobe.

**Method:** Cup on Tinggong point for 10–15 times by using the flash cupping method. Do not retain the cup. Then perform moxibustion with a moxa stick for 3–5 minutes until warmth is felt.

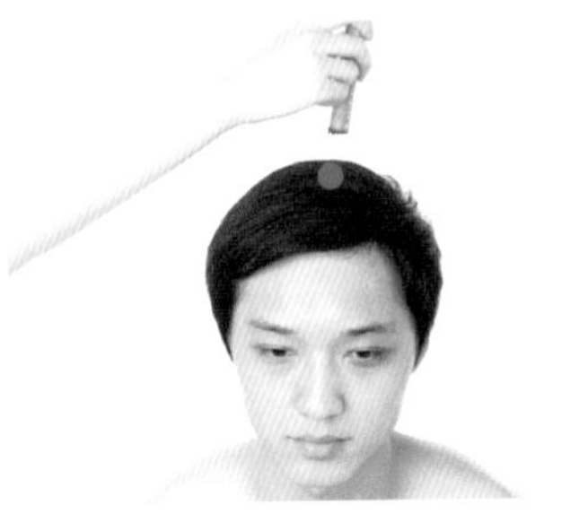

### 4. Baihui Point

**Location:** On the head, 5 cun superior to the anterior hairline, on the anterior midline.

**Method:** Cup on Baihui point for 10–15 times by using the flash cupping method. Do not retain the cup. Then perform moxibustion with a moxa stick for 3–5 minutes until warmth is felt.

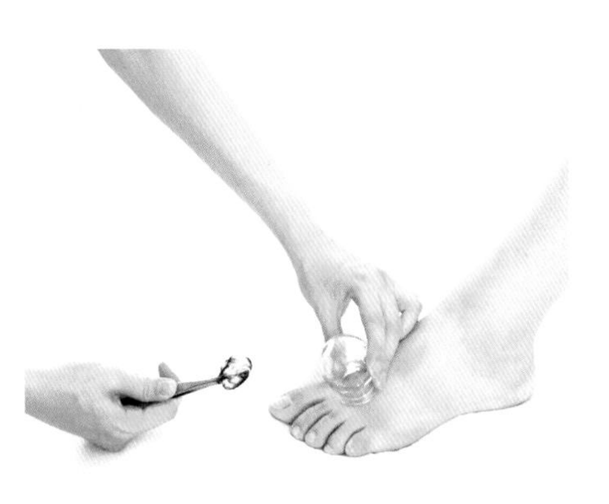

### 5. Taichong Point

**Location:** On the foot in a notch between the first and second metatarsal bones.

**Method:** First knead Taichong point with the thumb pulp for 2–3 minutes until a feeling of soreness and swelling is present. Then select and apply a cup of appropriate size to the point, retaining the cup for 10–15 minutes.

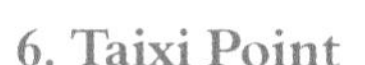

### 6. Taixi Point

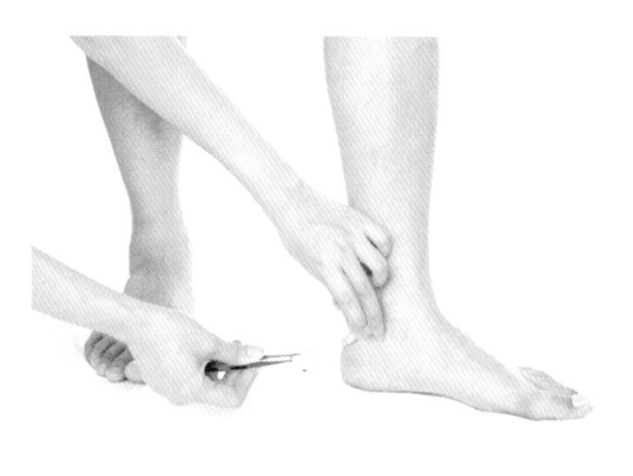

**Location:** In a cavity between the medial malleolus and Achilles tendon.

**Method:** First knead Taixi point with the thumb pulp for 2–3 minutes until a feeling of soreness and swelling is present, and then select a cup of appropriate size and apply it to the point, retaining the cup for 10–15 minutes. Then perform moxibustion with a moxa stick for 3–5 minutes until warmth is felt.

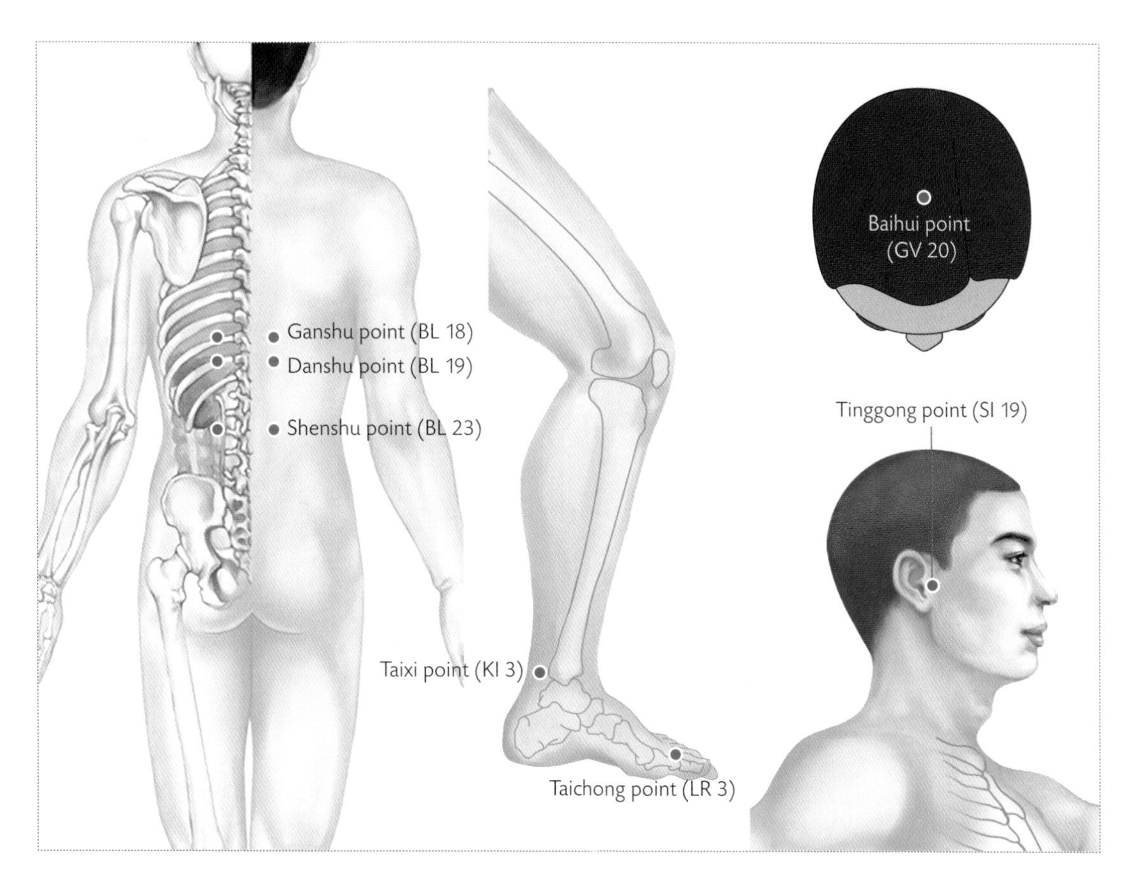

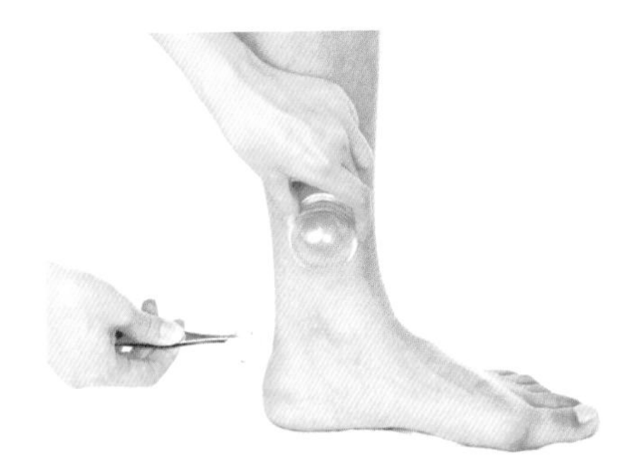

### 7. Sanyinjiao Point

**Location:** At the rear edge of the shinbone, 3 cun above the ankle.

**Method:** First knead Sanyinjiao point with the thumb pulp for 2–3 minutes, and then select and apply a cup of appropriate size to the point, retaining the cup for 10–15 minutes. Then perform moxibustion with a moxa stick for 3–5 minutes until warmth is felt.

### 8. Waiguan Point

**Location:** In the middle on the outside of the arm, between the ulna and radius about 2 cun away from the horizontal line of the wrist joint.

**Method:** First knead Waiguan point with the thumb pulp for 2–3 minutes, until a feeling of soreness and swelling is present, and then select and apply a cup of appropriate size to the point, retaining the cup for 10–15 minutes.

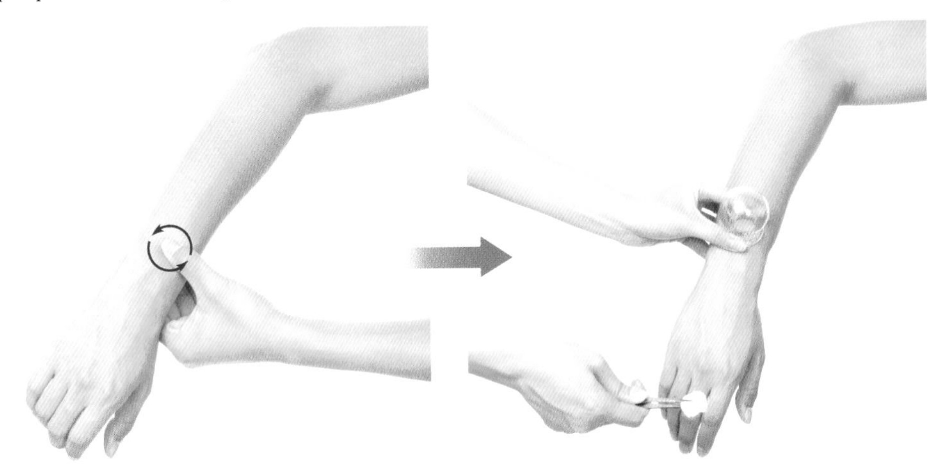

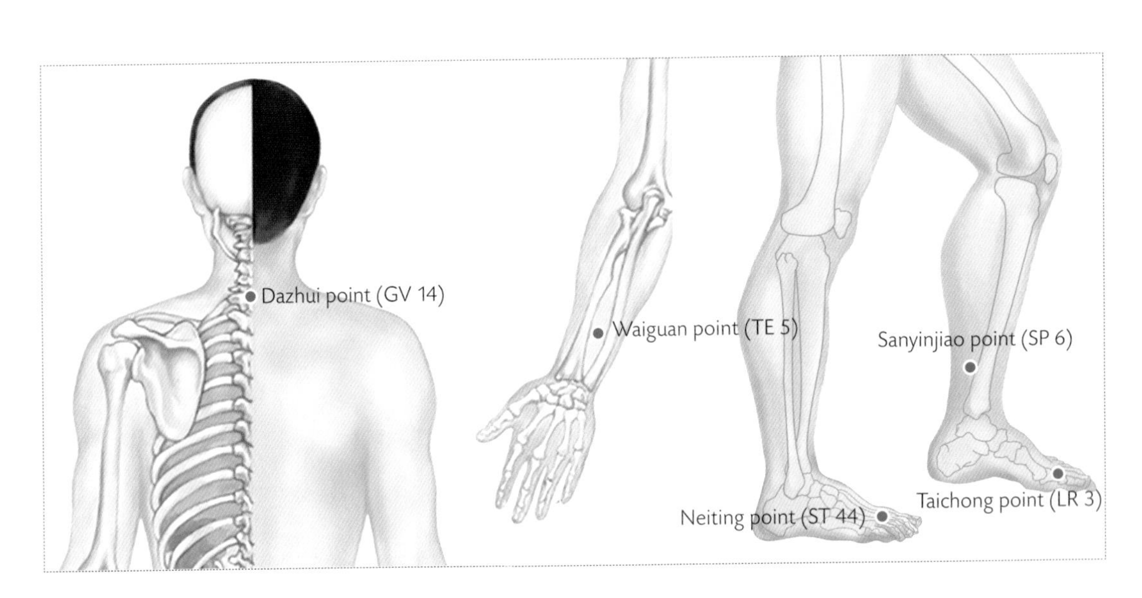

# 3 Nose Bleeding

Nose bleeding generally breaks out acutely, usually on one side, and sometimes on both sides. The bleeding amount is different, with only some blood in nasal discharge in moderate cases, hemorrhagic shock in severe cases. Anemia can happen in recurrence of bleeding.

To prevent and control nose bleeding, in dry seasons, people should drink more water and less alcohol, eat less spicy or heat-inducing food, but more food that lowers the body heat, such as bitter gourd, green bean soup, and watermelon. Do not pick nostrils. Once the nose bleeds, one may use clean absorbent cottons to fill the nasal cavity to stop bleeding, or use fingers to press both sides of the nosewing in the absence of absorbent cottons.

The cupping should be performed on Dazhui, Taichong, Neiting, Yintang, and Hegu points.

## Cupping Methods

### 1. Dazhui Point

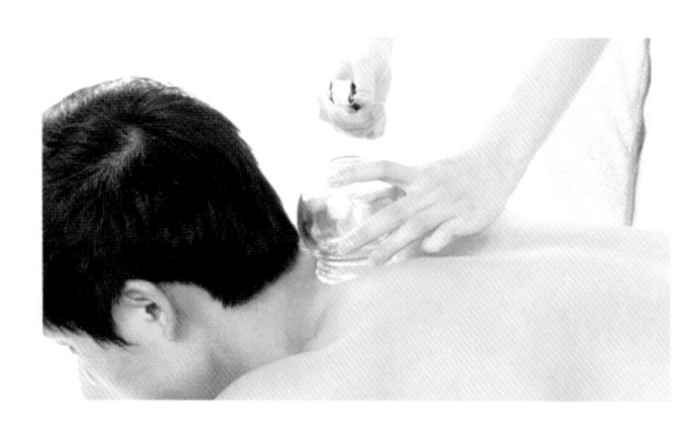

**Location:** Under the spinous process of the seventh cervical vertebrae.

**Method:** Select a cup of appropriate size and apply it to Dazhui point. Retain the cup for 10–15 minutes.

### 2. Taichong Point

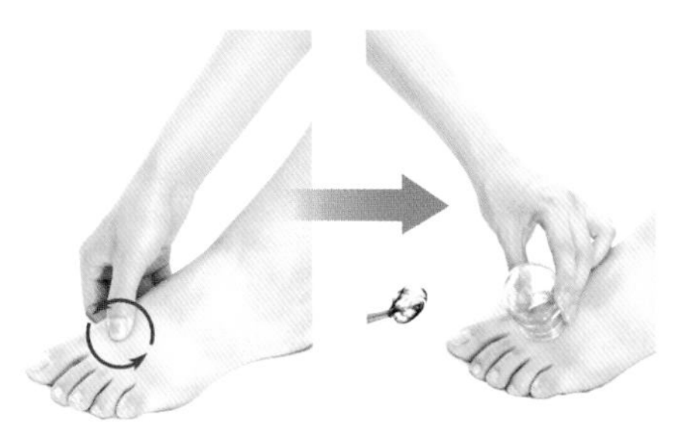

**Location:** On the foot in a notch between the first and second metatarsal bones.

**Method:** First knead Taichong point with the thumb pulp for 2–3 minutes until a feeling of soreness and swelling is present. Then select and apply a cup of appropriate size to the point, retaining the cup for 10–15 minutes.

### 3. Neiting Point

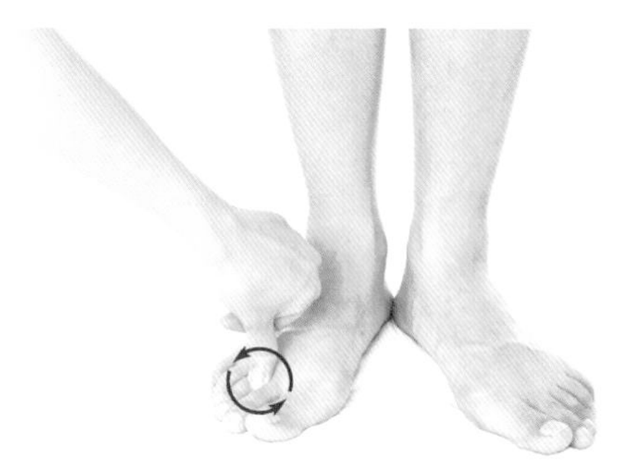

**Location:** On the dorso-ventral boundary of the foot, in the rear of the toe web between the second and third toe.

**Method:** First knead Neiting point with the thumb pulp for 2–3 minutes until a feeling of soreness and swelling is present. Then select and apply a cup of appropriate size to the point, retaining the cup for 10–15 minutes.

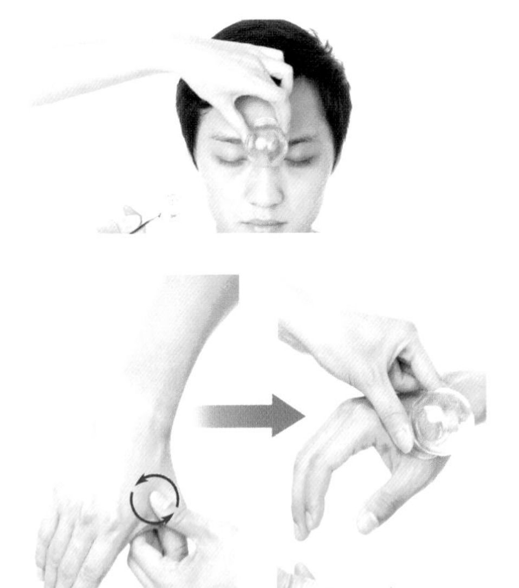

### 4. Yintang Point

**Location:** At the central point right between the eyebrows.

**Method:** First, apply a cold towel to Yintang point, and then select and apply a small cup, retaining the cup for 5–10 minutes.

### 5. Hegu Point

**Location:** In the highest point on the back of the hand between the thumb base and the base of the index finger (in the webbing between these two fingers).

**Method:** First knead Hegu point with the thumb pulp for 2–3 minutes until a feeling of soreness and swelling is present. Then select and apply a cup of appropriate size to the point, retaining the cup for 10–15 minutes.

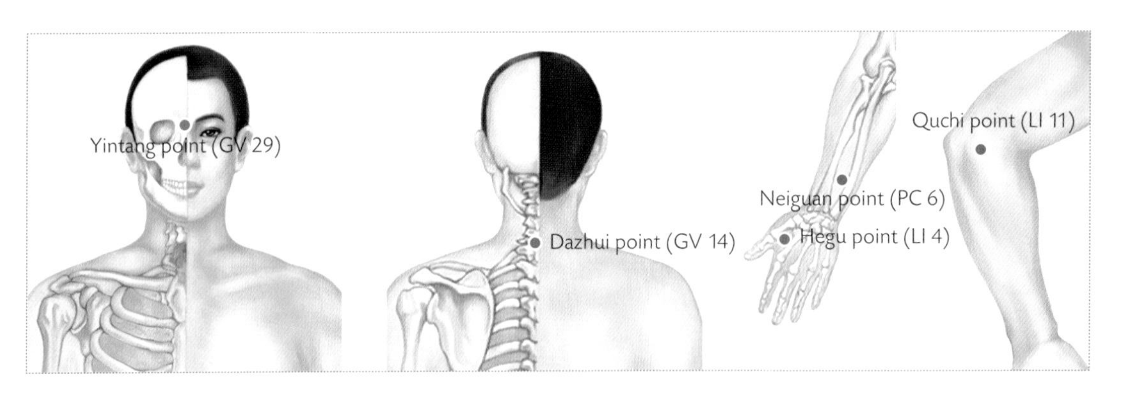


# 4 Tonsillitis

Tonsillitis is divided into acute and chronic tonsillitis, with symptoms including sore throat and throat discomfort. Acute tonsillitis may also be accompanied by fear of cold, fever, headache, and other discomforts.

Attention should be paid in daily life to keep the mouth clean. Patients should also actively participate in outdoor sports to enhance physical fitness and reduce the probability of tonsillitis onset. Patients who are receiving therapy cannot eat spicy and irritating food, and should take in light food and drinks.

Cupping can be applied to two groups of points, one group a day and two groups in turn, until the symptoms are alleviated or disappear. The first group includes Dazhui, Quchi, and Neiguan points. The second group includes Feishu, Shenshu, and Pishu points.

## Cupping Methods

### The First Group of Points

#### 1. Dazhui Point

**Location:** Under the spinous process of the seventh cervical vertebrae.

**Method:** Select a cup of appropriate size and apply it to Dazhui point. Retain the cup for 10–15 minutes.

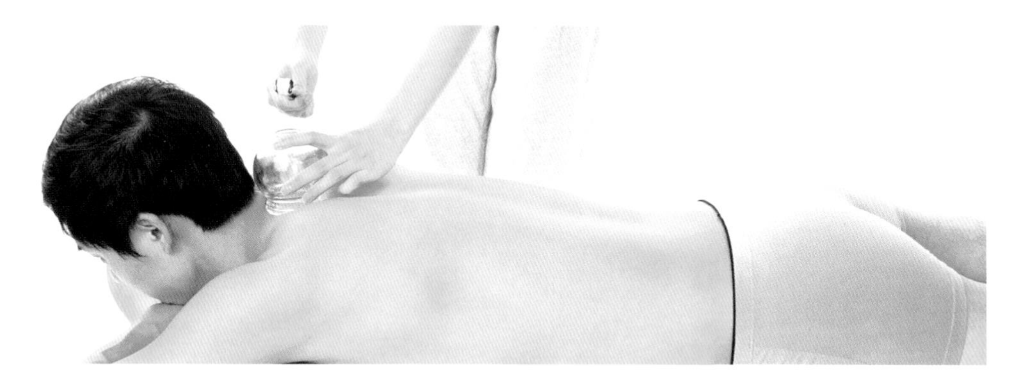

#### 2. Quchi Point

**Location:** With the elbow bent halfway, on the outer side of the cubital transverse crease.

**Method:** Select a cup of appropriate size and apply it to Quchi point. Retain the cup for 10–15 minutes.

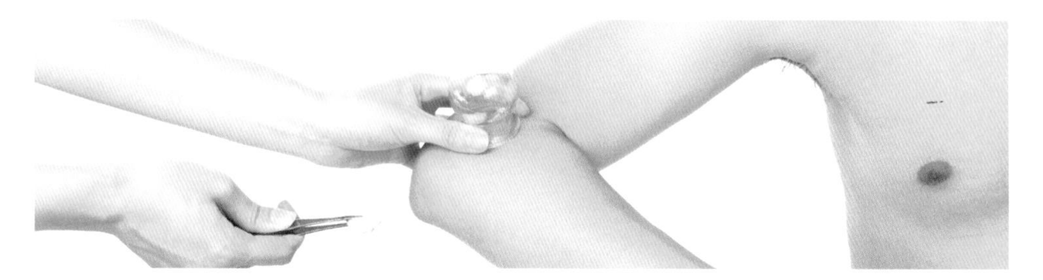

#### 3. Neiguan Point

**Location:** Between the two tendons about 2 cun above the wrist joint bend.

**Method:** First knead Neiguan point with the thumb pulp, and then select and apply a cup of appropriate size to the point, retaining the cup for 10–15 minutes.

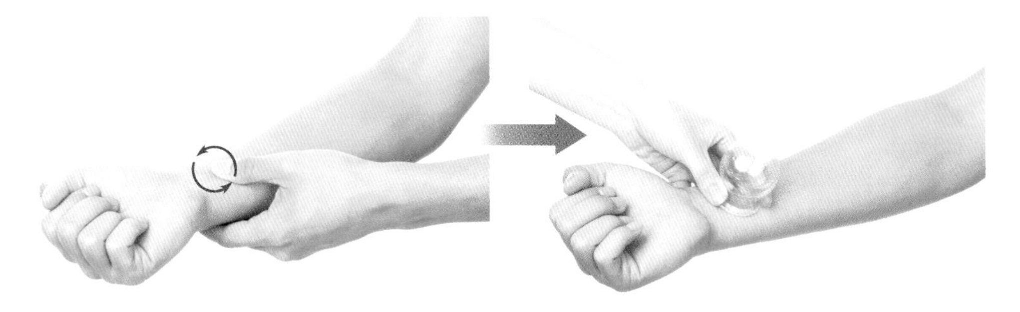

## The Second Group of Points

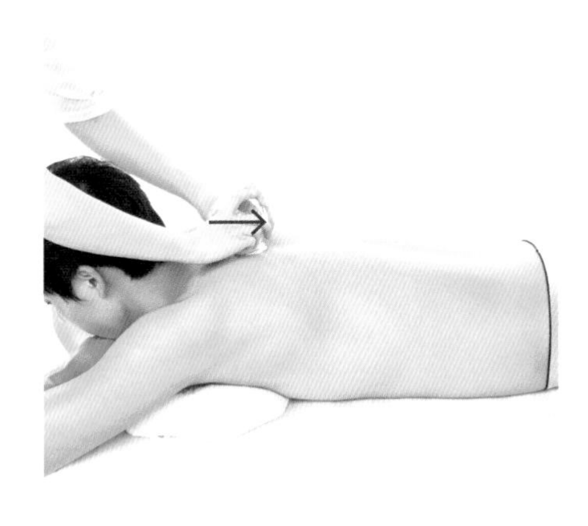

### 1. Feishu Point

**Location:** 1.5 cun beside the third thoracic vertebra on the inner side of the scapula.

**Method:** Use the moving cupping method by moving the cup on the bladder meridian on the back by segment along the meridian. Move the cup several times mainly on Feishu point, and repeatedly push and pull on the point back and forth, until the skin becomes red. The cup may be retained on the abovementioned point for 10–15 minutes after the moving cupping.

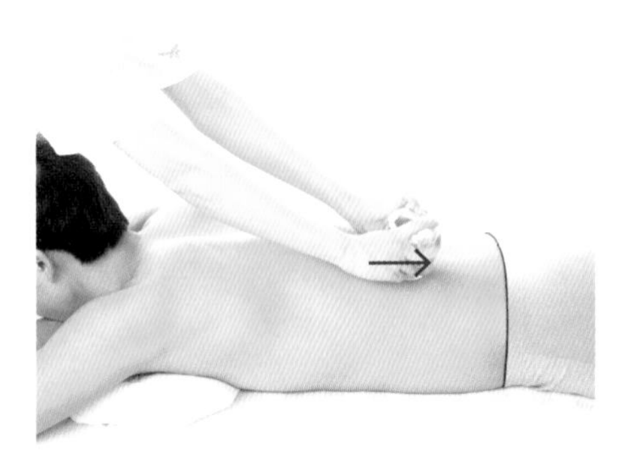

### 2. Shenshu Point

**Location:** 1.5 cun horizontally from the second lumbar spinal process.

**Method:** Use the moving cupping method. Move the cup on the bladder meridian on the back by segment along the meridian, and move it several times mainly on the Shenshu point. Repeatedly push and pull on the point back and forth, until the skin becomes red. The cup may be retained on the abovementioned point for 10–15 minutes after the moving cupping.

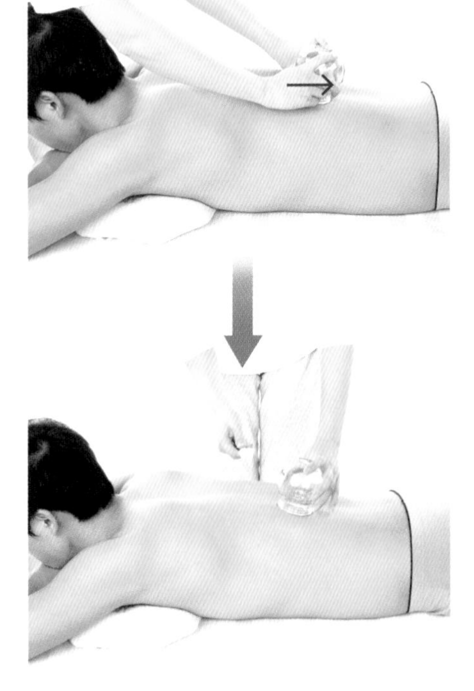

### 3. Pishu Point

**Location:** 1.5 cun away horizontally from the eleventh thoracic vertebra.

**Method:** Use the moving cupping method. Move the cup on the bladder meridian on the back by segment along the meridian, and move it several times mainly on the Pishu point. Repeatedly push and pull on the point back and forth, until the skin becomes red. The cup may be retained on the abovementioned point for 10–15 minutes after the moving cupping. With the cup removed, perform moxibustion with a moxa stick for 3–5 minutes until warmth is felt.

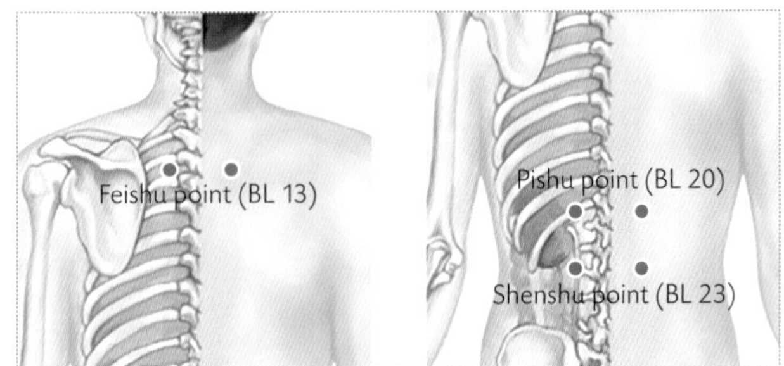

# 5 Chronic Pharyngitis

This disease has symptoms that include foreign body sensation in the throat, itching, burning, dry, slight pain, dry cough, inability to cough clean because of too many sputa, and other discomforts. The patient is prone to nausea and vomit when brushing or rinsing the mouth, or speaking too much, and feeling fatigue during speaking.

To prevent recurrent infection, one should speak less, and reduce tobacco, alcohol, spicy food, and avoid dust after catching a cold. Rinse the mouth with saline to keep your mouth hygienic.

The cupping should be applied mainly to Dingchuan, Dazhui, Feishu, Zhaohai, Shaoshang, and Quchi points.

## Cupping Methods

### 1. Dingchuan, Dazhui and Feishu Points

**Location:** Dingchuan point is 0.5 cun away from the spinous process of the seventh cervical vertebra; Dazhui point is under the spinous process of the seventh cervical vertebrae; Feishu point is 1.5 cun beside the third thoracic vertebra on the inner side of the scapula.

**Method:** Use the moving cupping method. Select a cup of appropriate size and move it continuously on the neck from Dingchuan and Dazhui points to Feishu point, until the skin becomes red. Cup on Dingchuan, Dazhui, and Feishu points after the moving cupping, and retain the cup for 10–15 minutes.

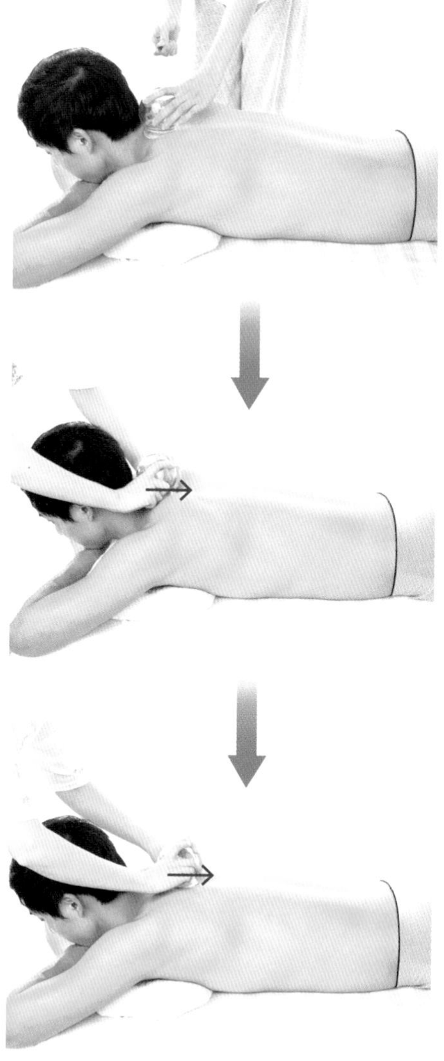

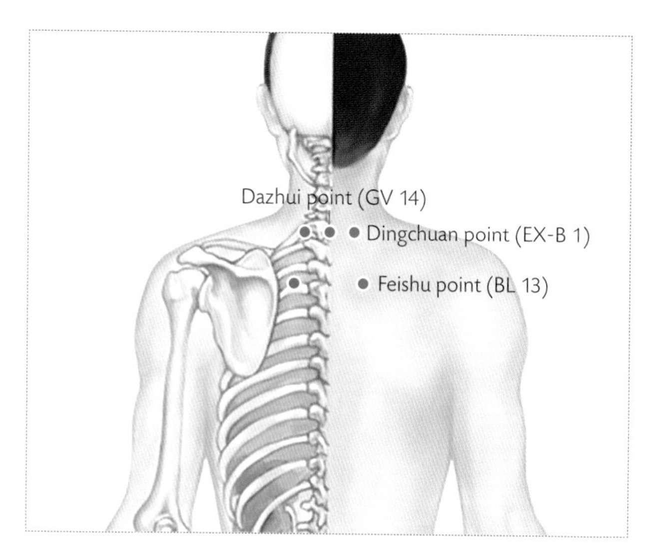

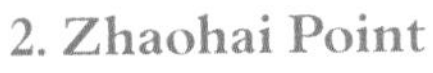

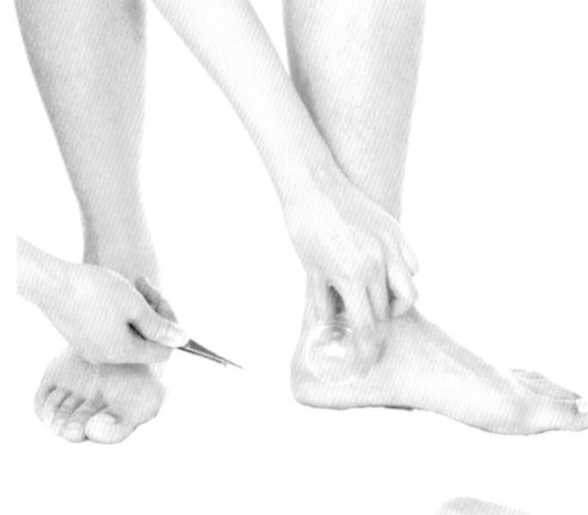

### 2. Zhaohai Point

**Location:** In a cavity below the protruding point in the interior of the ankle.

**Method:** Select and apply a cup to the point, retaining the cup for 10–15 minutes.

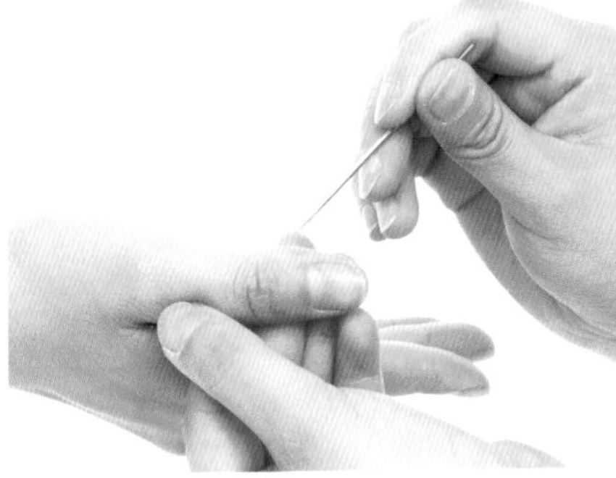

### 3. Shaoshang Point

**Location:** On the thumb, radial to the distal phalanx, 0.1 cun proximal to the corner of the nail.

**Method:** Use a three-edged needle to prick Shaoshang point until it bleeds, and squeeze 5–10 drops of blood. Acupuncture with a three-edged needle should be performed by professionals, and should not be operated by patients themselves.

### 4. Quchi Point

**Location:** With the elbow bent halfway, on the outer side of the cubital transverse crease.

**Method:** Select a cup of appropriate size and apply it to Quchi point. Retain the cup for 10–15 minutes.

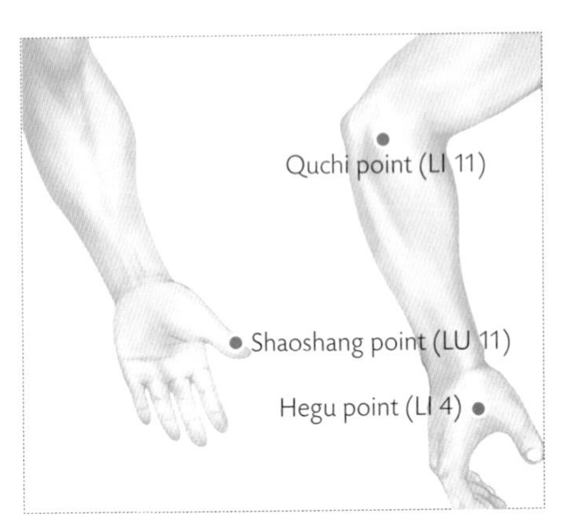


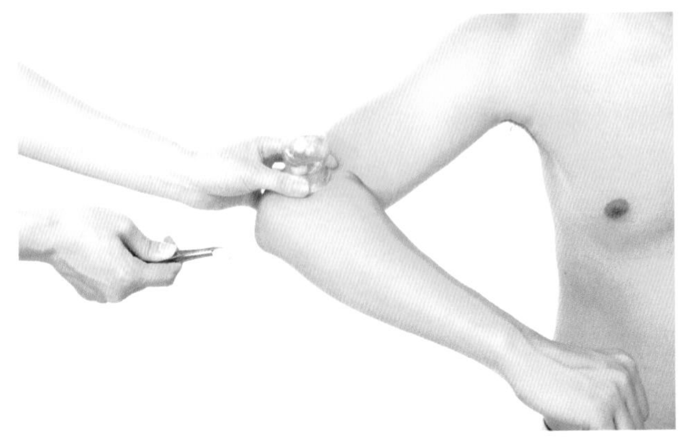

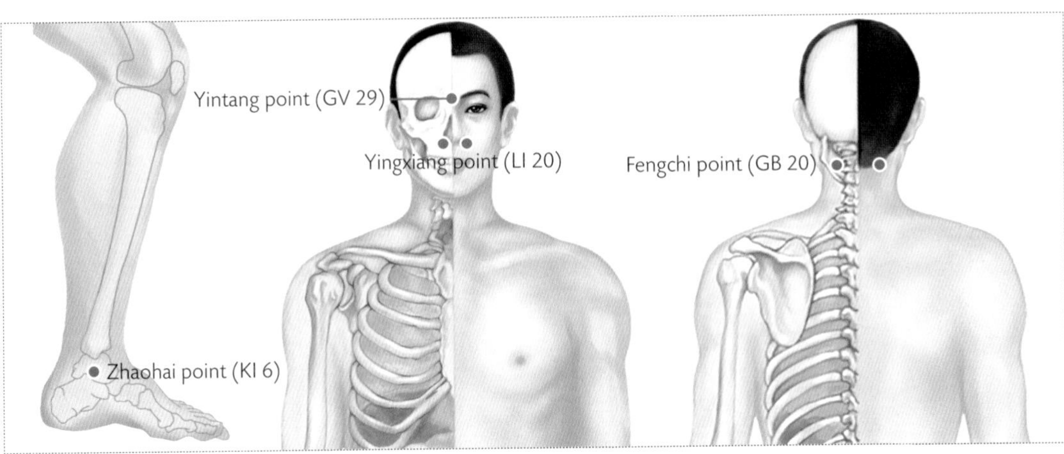

# 6 Nasosinusitis

Patients feel nasal congestion as there are plenty of mucopurulent or purulent discharge in the nose, associated with headaches that may occur on the forehead, eyebrows, or occiput, local pain in sinus, weakened sense of smell, or loss of smell.

To prevent this disease, patients should pay attention to nasal cavity hygiene, and develop a good healthy habit of washing the nose in the morning and evening. Washing face with cold water every morning may effectively enhance the disease resistance of nasal mucus. One can also massage the nose at ordinary times. Avoid smoking, drinking, and eating spicy food, and take more rest at the time of attack. Bedrooms of patients should be bright and kept indoor air flowing, but should avoid direct exposure to wind and direct sunlight.

The cupping should be applied to Hegu, Yingxiang, Fengchi, Yintang, and Dazhui points.

## Cupping Methods

### 1. Hegu Point

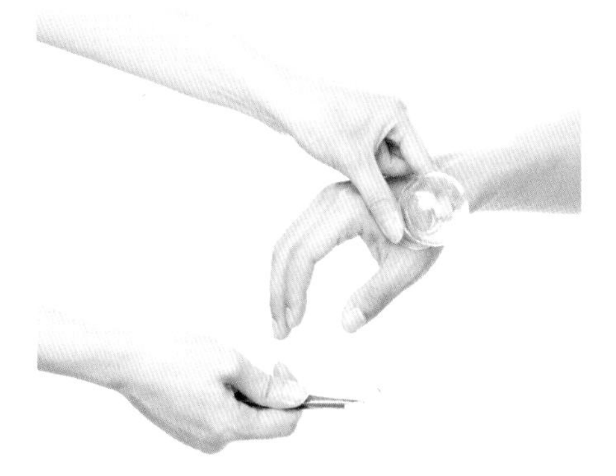

**Location:** In the highest point on the back of the hand between the thumb base and the base of the index finger (in the webbing between these two fingers).

**Method:** First knead Hegu point with the thumb pulp for 2–3 minutes until soreness and swelling is felt, and then select and apply a cup of appropriate size to the point, retaining the cup for 10–15 minutes.

### 2. Yingxiang Point

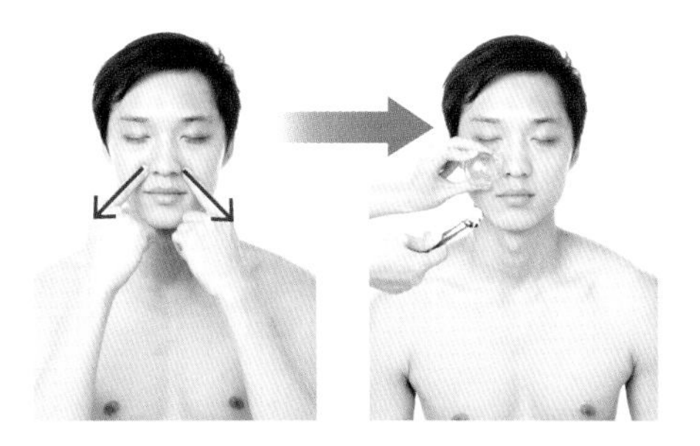

**Location:** Beside the wing of the nose, 0.5 cun away, in the nasolabial groove.

**Method:** First, rub Yingxiang point along both sides of the nosewing towards the nasion with the index finger for 2–3 minutes, and then select and apply a small cup to the point, retaining the cup for 5–10 minutes.

### 3. Yintang Point

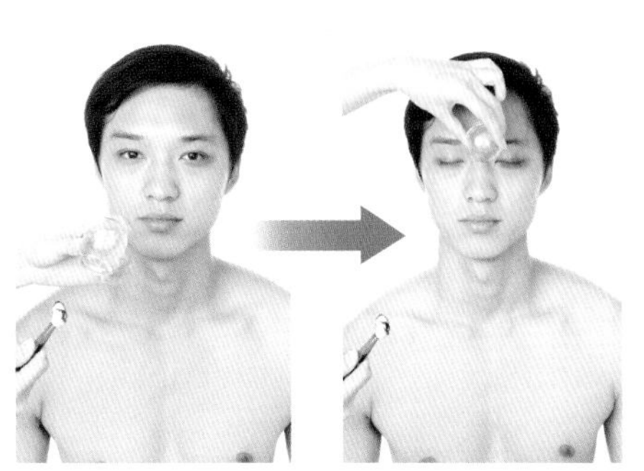

**Location:** At the central point right between the eyebrows.

**Method:** Cup on Yintang point for 10–15 times by using the flash cupping method. Then apply a cup to the point, retaining the cup for 10–15 minutes.

### 4. Fengchi Point

**Location:** In the depression on both sides of the

large tendon behind the nape of the neck, next to the lower edge of the skull.

**Method:** First knead Fengchi point with the thumb pulp for 2–3 minutes, until a feeling of soreness and swelling is present. Then select a cup of appropriate size and apply it to the point, retaining the cup for 10–15 minutes.

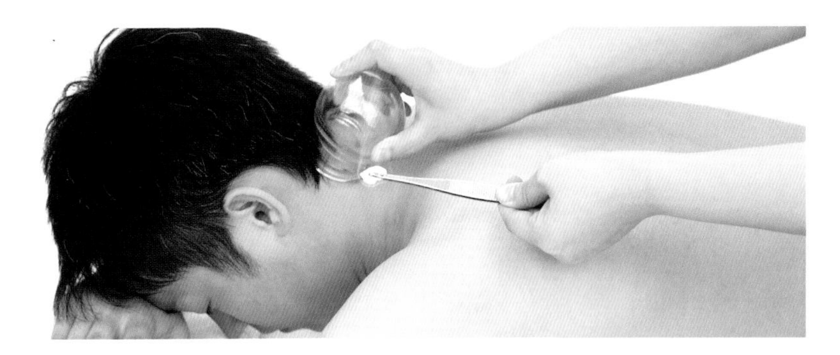

### 5. Dazhui Point

**Location:** Under the spinous process of the seventh cervical vertebrae.

**Method:** Select a cup of appropriate size and apply it to Dazhui point. Retain the cup for 10–15 minutes.

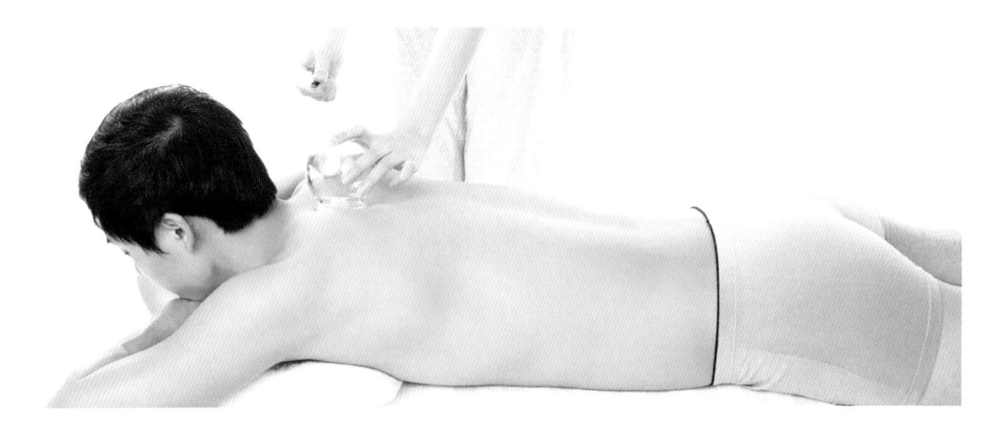

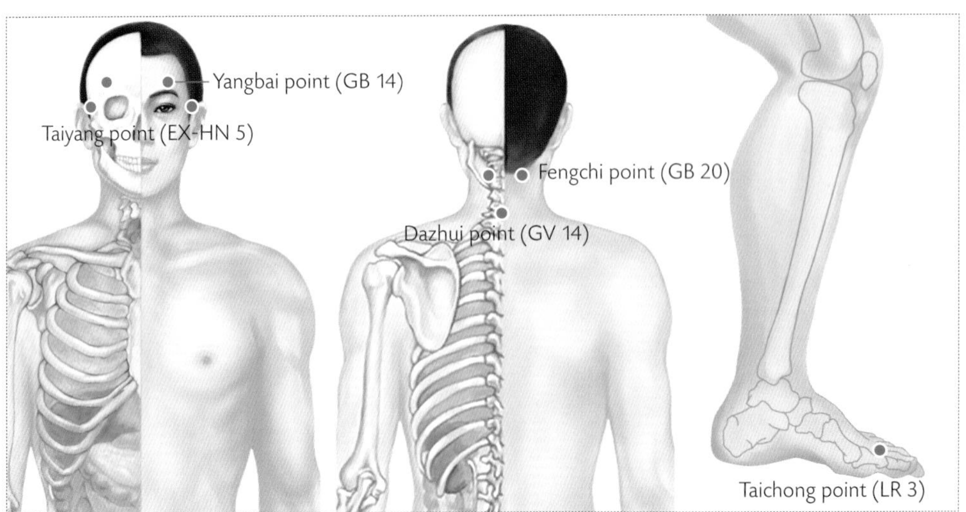

# 7 Stye

Stye, i.e., hordeolum, includes symptoms like eyelid itching and redness, with a touchable small induration in wheat-like shape and with obvious tenderness. Local swelling and pain can aggravate and gradually develop into pus, and the symptoms will be alleviated after the pus is discharged following ulceration or cutting of pus head.

To prevent stye, one should pay attention to eye hygiene, and do not rub eyes with the hands to avoid bringing bacteria into the eyes and causing infection. Do not squeeze pus head when it appears, so as not to cause infection. One can prick the ear tip to bleed 5–10 drops to quickly alleviate the symptoms. A professional physician may be invited to practice this method.

The cupping should be performed on the Taiyang, Yangbai, Dazhui, Ganshu, Weishu, and Taichong points.

## Cupping Methods

### 1. Taiyang Point

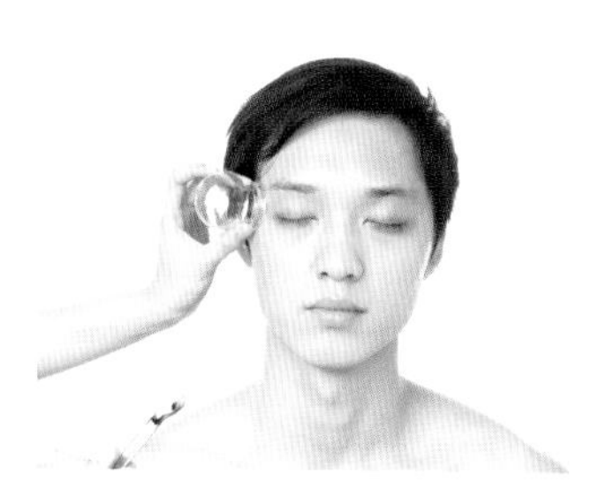

**Location:** In the depression about 1 cun behind the space between the outer tip of the brow and outer eye corner.

**Method:** Select a cup of appropriate size and cup on Taiyang point using the flash cupping method for 10–15 times.

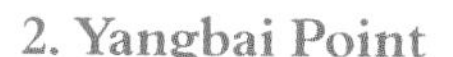

### 2. Yangbai Point

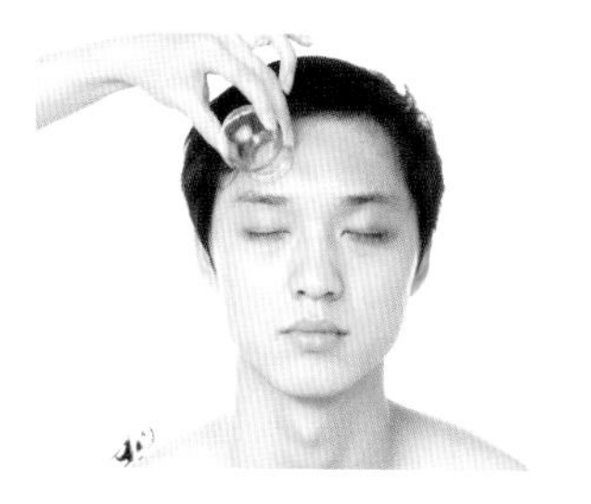

**Location:** Directly in line with the pupil, 1 cun above the eyebrow on the forehead.

**Method:** Select a cup of appropriate size and cup on Yangbai point using the flash cupping method for 10–15 times.

### 3. Dazhui Point

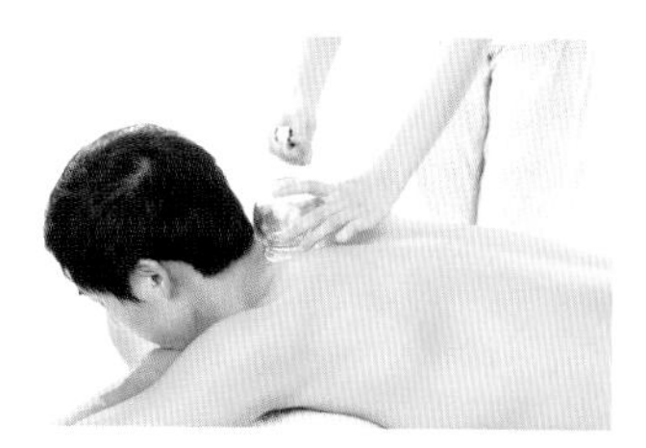

**Location:** Under the spinous process of the seventh cervical vertebrae.

**Method:** Select a cup of appropriate size and apply it to Dazhui point. Retain the cup for 10–15 minutes.

### 4. Taichong Point

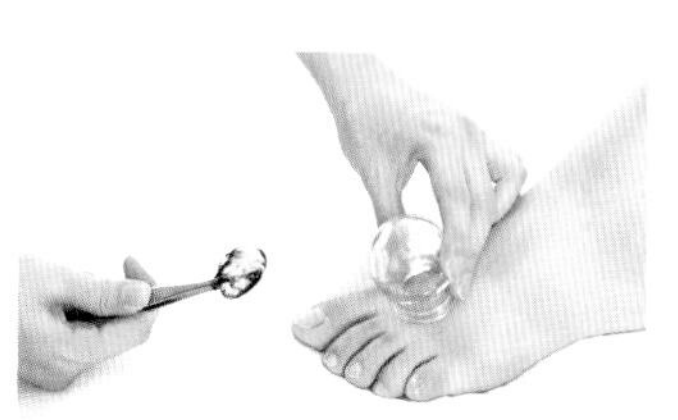

**Location:** On the foot in a notch between the first and second metatarsal bones.

**Method:** Select a cup of appropriate size and apply it to Taichong point. Retain the cup for 10–15 minutes.

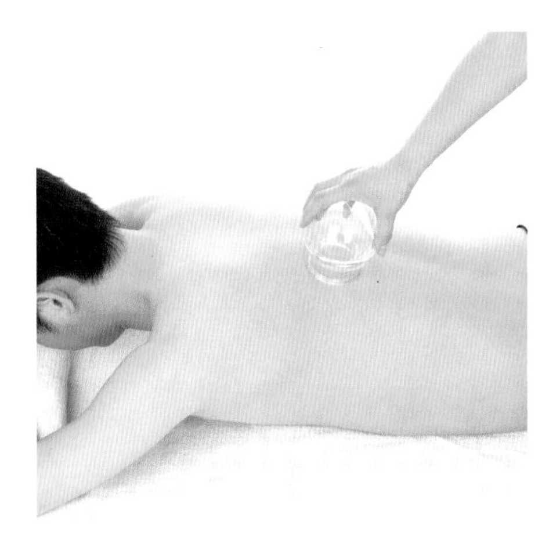

### 5. Ganshu and Weishu Points

**Location:** Ganshu point is 1.5 cun away from the ninth thoracic spinal process on the inner side of the scapula; Weishu point is about 1.5 cun below the spinous process of the twelfth thoracic vertebra.

**Method:** Use the moving cupping method. Move the cup on the bladder meridian on the back by segment along the meridian, and move the cup several times mainly on Ganshu and Weishu points. Repeatedly push and pull on the points back and forth, until the skin becomes red. The cup may be retained on the abovementioned points for 10–15 minutes after the moving cupping.

**Ear Tip**

Namely the Erjian point, on the top of the auricle, or the tip of the auricle when folding the ears forward. This point is helpful for curing redness, swelling and pain of eyes, headache, throat pain, etc.

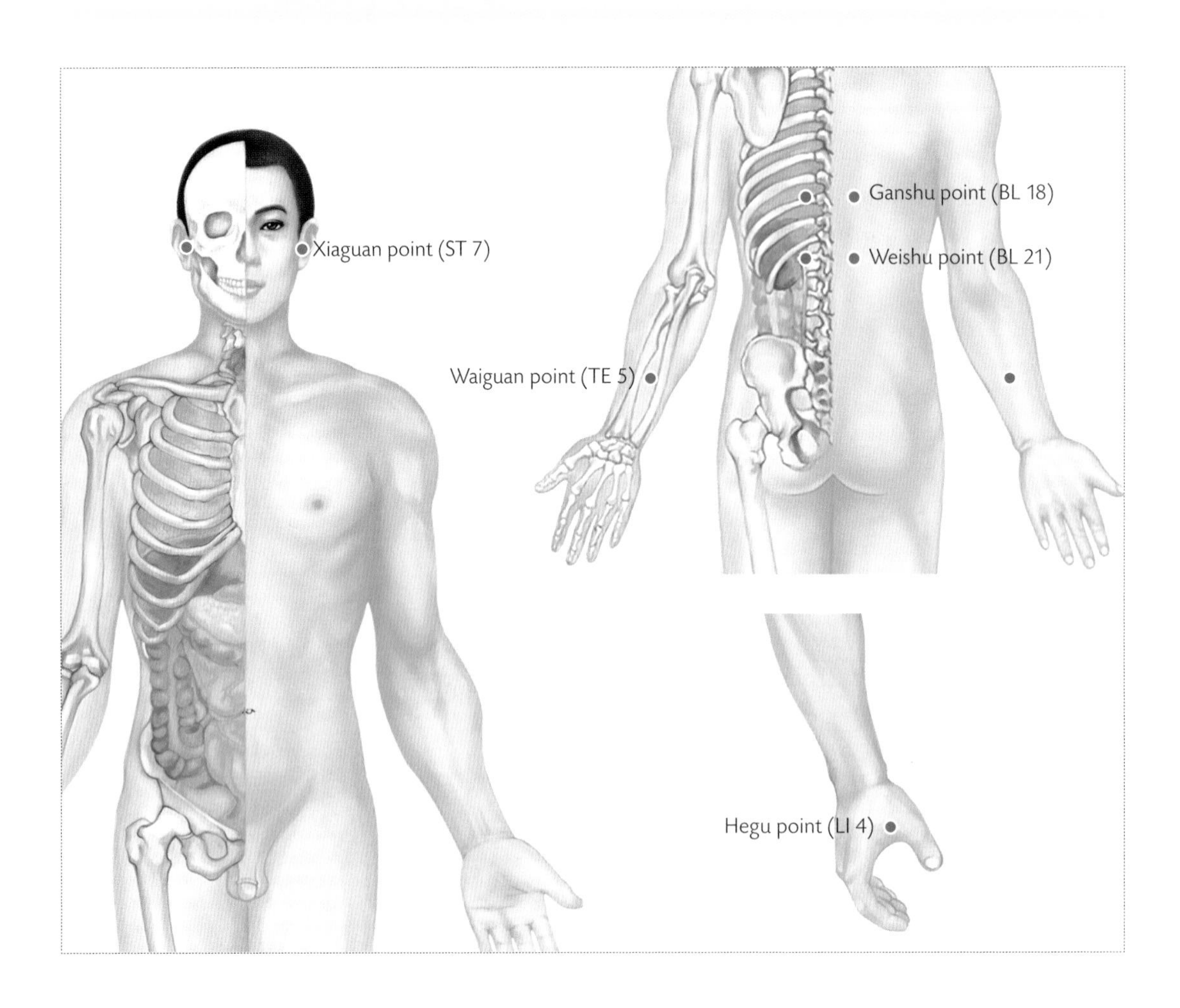

# 8 Temporomandibular Joint Dysfunction

Patients feel pain and soreness, snapping, and movement disorders on the lower jaw, and obvious joint soreness or pain when chewing.

During treatment, patients should ease the mind, eat mainly thin and soft food, do not chew food that is too hard, increase nutrition and try to enhance disease resistance.

The cupping should be applied to Ashi, Xiaguan, Hegu, and Waiguan points.

## Cupping Methods

### 1. Ashi Point

**Location:** Painful point.

**Method:** First, knead Ashi point with the palm heel for 2–3 minutes until soreness and swelling is felt, and then cup the point before retaining the cup for 15–20 minutes.

### 2. Xiaguan Point

**Location:** In the depression at the hairline in front of the ear; it can be felt when the mouth is closed and creases when the mouth is open.

**Method:** First, knead Xiaguan point with the thumb pulp for 2–3 minutes until soreness and swelling is felt, and then cup the point before retaining the cup for 10–15 minutes.

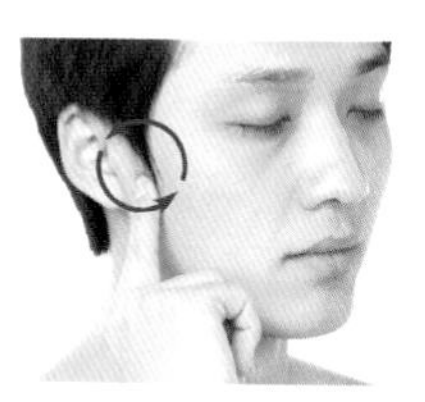

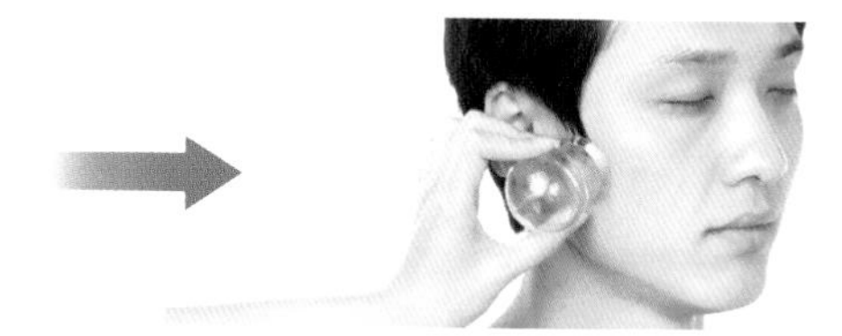

### 3. Hegu Point

**Location:** In the highest point on the back of the hand between the thumb base and the base of the index finger (in the webbing between these two fingers).

**Method:** First knead Hegu point with the thumb pulp for 2–3 minutes, and then select and apply a cup of appropriate size to the point, retaining the cup for 10–15 minutes.

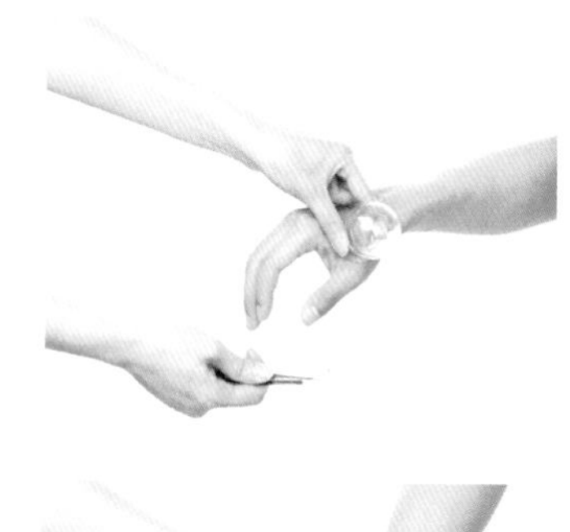

### 4. Waiguan Point

**Location:** In the middle on the outside of the arm, between the ulna and radius about 2 cun away from the horizontal line of the wrist joint.

**Method:** Select an appropriate cup and apply it to Waiguan point, retaining the cup for 10–15 minutes.

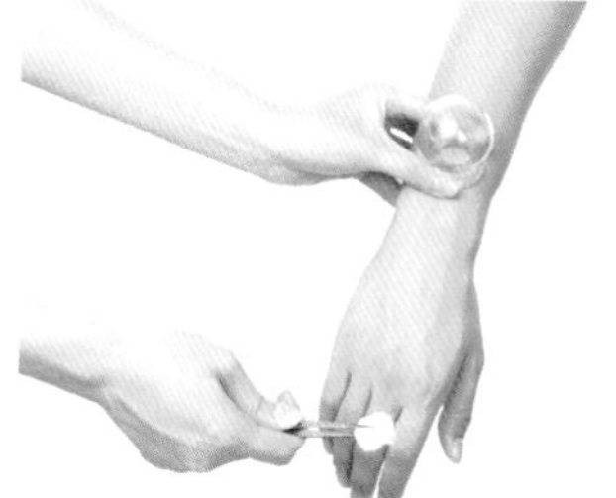

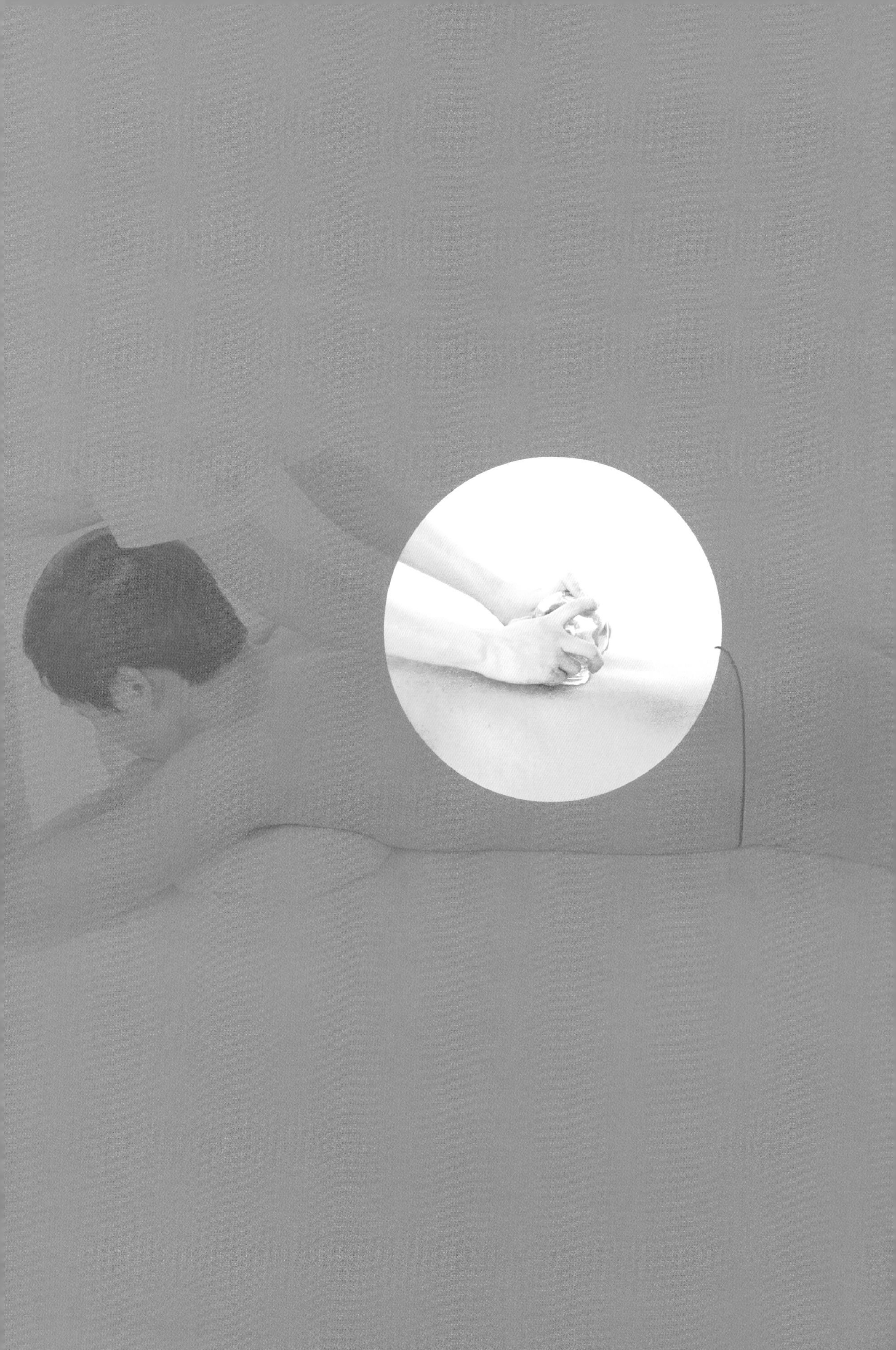

# Chapter Eight
## Skin Diseases

The health of the skin directly affects the beauty of a person. Skin problems are not only unbearable, but also make some people feel self-conscious. But the skin is the exposed outermost protective layer of the body, prone to be stimulated and infected. Therefore, skin disease should be given attention and treated timely. This chapter will introduce how to eliminate the problems caused by skin diseases through cupping.

## 1 Alopecia Areata

Patients have symptom of sudden appearance of hair loss in a round or oval form, with a clear boundary. In minor cases, hair loss only appears in one or several areas, and in more serious cases, hair will fall completely in a short time, and eyebrows, beard, armpit hair, and pubic hair may also fall in severe cases.

Patients should pay attention to balance work and rest in daily life, keep ease of the mind, and avoid being worried, pessimistic, and angry. For the diet, they may eat more polygonum multiflorum powder, lilies, lotus seeds, spina date seeds, walnuts, and other food replenishing essence and blood. Besides cupping, gingers can also be used to rub the alopecia areata areas.

During cupping, it should be done mainly on the local alopecia areata areas, supplemented by one group of points every day, two groups in turn, until the symptoms disappear. The first group includes Fengchi, Xinshu, Geshu, Ganshu, and Pishu points. The second group includes Zusanli, Sanyinjiao, and Xuehai points.

### Cupping Methods

#### Local Alopecia Areata Area

**Method:** Select a cup of appropriate size and apply it to local alopecia areata area using the flash cupping method for 15–20 times. Do not retain the cup.

#### The First Group of Points

#### 1. Xinshu, Geshu, Ganshu and Pishu Points

**Location:** Xinshu point is under the fifth thoracic vertebra on the inner side of the scapula, 1.5 cun horizontally away; Geshu point is 1.5 cun away from the spinous process of the seventh thoracic vertebra; Ganshu point is 1.5 cun away from the ninth thoracic spinal process on the inner side of the scapula; Pishu point is 1.5 cun away horizontally from the eleventh thoracic vertebra.

**Method:** Use the moving cupping method. Move the cup on the bladder meridian on the back by segment along the meridian, and move the cup several times mainly on Xinshu, Geshu, Ganshu and Pishu points. Repeatedly push and pull on the points back and forth, until the skin becomes red. The cup may be retained on the abovementioned points for 10–15 minutes after the moving cupping.

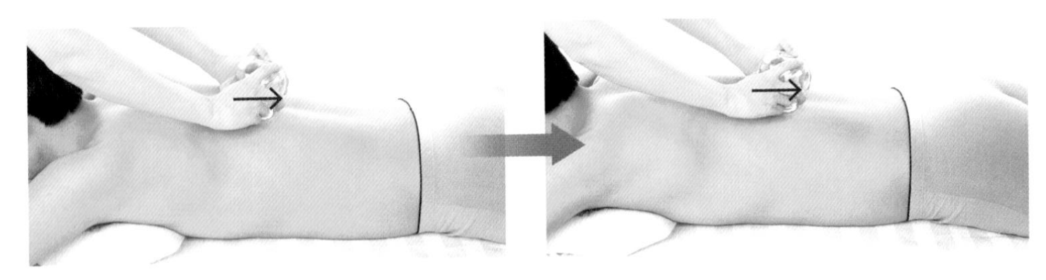

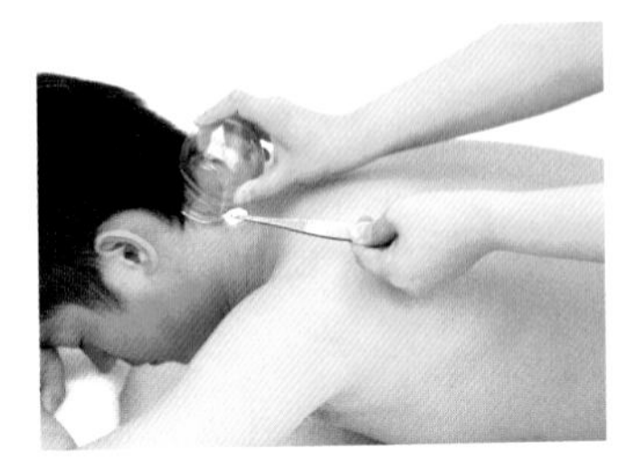

### 2. Fengchi Point

**Location:** In the depression on both sides of the large tendon behind the nape of the neck, next to the lower edge of the skull.

**Method:** First knead Fengchi point with the thumb pulp for 2–3 minutes. Then apply a cup to the point, retaining the cup for 10–15 minutes.

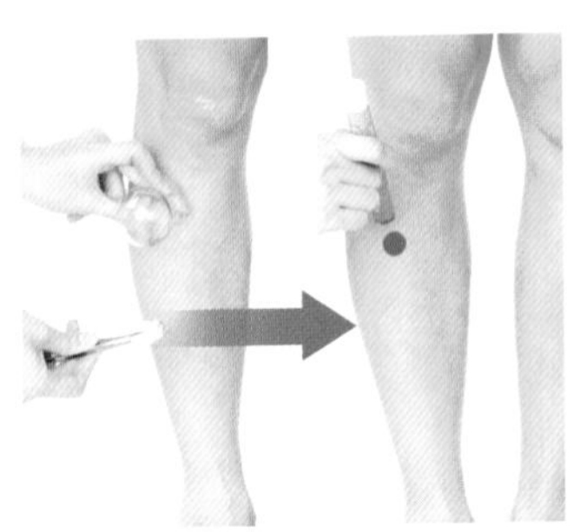

## The Second Group of Points

### 1. Zusanli Point

**Location:** About 3 cun below the knee on the outer side of the tibia.

**Method:** Select and apply a cup of appropriate size to Zusanli point, retaining the cup for 10–15 minutes. With the cup removed, perform moxibustion with a moxa stick for 3–5 minutes.

### 2. Sanyinjiao Point

**Location:** At the rear edge of the shinbone, 3 cun above the ankle.

**Method:** Select and apply a cup of appropriate size to Sanyinjiao point, retaining the cup for 10–15 minutes. With the cup removed, perform moxibustion with a moxa stick for 3–5 minutes.

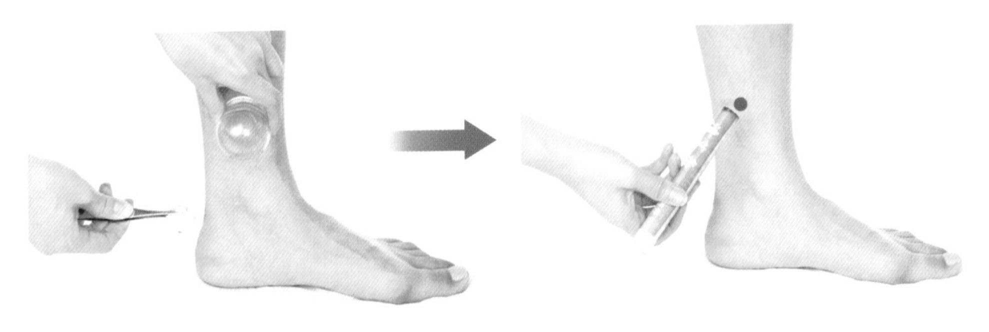

**3. Xuehai Point**

**Location:** In a cavity about 2 cun away from the inner upper corner of the patella, when the knee is bent.

**Method:** Select and apply a cup of appropriate size to Xuehai point, retaining the cup for 10–15 minutes. With the cup removed, perform moxibustion with a moxa stick for 3–5 minutes until warmth is felt.

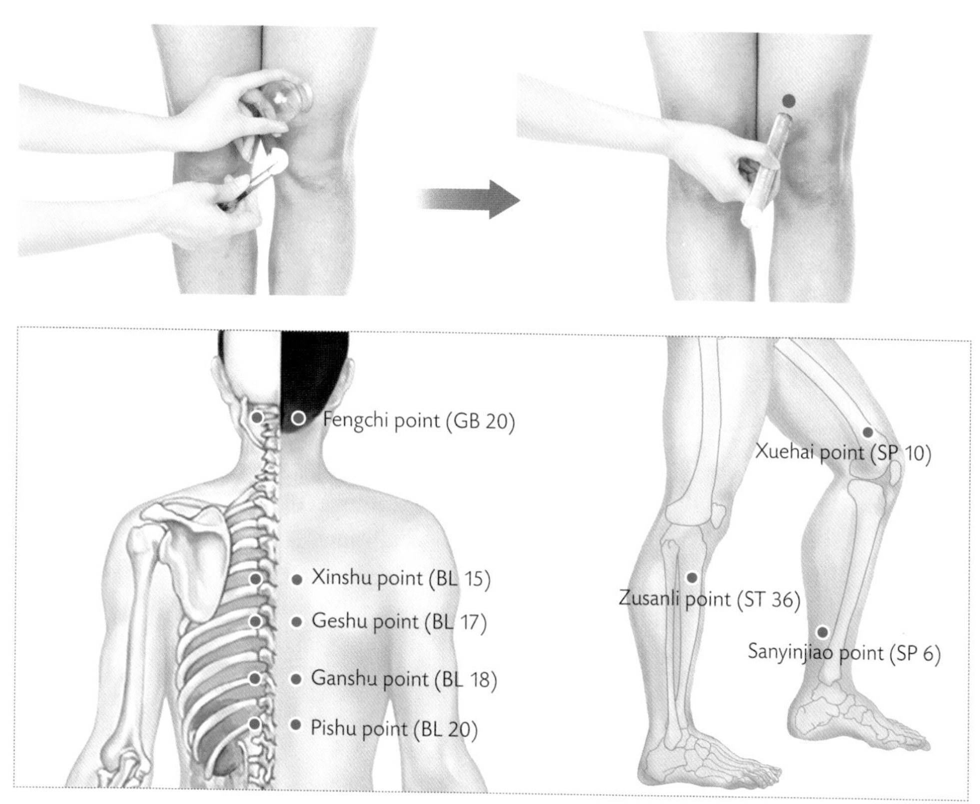


# 2 Eczema

This disease mostly occurs with children, often on the head, the face, behind the ears, on four limbs, hands, feet, genitals, anal, and other parts. The affected parts will itch, and some will appear skin ulcers, with much exudate, being recurrent and persistent, and with skin pigmentation and scars.

Eczema parts with exudate should be washed as little as possible, and be kept dry, and avoid or have little contact with chemical cleaning supplies. Patients should choose more food that can clear heat and promote diuresis, such as green beans, red beans, white gourd, cucumber, lettuce, and eat less fish, onions, garlic, pepper, shrimp, beef, and mutton and irritating food.

The cupping should be applied mainly to local skin lesions, and may choose one group of points for cupping therapy every day, two groups in turn, until the symptoms disappear. The first group includes Geshu, Weishu, Dazhui, and Quchi points, and the second group includes Yinlingquan, Fenglong, and Weizhong points.

## Cupping Methods

### Skin Lesions

**Method:** Select a cup of appropriate size, and apply it to the affected skin by using the flash cupping method, until the skin becomes red. In severe cases, first disinfect the affected area with 75% alcohol, and lightly knock the affected skin with a plum-blossom needle before flash cupping.

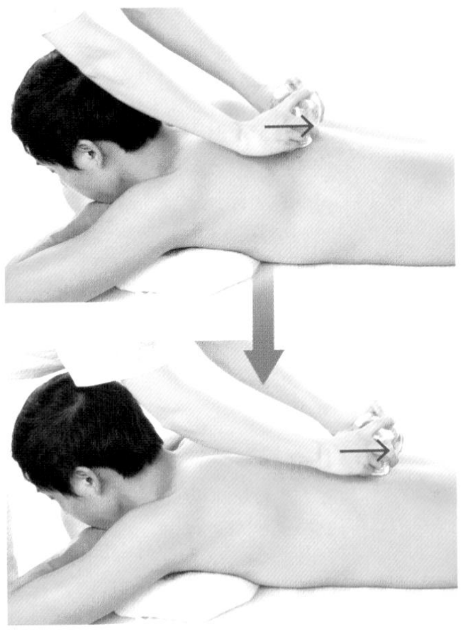

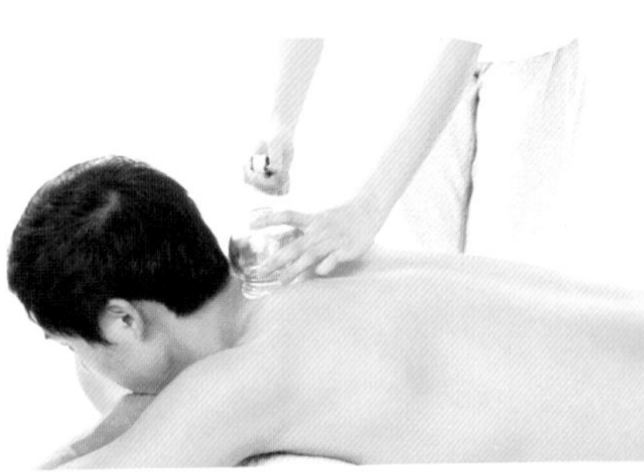

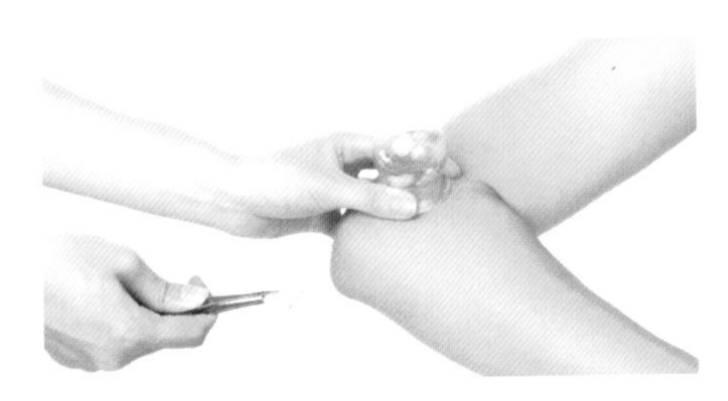

### The First Group of Points

#### 1. Geshu and Weishu Points

**Location:** Geshu point is 1.5 cun away from the spinous process of the seventh thoracic vertebra; Weishu point is about 1.5 cun below the spinous process of the twelfth thoracic vertebra.

**Method:** Use the moving cupping method. Move the cup on the bladder meridian on the back by segment along the meridian, and move the cup several times mainly on Geshu and Weishu points. Repeatedly push and pull on the points back and forth, until the skin becomes red. The cup may be retained on the abovementioned points for 10–15 minutes after the moving cupping.

#### 2. Dazhui Point

**Location:** At the rear edge of the shinbone, 3 cun above the ankle.

**Method:** First, disinfect the skin on the point with 75% alcohol, pierce Dazhui point with a three-edged needle and prick the white fibre under the skin. Then cup on the point immediately, retaining the cup for 5 minutes. This method should be done by professionals.

#### 3. Quchi Point

**Location:** With the elbow bent halfway, on the outer side of the cubital transverse crease.

**Method:** Select a cup of appropriate size and apply it to Quchi point. Retain the cup for 10–15 minutes.

## The Second Group of Points

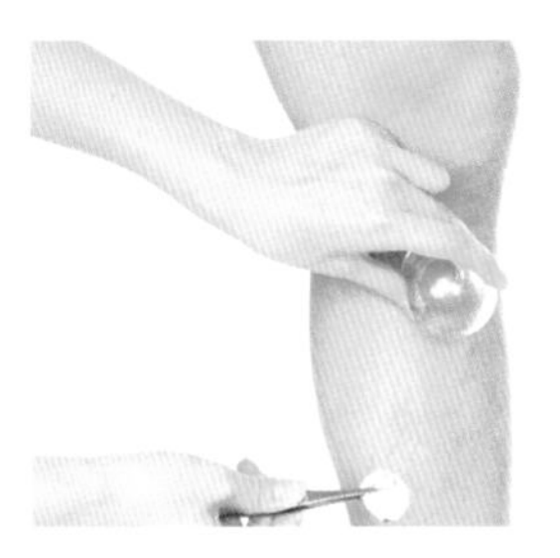

### 1. Yinlingquan Point

**Location:** In the depression on the inner edge of the shinbone below the knee.

**Method:** Select a cup of appropriate size and apply it to Yinlingquan point. Retain the cup for 10–15 minutes.

### 2. Fenglong Point

**Location:** 8 cun above the ankle tip.

**Method:** First knead the Fenglong point with the thumb pulp for 2–3 minutes, and then select and apply a cup of appropriate size to the point, retaining the cup for 10–15 minutes.

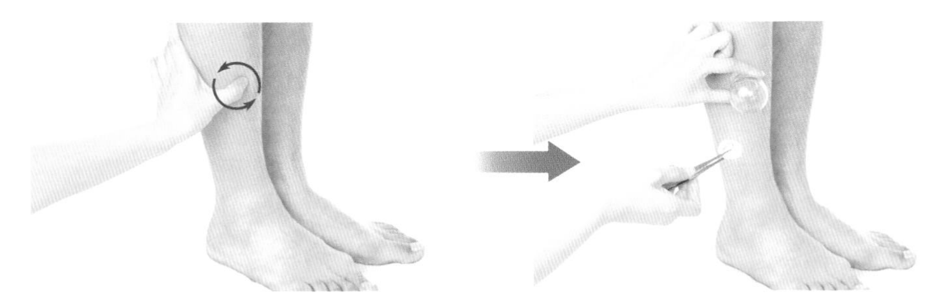

### 3. Weizhong Point

**Location:** Right in the middle of popliteal crease (at the back of the knee).

**Method:** First, disinfect the skin on the point with 75% alcohol, and lightly pierce Weizhong point with a plum-blossom needle, until the skin becomes red. Then do cupping using the flash cupping method.

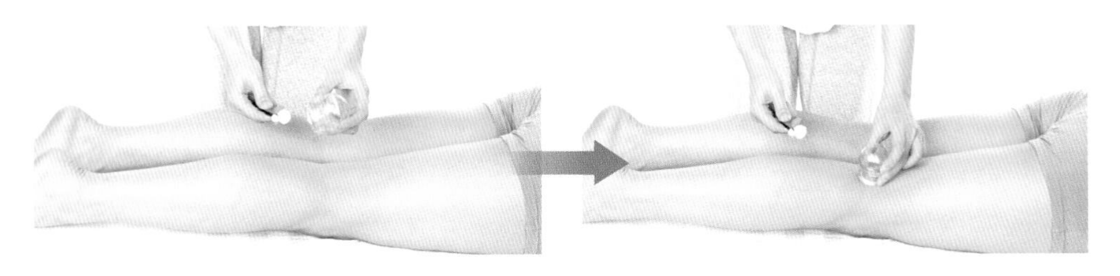

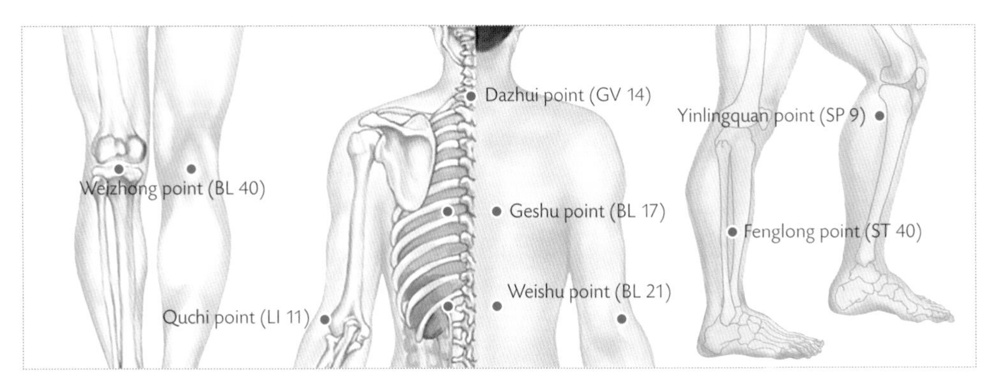

# 3 Chloasma

Chloasma is particularly common in women, and often appears on the forehead, eyebrows, cheeks, back of nose, lips, and other facial parts. Black spots appear on the face, level to the skin, in dust-like, light brown or light black color, without itching.

Patients should pay attention to sun protection, prevent various ionizing radiation, and reduce exposure of the skin to the daylight, computer and other occasions with radiation. They should drink more water, eat more vegetables and fruits like tomatoes, cucumbers, strawberries, peaches, etc., and avoid eating irritating food. They should also pay attention to get enough rest and ensure adequate sleep, and choose the right cosmetics, but should not use "freckle cream" containing a variety of harmful substances for eliminating freckles.

The cupping should be applied to Zhongwan, Qihai, Feishu, Shenshu, Weishu, and Ganshu points.

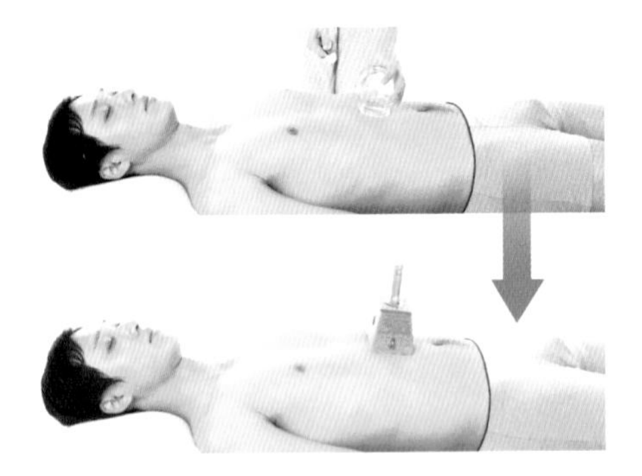

## Cupping Methods

### 1. Zhongwan Point

**Location:** On the upper abdomen, 4 cun above the center of the umbilicus, on the anterior midline.

**Method:** Select a cup of appropriate size and apply it to Zhongwan point. Retain the cup for 10–15 minutes. With the cup removed, perform moxibustion with a moxa box for 3–5 minutes until warmth is felt.

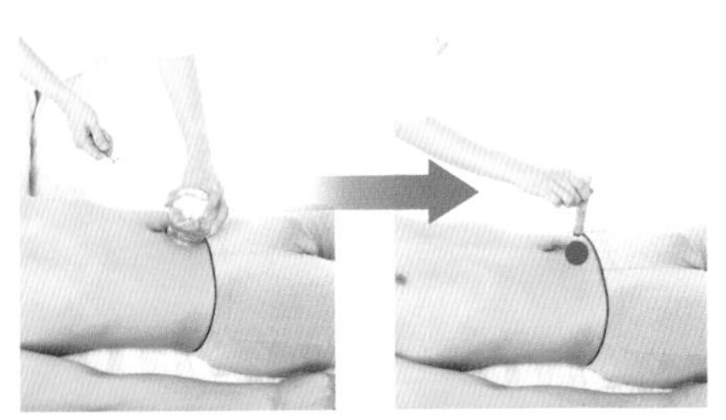

### 2. Qihai Point

**Location:** About 1.5 cun below the navel.

**Method:** Select a cup of appropriate size and apply it to Qihai point. Retain the cup for 10–15 minutes. With the cup removed, perform moxibustion with a moxa stick for 3–5 minutes until warmth is felt.

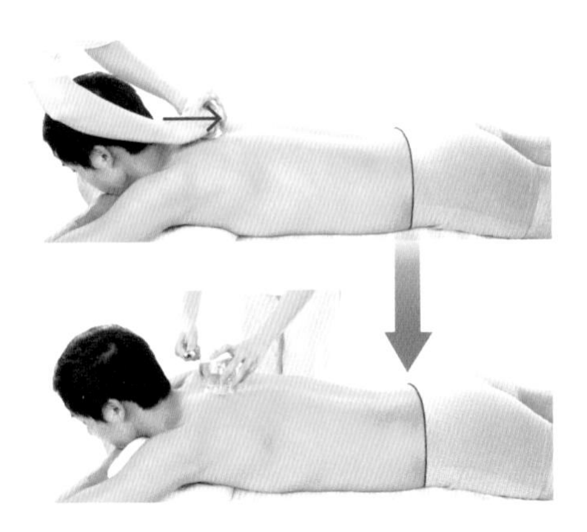

### 3. Feishu Point

**Location:** 1.5 cun beside the third thoracic vertebra on the inner side of the scapula.

**Method:** Use the moving cupping method. Move the cup on the bladder meridian on the back by segment along the meridian, and move the cup several times mainly on Feishu point. Repeatedly push and pull on the point back and forth, until the skin becomes red. The cup may be retained on the abovementioned point for 10–15 minutes after the moving cupping.

### 4. Shenshu Point

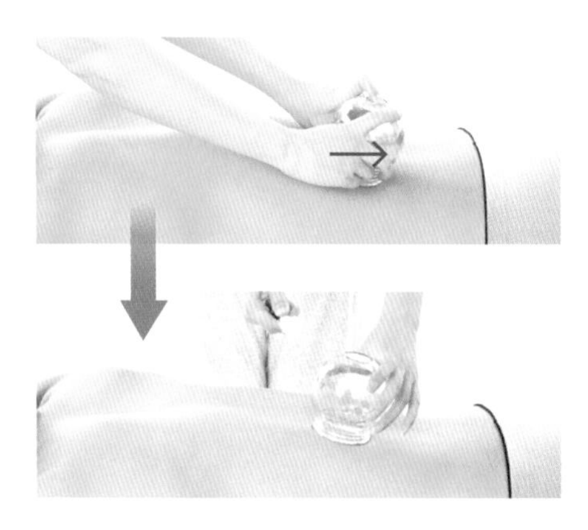

**Location:** 1.5 cun horizontally from the second lumbar spinal process.

**Method:** Use the moving cupping method. Move the cup on the bladder meridian on the back by segment along the meridian, and move the cup several times mainly on Shenshu point. Repeatedly push and pull on the point back and forth, until the skin becomes red. The cup may be retained on the abovementioned point for 10–15 minutes after the moving cupping.

### 5. Weishu Point

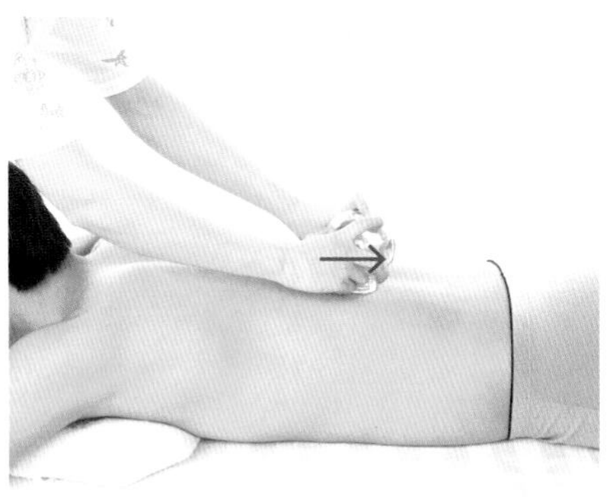

**Location:** About 1.5 cun below the spinous process of the twelfth thoracic vertebra.

**Method:** Use the moving cupping method. Move the cup on the bladder meridian on the back by segment along the meridian, and move the cup several times mainly on Weishu point. Repeatedly push and pull on the point back and forth, until the skin becomes red. The cup may be retained on the abovementioned point for 10–15 minutes after the moving cupping.

### 6. Ganshu Point

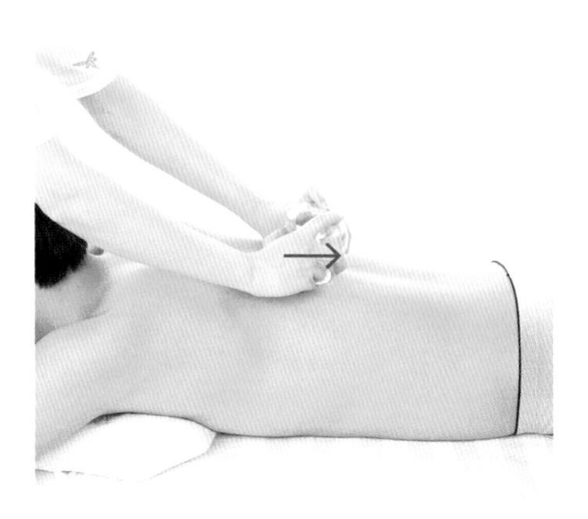

**Location:** 1.5 cun away from the ninth thoracic spinal process on the inner side of the scapula.

**Method:** Use the moving cupping method. Move the cup on the bladder meridian on the back by segment along the meridian, and move the cup several times mainly on Ganshu point. Repeatedly push and pull on the point back and forth, until the skin becomes red. The cup may be retained on the abovementioned point for 10–15 minutes after the moving cupping.

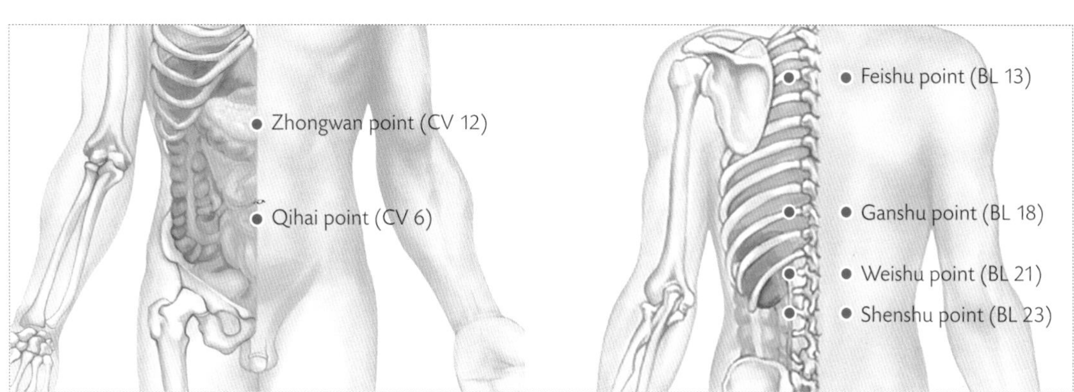

# 4 Urticaria

Urticaria has manifestations including different sizes and indefinite number of red and unbearably itchy pimples on various parts of the skin. They may disappear within several hours, without any marks, but may happen several times within a day.

As this disease is mostly caused by allergies, patients should avoid contacting with allergens at ordinary times, pay attention to rest, and avoid invasion of external evils of wind, cold, dampness and heat. See a doctor immediately if laryngeal edema, chest tightness, and difficult breathing occur during the attack of urticaria.

The cupping should be performed on Dazhui, Quchi, Fengchi, Xuehai, Feishu, and Geshu points.

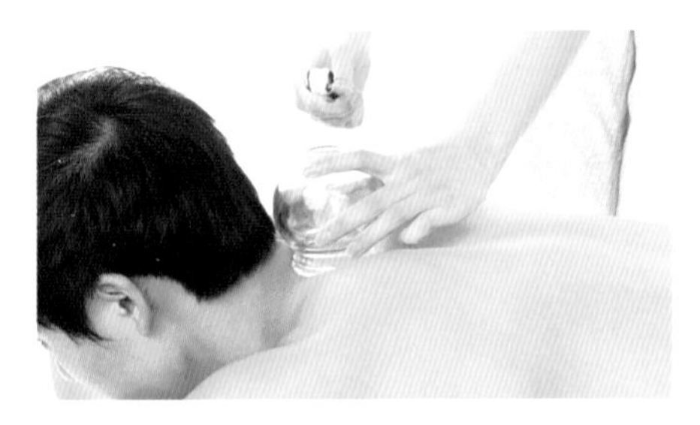

## Cupping Methods

### 1. Dazhui Point

**Location:** Under the spinous process of the seventh cervical vertebrae.

**Method:** Select a cup of appropriate size and apply it to Dazhui point. Retain the cup for 10–15 minutes.

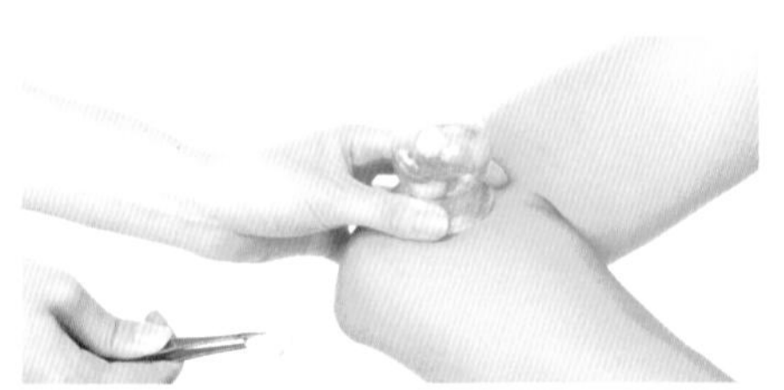

### 2. Quchi Point

**Location:** With the elbow bent halfway, on the outer side of the cubital transverse crease.

**Method:** Select a cup of appropriate size and apply it to Quchi point. Retain the cup for 10–15 minutes.

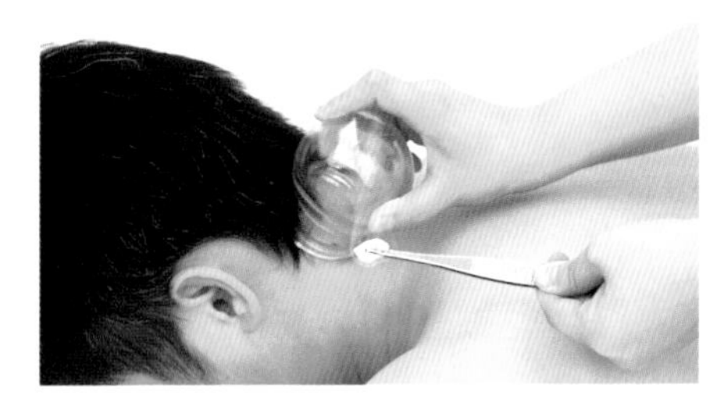

### 3. Fengchi Point

**Location:** In the depression on both sides of the large tendon behind the nape of the neck, next to the lower edge of the skull.

**Method:** Select a cup of appropriate size and apply it to Fengchi point, retaining the cup for 10–15 minutes.

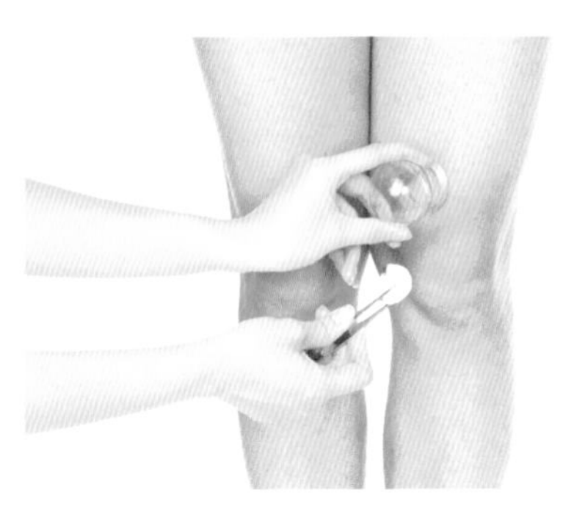

### 4. Xuehai Point

**Location:** In a cavity about 2 cun away from the inner upper corner of the patella, when the knee is bent.

**Method:** Select and apply a cup of appropriate size to Xuehai point, retaining the cup for 5–10 minutes.

### 5. Feishu Point

**Location:** At the point 1.5 cun beside the third thoracic vertebra on the inner side of the scapula.

**Method:** Select a cup of appropriate size and apply it to Feishu point by using the flash cupping method for 15–20 times. Then retain the cup for 5 minutes.

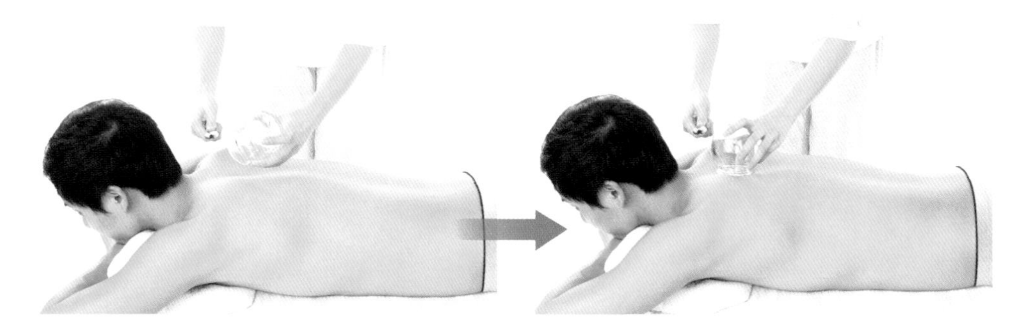

### 6. Geshu Point

**Location:** At the point 1.5 cun away from the spinous process of the seventh thoracic vertebra.

**Method:** Select a cup of appropriate size and apply it to Geshu point by using the flash cupping method for 15–20 times. Then retain the cup for 5 minutes.

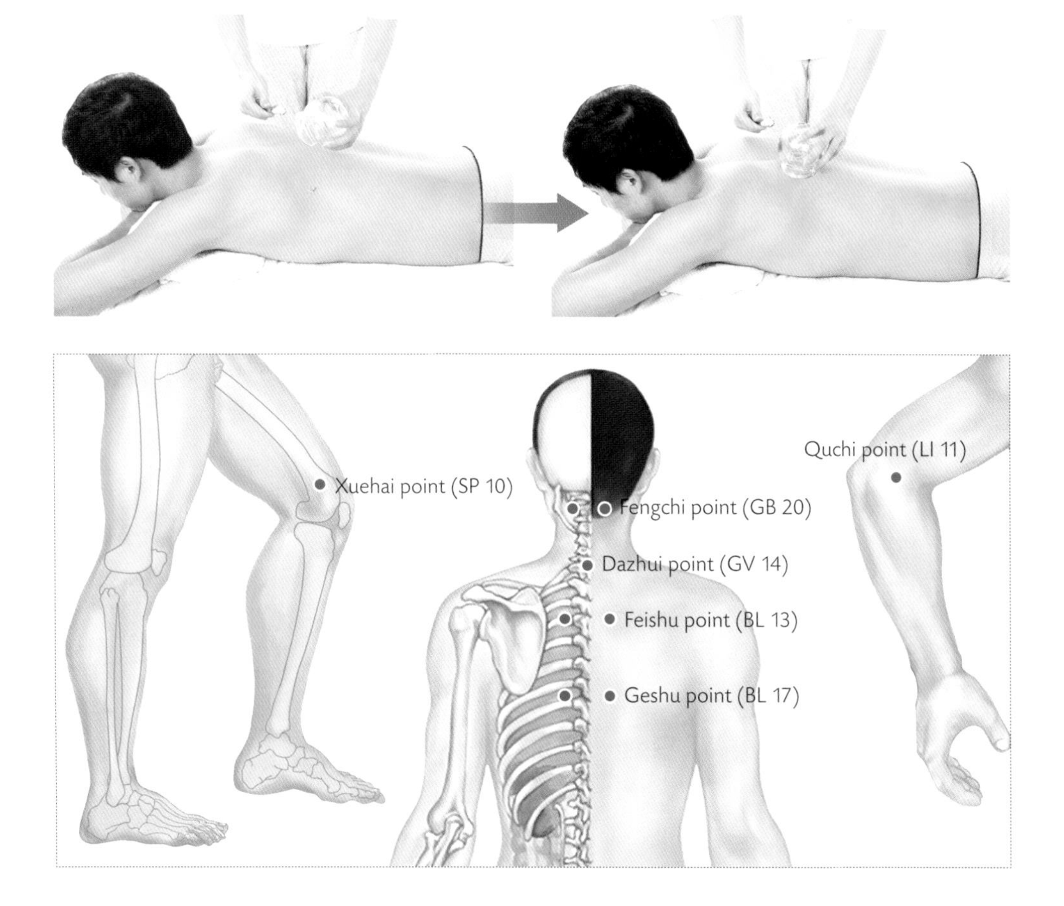

# 5 Neurodermatitis

This disease is particularly common in the adults, mainly manifested by light red flat papules, in round or polygonal shape, which can be very dense. Patients consciously feel an unbearable paroxysmal itching, which can aggravate at night.

Neurodermatitis can be affected by a variety of factors, such as irregular life, poor sleep, female menstrual disorders, indigestion, constipation, etc. These factors may aggravate the symptoms. Therefore, people should receive active treatment and maintenance when there is an abnormality in these respects. Try to avoid fish, shrimp, seafood, beef, mutton, spicy and irritating food, eat more fruits and vegetables, and avoid alcohol consumption. Patients should avoid the use of antiperspirants, and try to avoid the use of hormones containing ointment to avoid the formation of hormone-dependent dermatitis.

The cupping should be applied to local affected parts, associated with Xuehai, Feishu, and Geshu points.

## Cupping Methods

### 1. Affected Parts

**Method:** Select a cup of appropriate size and apply it to the affected skin by using the flash cupping method, until the skin becomes red. In severe cases, first disinfect the affected area with 75% alcohol, and lightly knock the affected skin with a plum-blossom needle, before using the flash cupping method. (This method should be operated by a physician.)

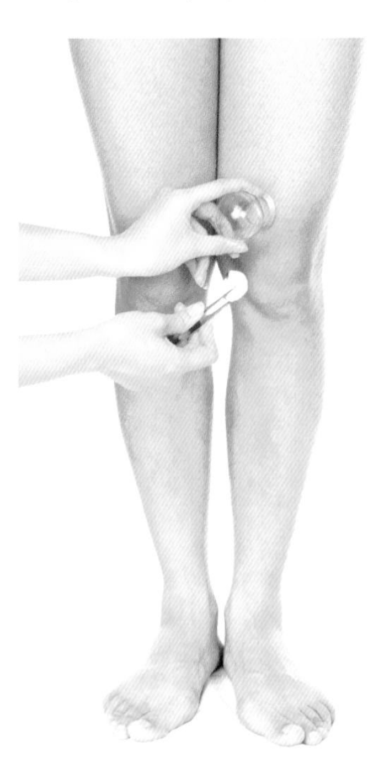

### 2. Xuehai Point

**Location:** In a cavity about 2 cun away from the inner upper corner of the patella, when the knee is bent.

**Method:** Select and apply a cup of appropriate size to Xuehai point, retaining the cup for 10–15 minutes.

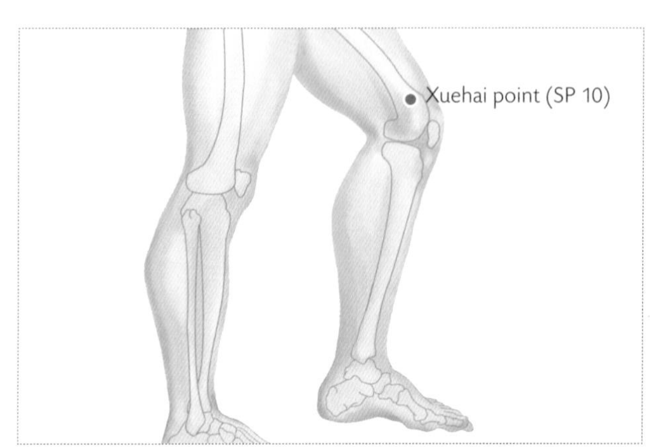

### 3. Geshu and Feishu Points

**Location:** Geshu point is 1.5 cun away from the spinous process of the seventh thoracic vertebra; Feishu point is 1.5 cun beside the third thoracic vertebra on the inner side of the scapula.

**Method:** Use the moving cupping method. Move the cup on the bladder meridian on the back by segment along the meridian, and move the cup several times mainly on Geshu and Feishu points. Repeatedly push and pull on the points back and forth, until the skin becomes red. The cup may be retained on the abovementioned points for 10–15 minutes after the moving cupping.

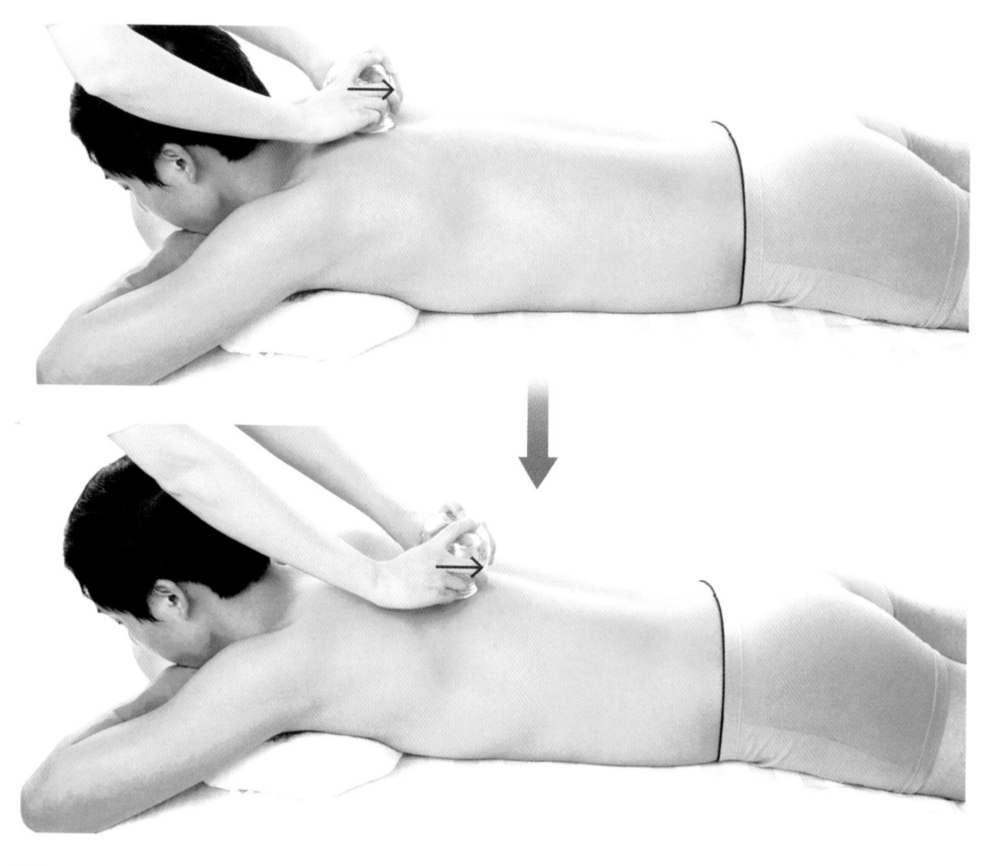

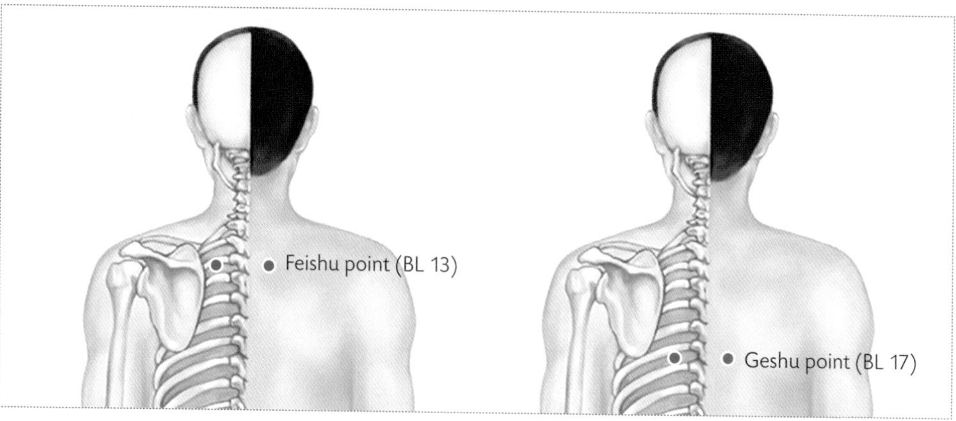

# 6 Acne

Acne commonly occurs during adolescence, mostly on the parts with rich sebaceous glands such as the face, the upper chest and the back, in a symmetrical distribution, manifested by follicular papules, pustules, nodules, cysts, blackheads, and scars, accompanied by seborrhea.

Patients should pay attention to skin hygiene, and avoid eating spicy and irritating food. Do not squeeze immature acne. Do not wash the face with soaps containing strong irritants.

The cupping should be applied to local affected parts, in conjunction with Dazhui, Xuehai, Geshu, Pishu, Weishu, and Dachangshu points.

## Cupping Methods

### 1. Affected Parts (Except for the Face)

**Method:** Select a cup of appropriate size and apply it to local affected part. Retain the cup for 10–15 minutes. If the acne is broken after the cup is removed, disinfect it with 75% alcohol.

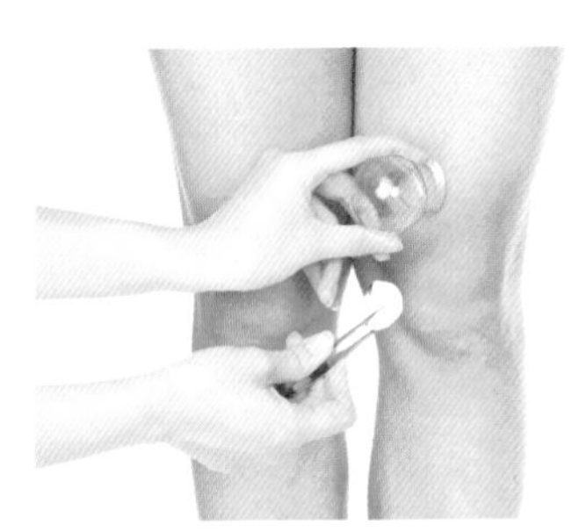

### 2. Xuehai Point

**Location:** In a cavity about 2 cun away from the inner upper corner of the patella, when the knee is bent.

**Method:** Select and apply a cup of appropriate size to Xuehai point, retaining the cup for 10–15 minutes.

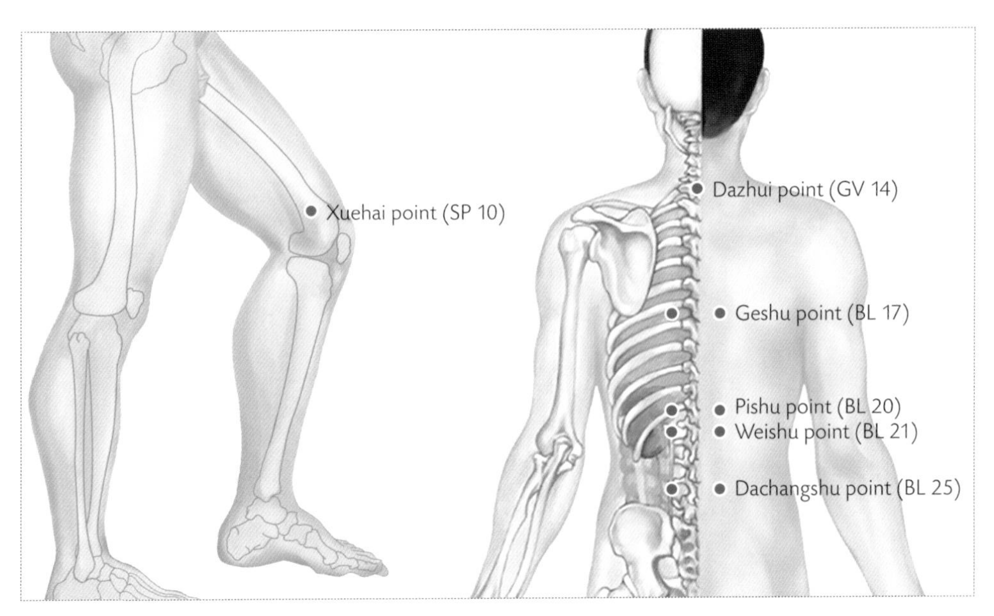

### 3. Dazhui Point

**Location:** Under the spinous process of the seventh cervical vertebrae.

**Method:** Select a cup of appropriate size and apply it to Dazhui point. Retain the cup for 10–15 minutes.

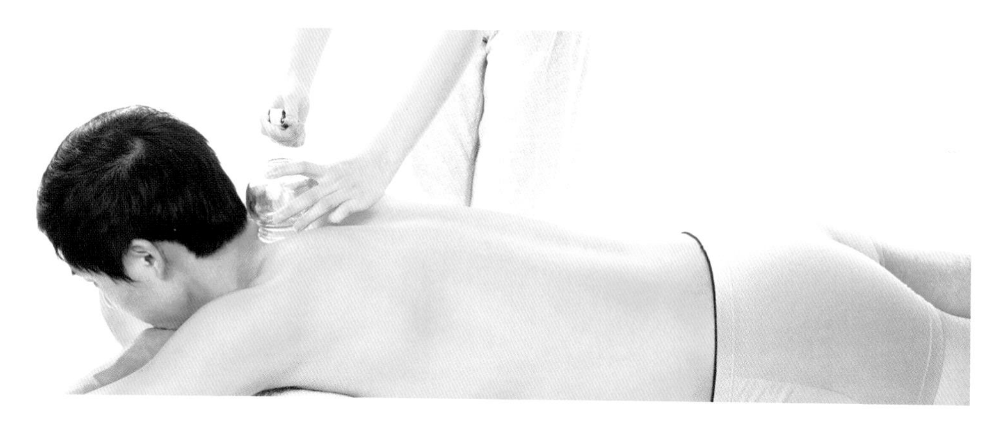

### 4. Geshu, Pishu, Weishu and Dachangshu Points

**Location:** Geshu point is 1.5 cun away from the spinous process of the seventh thoracic vertebra; Pishu point is 1.5 cun away horizontally from the eleventh thoracic vertebra; Weishu point is about 1.5 cun below the spinous process of the twelfth thoracic vertebra; Dachangshu point is about 1.5 cun away from the fourth lumbar vertebra on two sides.

**Method:** Use the moving cupping method. Move the cup on the bladder meridian on the back by segment along the meridian, and move the cup several times mainly on Geshu, Pishu, Weishu and Dachangshu points. Repeatedly push and pull on the points back and forth, until the skin becomes red. The cup may be retained on the abovementioned points for 10–15 minutes after the moving cupping.

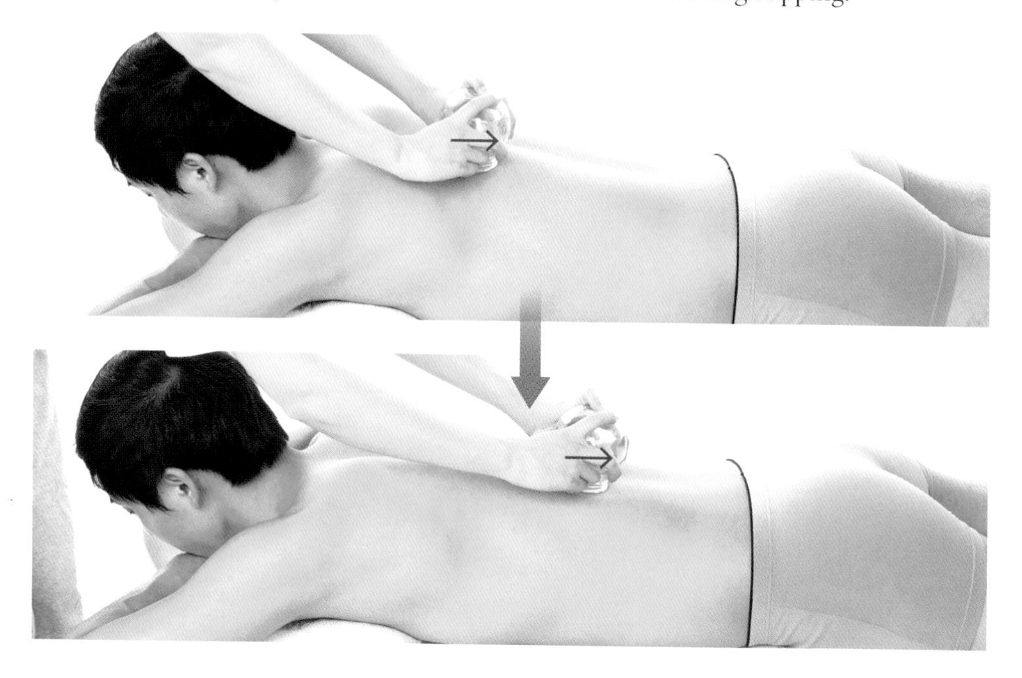

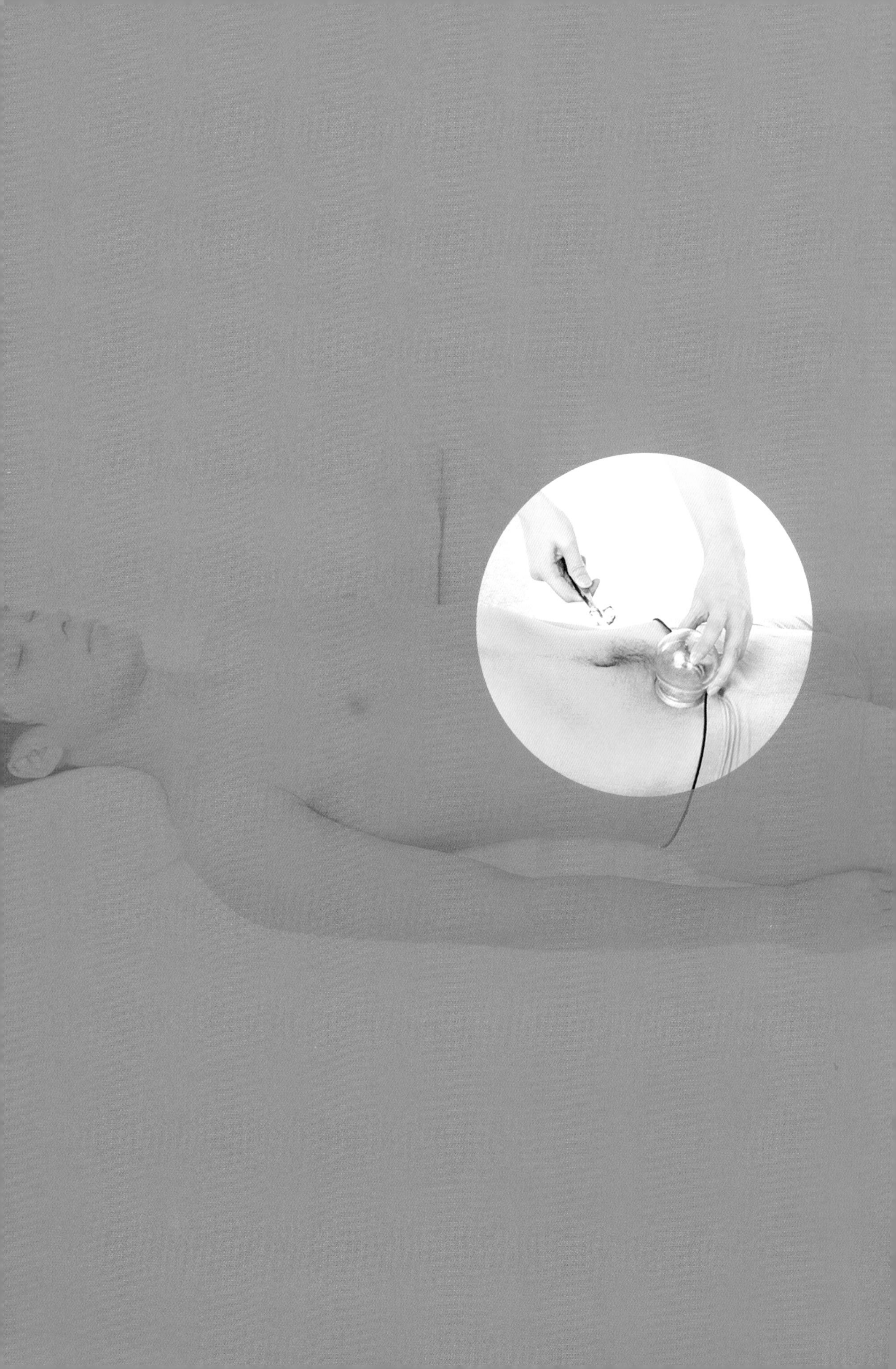

# Chapter Nine
## Male Diseases

Sometimes it is difficult to speak out when one suffers a disease. Male diseases have seriously affected many men's normal work and life, and can even lead to a psychological shadow for some of them. As a Traditional Chinese Medicine therapy, cupping can pose two-way regulation effects to the human body, and the disease can be alleviated through operation at home by oneself.

## 1 Prostatitis

Patients feel urinary tract burning and pain during urination, radiating to the glans, and accompanied by lower waist pain, loss of libido, ejaculation pain, premature ejaculation, and probable outflow of white secreta at urethral orifice after urination or defecation.

To prevent the disease, one should pay attention to having a moderate sexual life, and develop the habit of timely urination. Avoid drinking too much alcohol or eating a lot of spicy food, but eat more white gourds, red beans, bitter gourd, kelp, and other food that can clear heat and promote urination.

The cupping can be applied to two groups of points, one group a day and two groups in turn, until the symptoms are alleviated or disappear. The first group includes Pishu, Sanjiaoshu, Shenshu, Pangguangshu, Ciliao, Zusanli, Guanyuan, and Zhongji points, and the second group includes Sanyinjiao, Yinlingquan, Zhaohai, and Taixi points.

### Cupping Methods

**The First Group of Points**

#### 1. Zusanli Point

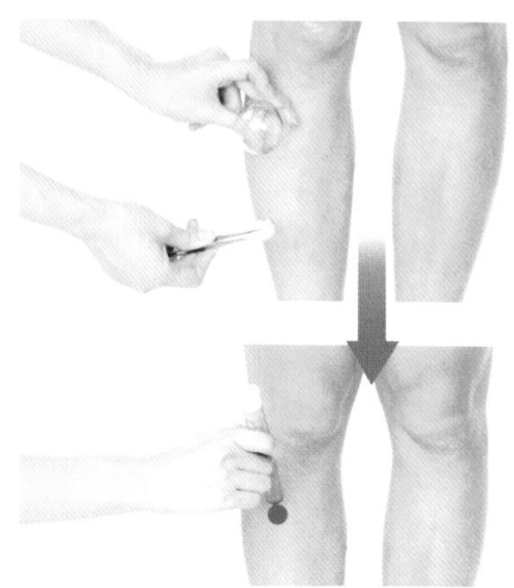

**Location:** About 3 cun below the knee on the outer side of the tibia.

**Method:** First knead Zusanli point with the thumb pulp for 2–3 minutes, and then select a cup of appropriate size and apply it to the point, retaining for 10–15 minutes. With the cup removed, perform moxibustion with a moxa stick for 3–5 minutes until warmth is felt.

### 2. Pishu, Sanjiaoshu, Shenshu, Pangguangshu and Ciliao Points

**Location:** Pishu point is 1.5 cun away horizontally from the eleventh thoracic vertebra; Sanjiaoshu point is 1.5 cun away from the spinous process of the first lumbar vertebra; Shenshu point is 1.5 cun horizontally from the second lumbar spinal process; Pangguangshu point is in the sacral area, at the same level as the second posterior sacral foramen, 1.5 cun lateral to the median sacral crest; Ciliao point is in the sacral region, in the second posterior sacral foramen.

**Method:** Use the moving cupping method. Move the cup on the bladder meridian on the back by segment along the meridian, and move it several times mainly on the Pishu, Sanjiaoshu, Shenshu, Pangguangshu and Ciliao points. Repeatedly push and pull on the points back and forth, until the skin becomes red. The cup may be retained on the abovementioned points for 10–15 minutes after the moving cupping.

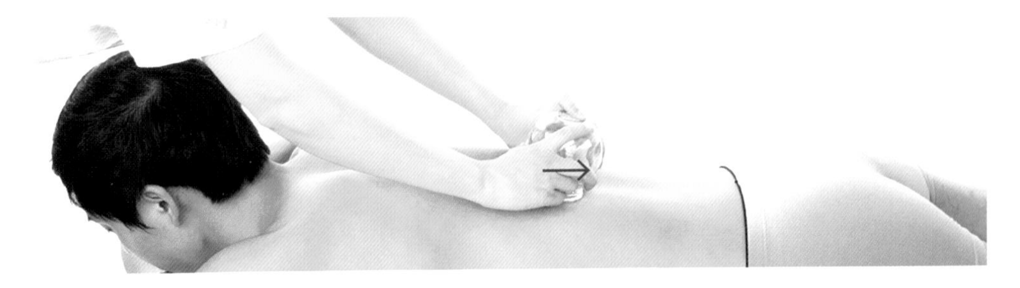

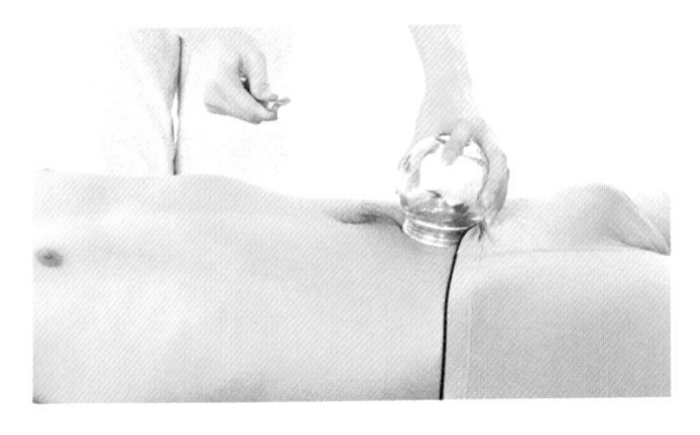

### 3. Guanyuan Point

**Location:** About 3 cun below the navel.

**Method:** First knead Guanyuan point with the thumb pulp for 2–3 minutes, and then select and apply a cup of appropriate size to the point, retaining the cup for 10–15 minutes. With the cup removed, perform moxibustion with a moxa stick for 3–5 minutes until warmth is felt.

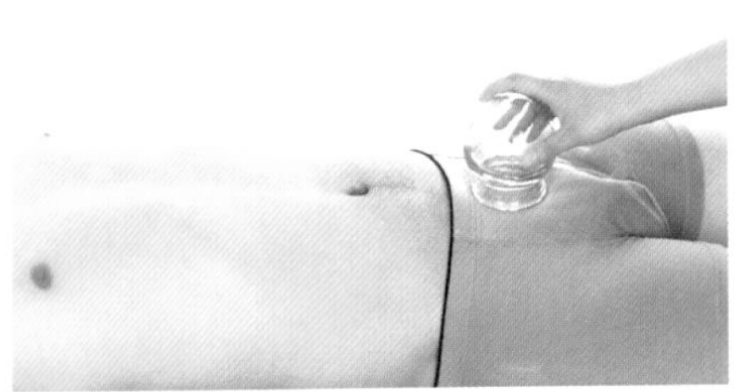

### 4. Zhongji Point

**Location:** On the lower abdomen, 4 cun below the center of the umbilicus, on the anterior midline.

**Method:** Cup this point, retaining the cup for 10–15 minutes. With the cup removed, perform moxibustion with a moxa stick for 3–5 minutes until warmth is felt.

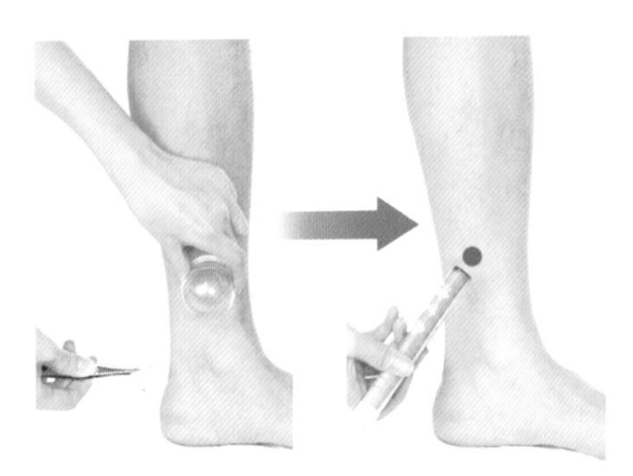

## The Second Group of Points

### 1. Sanyinjiao Point

**Location:** At the rear edge of the shinbone, 3 cun above the ankle.

**Method:** Select and apply a cup of appropriate size to the point, retaining the cup for 10–15 minutes. With the cup removed, perform moxibustion with a moxa stick for 3–5 minutes, until warmth is felt.

### 2. Yinlingquan Point

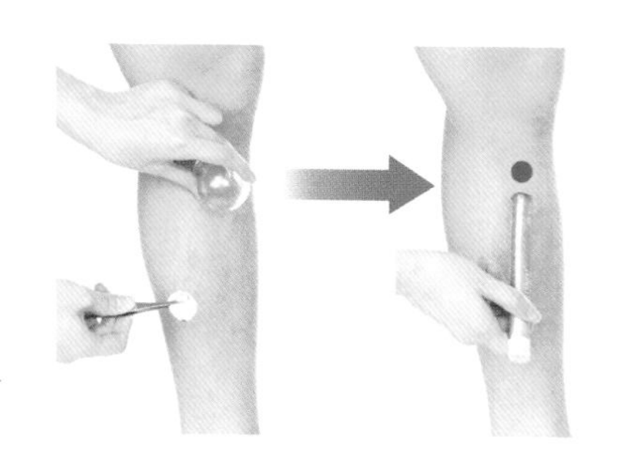

**Location:** In the depression on the inner edge of the shinbone below the knee.

**Method:** First knead Yinlingquan point with the thumb pulp for 2–3 minutes, and then cup this point, retaining the cup for 10–15 minutes. With the cup removed, perform moxibustion with a moxa stick for 3–5 minutes until warmth is felt.

### 3. Zhaohai Point

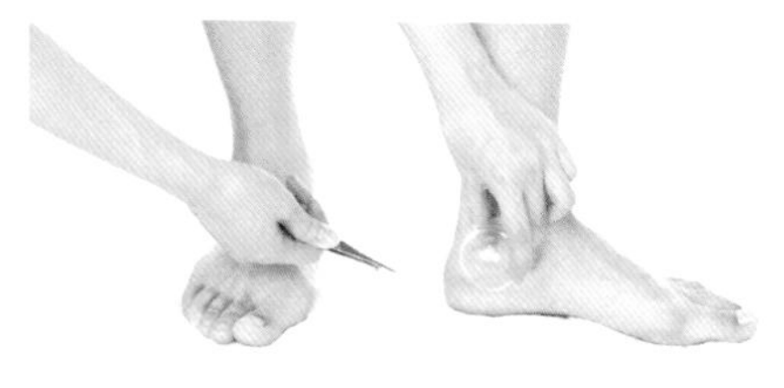

**Location:** In a cavity below the protruding point in the interior of the ankle.

**Method:** Select a cup of appropriate size and apply it to the point, retaining the cup for 10–15 minutes.

### 4. Taixi Point

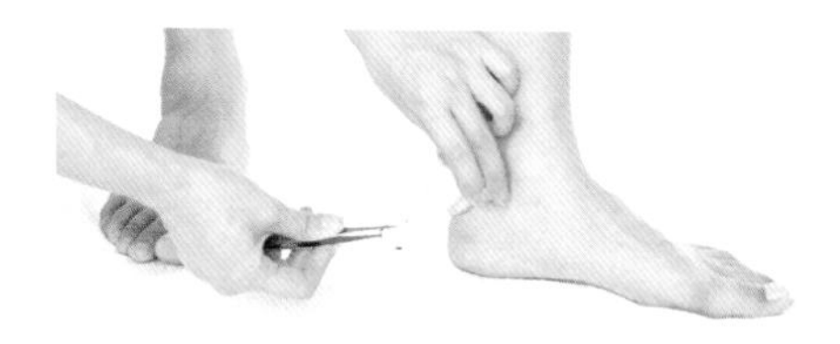

**Location:** In a cavity between the medial malleolus and Achilles tendon.

**Method:** Select a cup of appropriate size and apply it to the point, retaining the cup for 10–15 minutes.

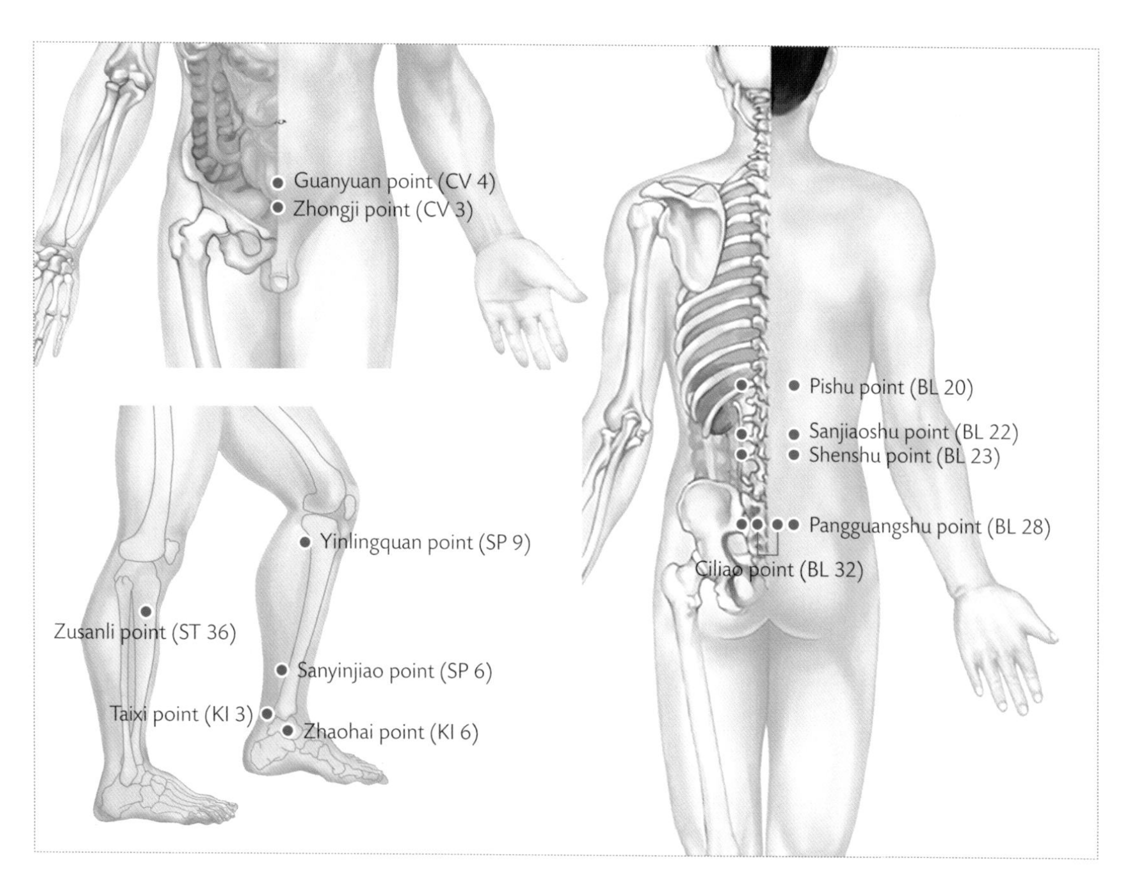

# 2 Prostatic Hyperplasia

Symptoms of the disease are manifested by frequent urination, urgency of urination, increased urination at night, urinary incontinence, decreased force of urination, urinary tract thinning and incomplete voiding, as well as hematuria and urinary retention in severe cases.

Patients should drink more water but less strong tea during the day, avoid drinking alcohol and smoking, eat less spicy and fatty food, drink less coffee, eat less citrus and other acidic food. Do not hold urine and avoid sitting for a long time. Massage the lower abdomen after urination, which can promote emptying of the bladder, and reduce residual urine.

The cupping can be applied to two groups of points, one group a day and two groups in turn, until the symptoms disappear. The first group includes Zhongji, Shuidao, Qihai, Ciliao, and Touwei points, and the second group mainly includes Sanyinjiao, Yongquan, Taixi, and Mingmen points.

## Cupping Methods

### The First Group of Points

#### 1. Shuidao Point

**Location:** 3 cun below the navel and two cun from the frontal middle line.

**Method:** Cup this point, retaining the cup for 10–15 minutes. With the cup removed, perform moxibustion with a moxa stick for 3–5 minutes until warmth is felt.

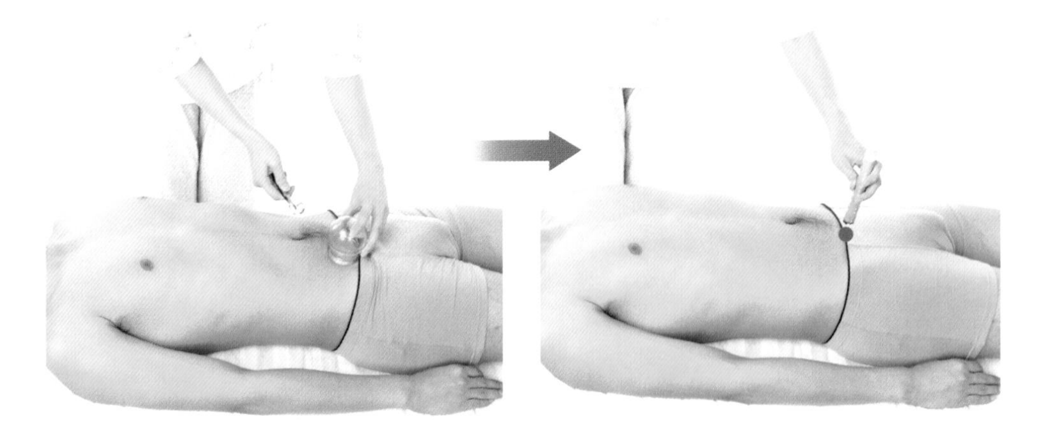

#### 2. Qihai and Zhongji Points

**Location:** Qihai point is about 1.5 cun below the navel; Zhongji point is 4 cun below the navel.

**Method:** First knead Qihai and Zhongji points with the thumb pulp for 2–3 minutes, and then select and apply a cup of appropriate size to the points, retaining the cup for 10–15 minutes. With the cup removed, perform moxibustion with a moxa stick for 3–5 minutes until warmth is felt.

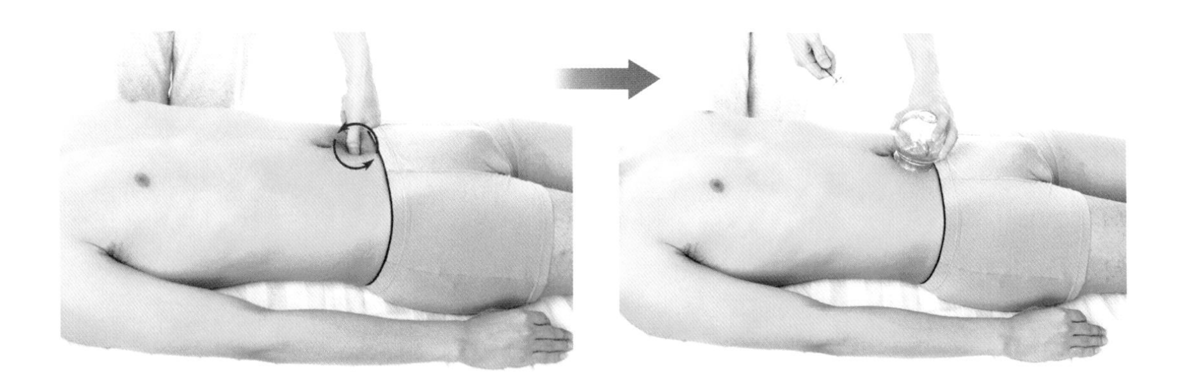

### 3. Ciliao Point

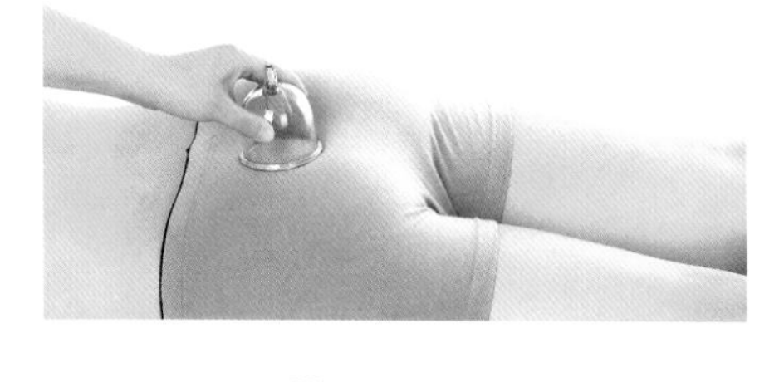

**Location:** In the sacral region, in the second posterior sacral foramen.

**Method:** Select a cup of appropriate size and apply it to Ciliao point. Retain the cup for 10–15 minutes.

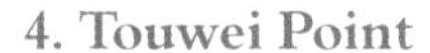

### 4. Touwei Point

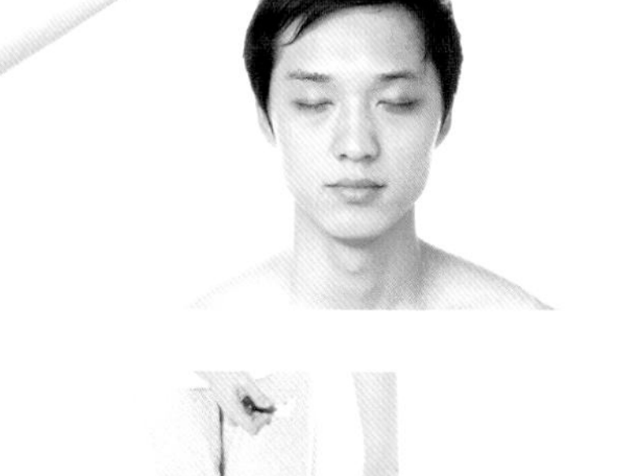

**Location:** Front of the head at the hairline, 0.5 cun from the center line on both sides.

**Method:** Select a cup of appropriate size and apply it to Touwei point by using the flash cupping method for 10–15 times. Do not retain the cup. Then perform moxibustion with a moxa stick for 3–5 minutes until warmth is felt.

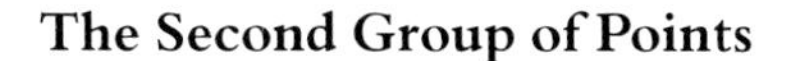

## The Second Group of Points

### 1. Mingmen Point

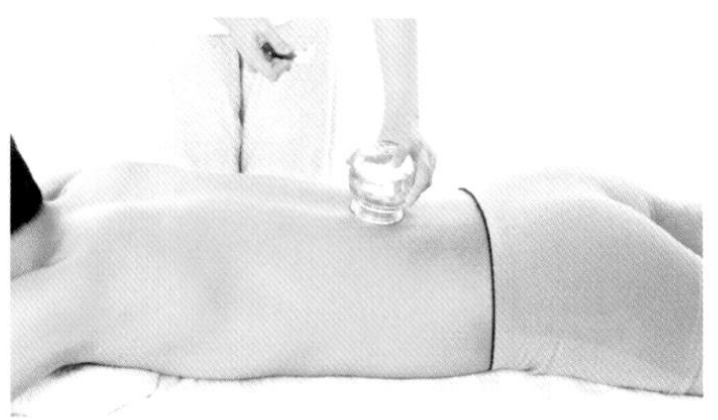

**Location:** In a cavity below the spinous process of the second cervical vertebra.

**Method:** Select a cup of appropriate size and apply it to the point, retaining the cup for 5–10 minutes.

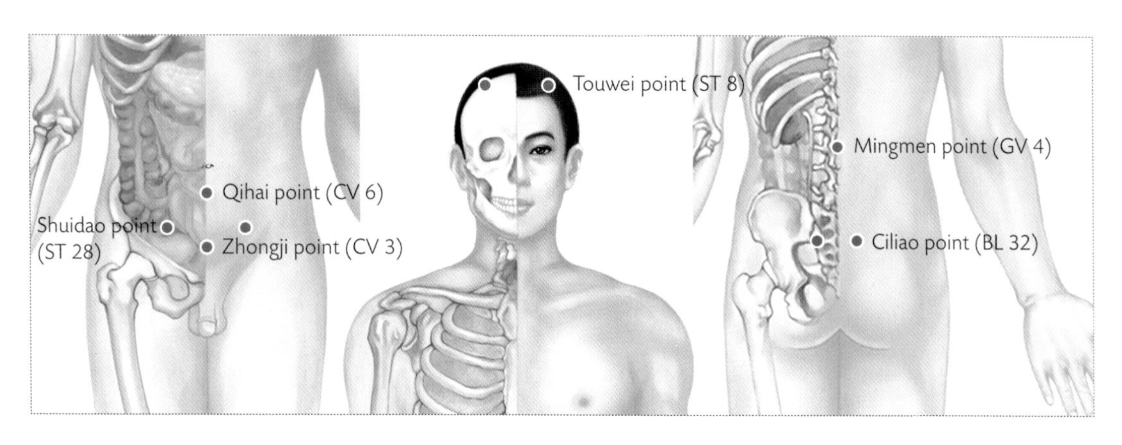

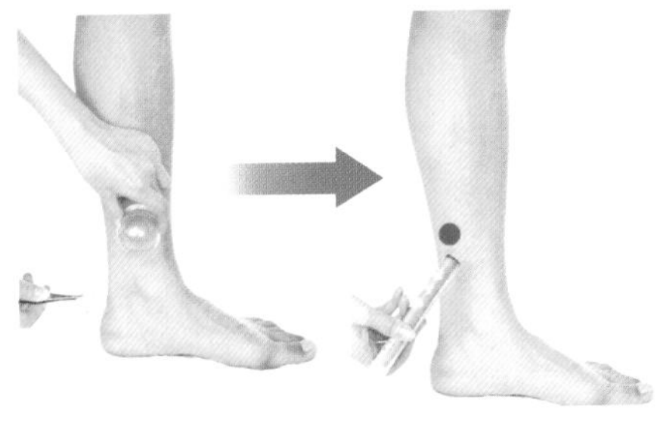

### 2. Sanyinjiao Point

**Location:** At the rear edge of the shinbone, 3 cun above the ankle.

**Method:** Select a cup of appropriate size and apply it to Sanyinjiao point, retaining the cup for 10–15 minutes. With the cup removed, perform moxibustion with a moxa stick for 3–5 minutes, until warmth is felt.

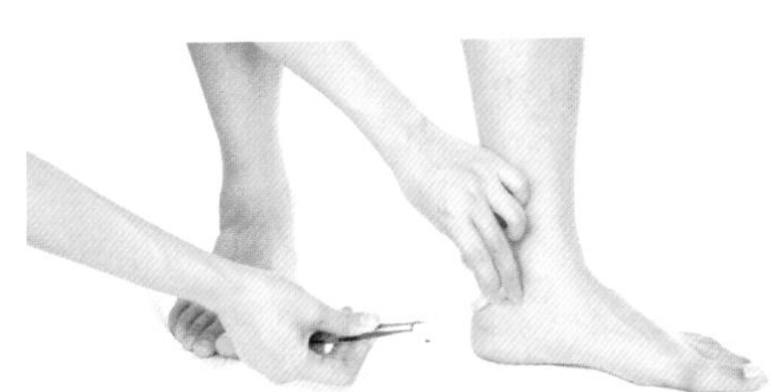

### 3. Taixi Point

**Location:** In a cavity between the medial malleolus and Achilles tendon.

**Method:** Select a cup of appropriate size and apply it to the point, retaining the cup for 10–15 minutes.

### 4. Yongquan Point

**Location:** In a depression in the front of the sole of the foot, about one-third of the way down from the toes.

**Method:** First knead Yongquan point with the palm for 2–3 minutes, until a feeling of heat is present. Then select a cup of appropriate size and apply it to the point, retaining the cup for 10–15 minutes. With the cup removed, perform moxibustion with a moxa stick for 3–5 minutes until warmth is felt.

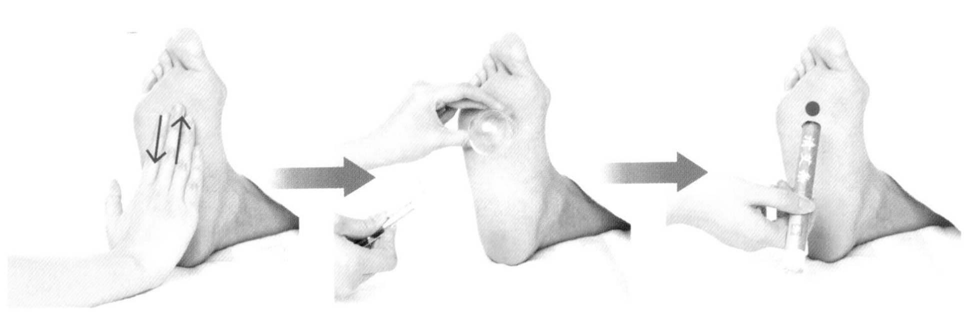

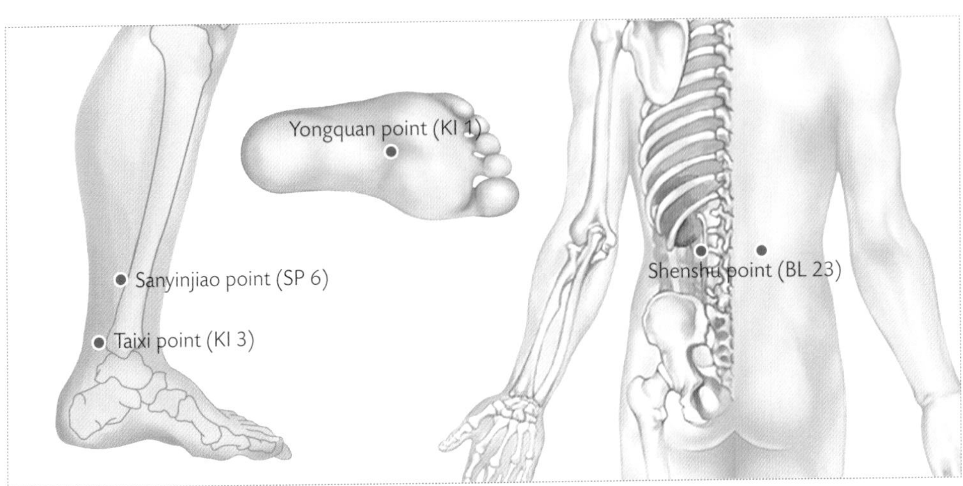

# 3 Premature Ejaculation

Premature ejaculation refers to an inharmonious sex life due to ejaculation before the penis entering the vagina, or early ejaculation after the penis entering the vagina for a short time or before women have reached orgasm.

The patient should prohibit himself from masturbation, and control sexual intercourse, take part in appropriate cultural and sports activities like listening to music or doing exercise, which can regulate the emotions, enhance physical fitness, and help prevent premature ejaculation. They should also adjust their emotions, and eliminate psychology states of tension, low self-esteem, and fear. Relax when having sex.

The cupping should be performed on Shenshu, Taixi, Guanyuan, Mingmen, and Yongquan points for premature ejaculation due to kidney deficiency, and on Sanyinjiao, Yinlingquan, Taichong, and Zhongji points for premature ejaculation due to damp heat.

## Cupping Methods

### For Premature Ejaculation Caused by Kidney Deficiency

#### 1. Shenshu Point

**Location:** Shenshu point is 1.5 cun horizontally from the second lumbar spinal process.

**Method:** Select and apply a cup of appropriate size to Shenshu point, retaining the cup for 10–15 minutes. With the cup removed, perform moxibustion with a moxa stick for 3–5 minutes until warmth is felt.

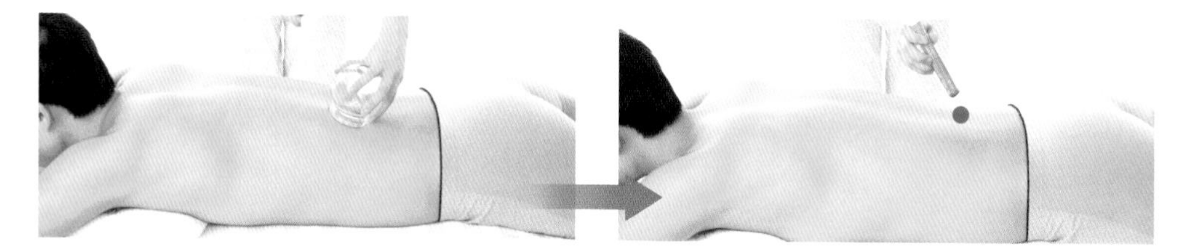

#### 2. Taixi Point

**Location:** In a cavity between the medial malleolus and Achilles tendon.

**Method:** Select and apply a cup of appropriate size to Taixi point, retaining the cup for 10–15 minutes. With the cup removed, perform moxibustion with a moxa stick for 3–5 minutes until warmth is felt.

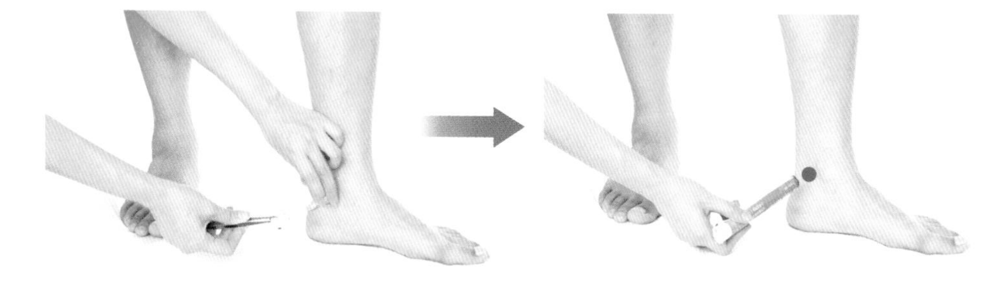

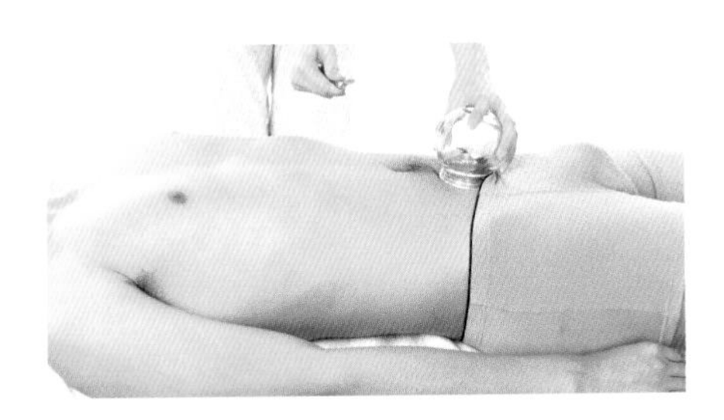

### 3. Guanyuan Point

**Location:** About 3 cun below the navel.

**Method:** Select and apply a cup of appropriate size to Guanyuan point, retaining the cup for 10–15 minutes. With the cup removed, perform moxibustion with a moxa stick for 3–5 minutes until warmth is felt.

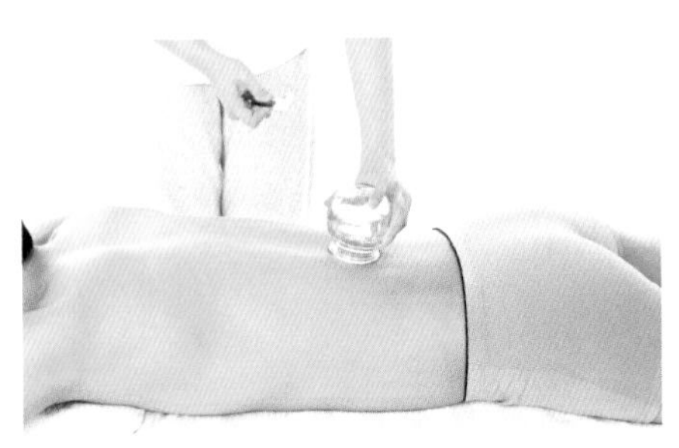

### 4. Mingmen Point

**Location:** In a cavity below the spinous process of the second cervical vertebra.

**Method:** Select and apply a cup of appropriate size to Mingmen point, retaining the cup for 10–15 minutes. With the cup removed, perform moxibustion with a moxa stick for 3–5 minutes until warmth is felt.

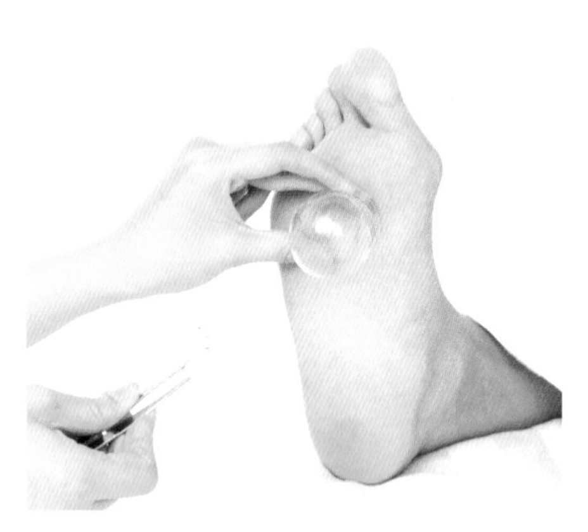

### 5. Yongquan Point

**Location:** In a depression in the front of the sole of the foot, about one-third of the way down from the toes.

**Method:** First knead Yongquan point with the palm for 2–3 minutes, until a feeling of heat is present. Then select a cup of appropriate size and apply it to the point, retaining the cup for 10–15 minutes. With the cup removed, perform moxibustion with a moxa stick for 3–5 minutes until warmth is felt.

## For Premature Ejaculation Caused by Damp Heat

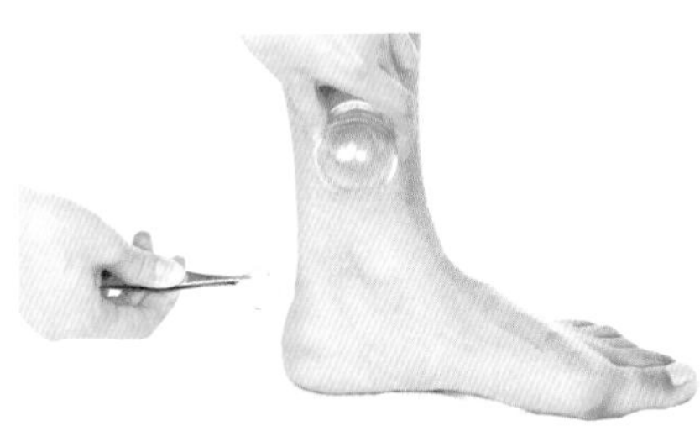

### 1. Sanyinjiao Point

**Location:** At the rear edge of the shinbone, 3 cun above the ankle.

**Method:** Select and apply a cup of appropriate size to the point, retaining the cup for 10–15 minutes.

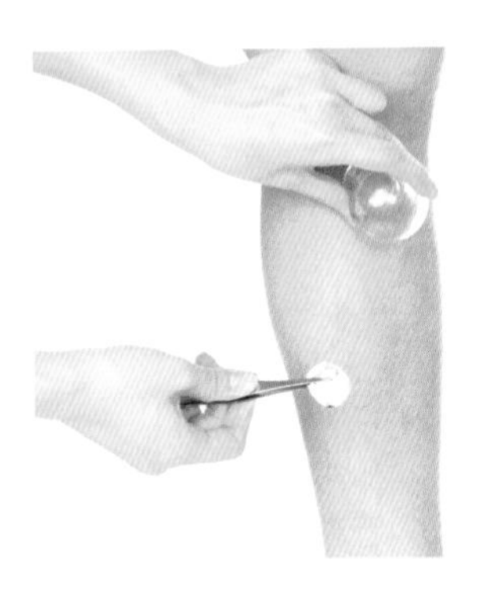

### 2. Yinlingquan Point

**Location:** In the depression on the inner edge of the shinbone below the knee.

**Method:** Select and apply a cup of appropriate size to the point, retaining the cup for 10–15 minutes.

### 3. Taichong Point

**Location:** On the foot in a notch between the first and second metatarsal bones.

**Method:** Select and apply a cup of appropriate size to the point, retaining the cup for 10–15 minutes.

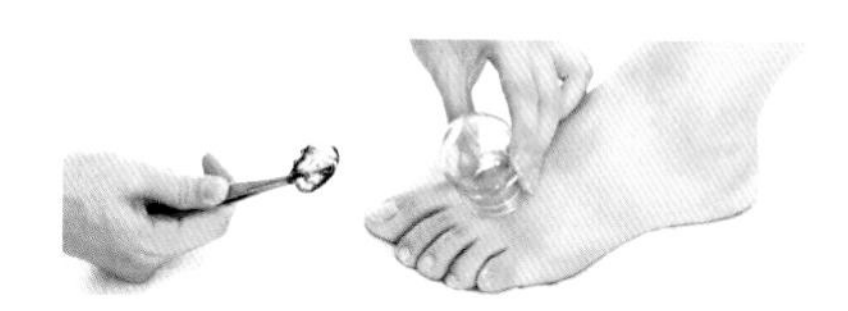

### 4. Zhongji Point

**Location:** On the lower abdomen, 4 cun below the center of the umbilicus, on the anterior midline.

**Method:** Select and apply a cup of appropriate size to the point, retaining the cup for 10–15 minutes.

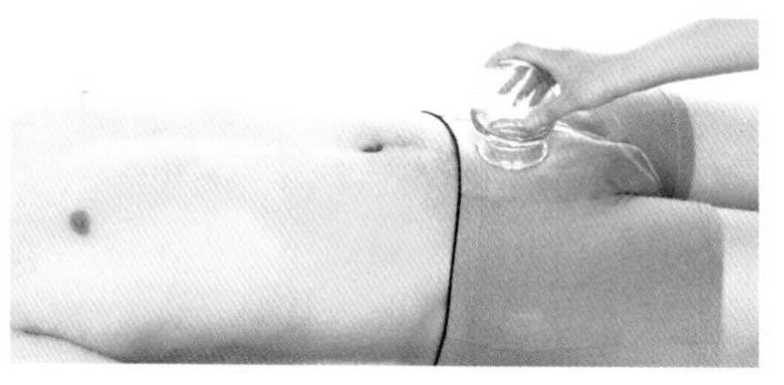

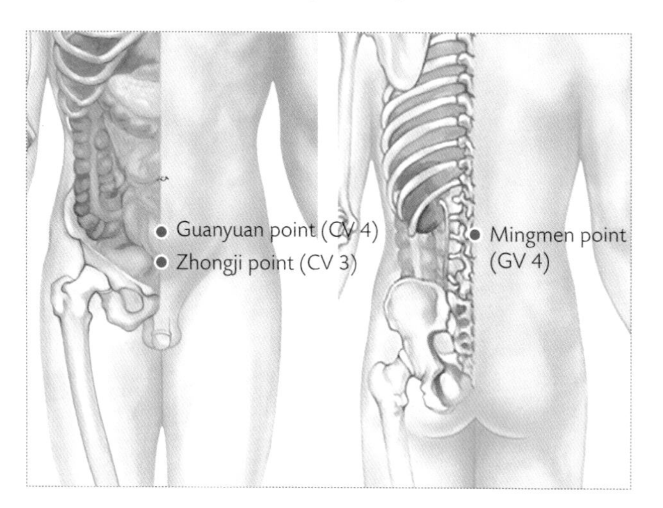


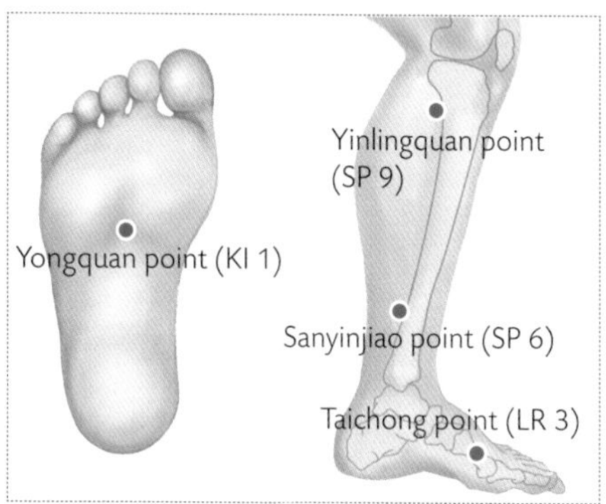


# 4 Impotence

Impotence, also known as erectile dysfunction, refers to an inability to erect or weak erection during sex, which leads to an unsatisfactory sex life.

The patient should eliminate psychological barriers, control sex life, pay attention to diet regulation, and eat more aphrodisiac food, but should not blindly believe the so-called "aphrodisiacs," or blindly use tonics. Actively carry out physical exercise to improve physical fitness.

The cupping should be performed on Mingmen, Guanyuan, Zhishi, Ciliao, Zusanli, Sanyinjiao, Yongquan, and Taixi points.

## Cupping Methods

### 1. Mingmen Point

**Location:** In a cavity below the spinous process of the second cervical vertebra.

**Method:** Select and apply a cup of appropriate size to the point, retaining the cup for 10–15 minutes. With the cup removed, perform moxibustion with a moxa stick for 3–5 minutes until warmth is felt.

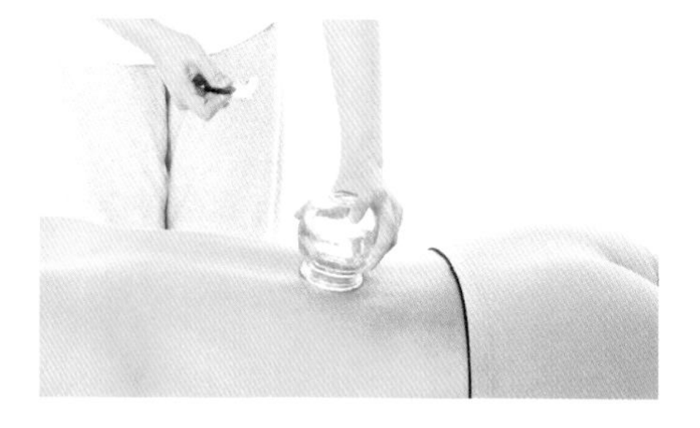

### 2. Guanyuan Point

**Location:** About 3 cun below the navel.

**Method:** Select and apply a cup of appropriate size to the point, retaining the cup for 10–15 minutes. With the cup removed, perform moxibustion with a moxa box for 3–5 minutes until warmth is felt.

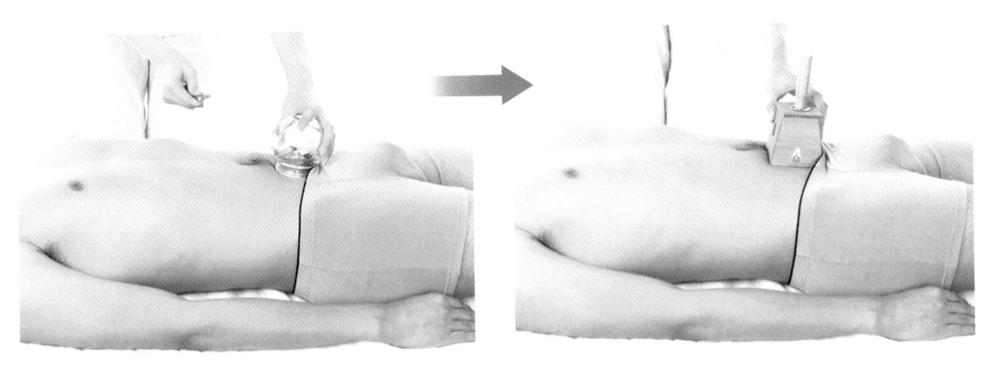

### 3. Zhishi Point

**Location:** 3 cun away from the spinous process of the second lumbar vertebra.

**Method:** Select and apply a cup of appropriate size to the point, retaining the cup for 10–15 minutes.

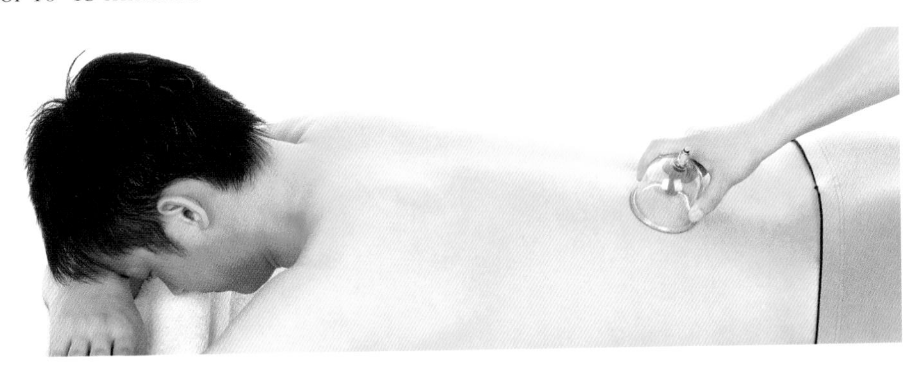

### 4. Yongquan Point

**Location:** In a depression in the front of the sole of the foot, about one-third of the way down from the toes.

**Method:** First knead Yongquan point with the palm for 2–3 minutes, until a feeling of heat is present. Then select a cup of appropriate size and apply it to the point, retaining the cup for 10–15 minutes. With the cup removed, perform moxibustion with a moxa stick for 3–5 minutes until warmth is felt.

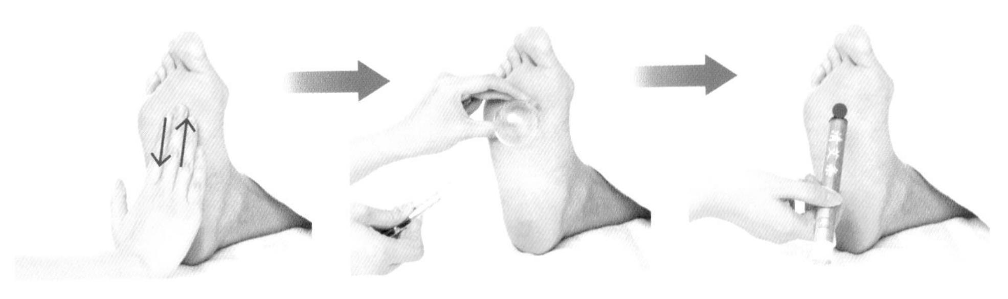

### 5. Ciliao Point

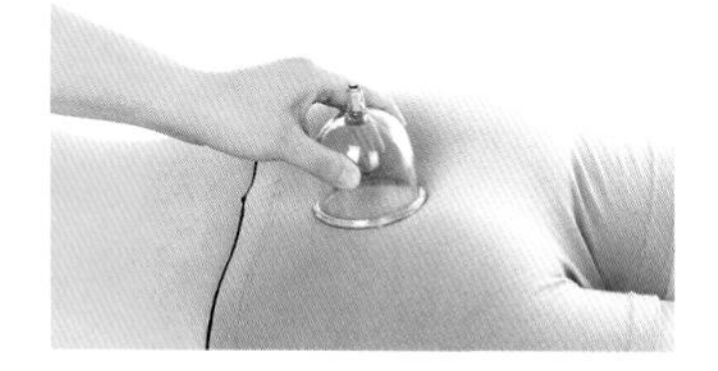

**Location:** In the sacral region, in the second posterior sacral foramen.

**Method:** Select a cup of appropriate size and apply it to Ciliao point. Retain the cup for 10–15 minutes.

### 6. Zusanli Point

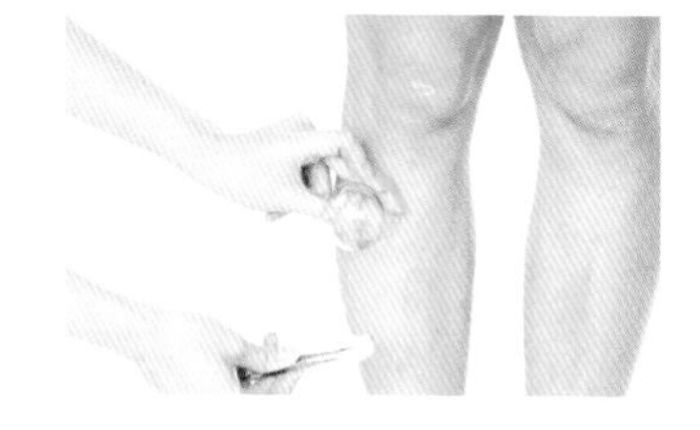

**Location:** About 3 cun below the knee on the outer side of the tibia.

**Method:** Cup this point, retaining the cup for 10–15 minutes. With the cup removed, perform moxibustion with a moxa stick for 3–5 minutes until warmth is felt.

### 7. Sanyinjiao Point

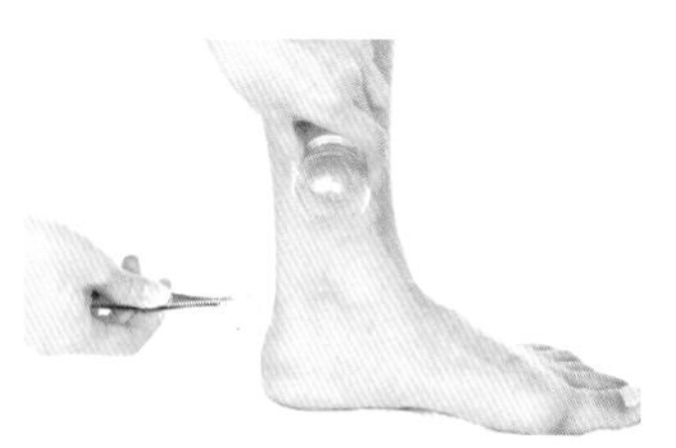

**Location:** At the rear edge of the shinbone, 3 cun above the ankle.

**Method:** Select and apply a cup of appropriate size to the point, retaining the cup for 10–15 minutes.

### 8. Taixi Point

**Location:** In a cavity between the medial malleolus and Achilles tendon.

**Method:** Select a cup of appropriate size and apply it to the point, retaining the cup for 10–15 minutes. With the cup removed, perform moxibustion with a moxa stick for 3–5 minutes until warmth is felt.

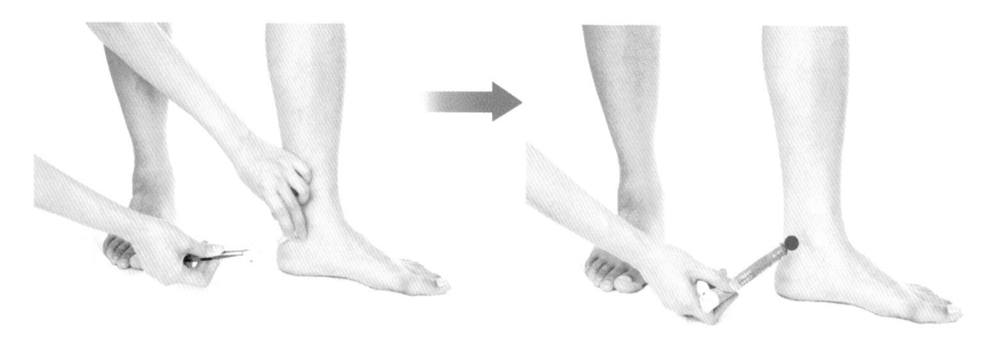

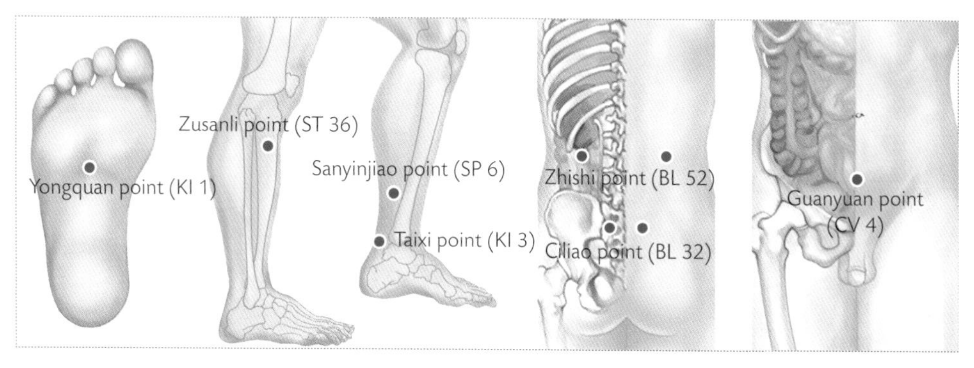

# 5 Male Infertility

The disease refers to the female infertility due to the reasons of the male after the couple has lived together for more than a year, without taking any contraceptive measures.

Couples should pay attention to premarital physical examination, for early detection and early treatment. Men should avoid frequent exposure to radioactive substances and poisons, and strictly follow the operation procedures if required by the work.

The cupping should be performed on Pishu, Shenshu, Pangguangshu, Guanyuan, Zusanli, and Taixi points.

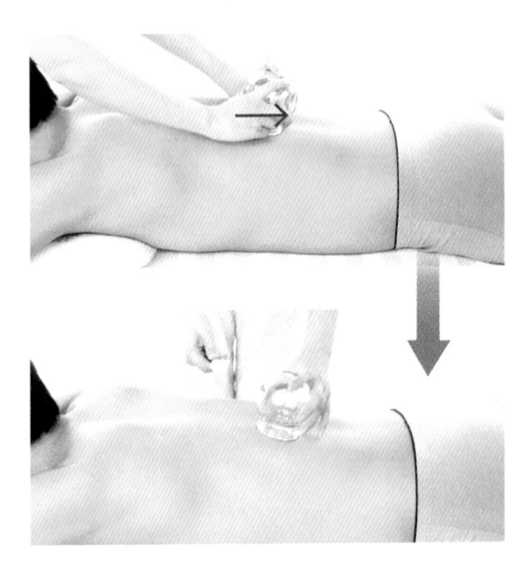

## Cupping Methods

### 1. Pishu Point

**Location:** 1.5 cun away horizontally from the eleventh thoracic vertebra.

**Method:** Use the moving cupping method. Move the cup on the bladder meridian on the back by segment along the meridian, and move it several times mainly on the Pishu point. Repeatedly push and pull on the point back and forth, until the skin becomes red. The cup may be retained on the abovementioned point for 10–15 minutes after the moving cupping. With the cup removed, perform moxibustion with a moxa stick for 3–5 minutes until warmth is felt.

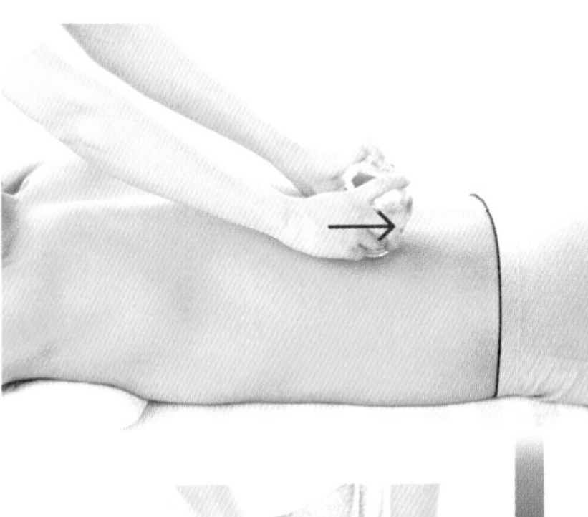

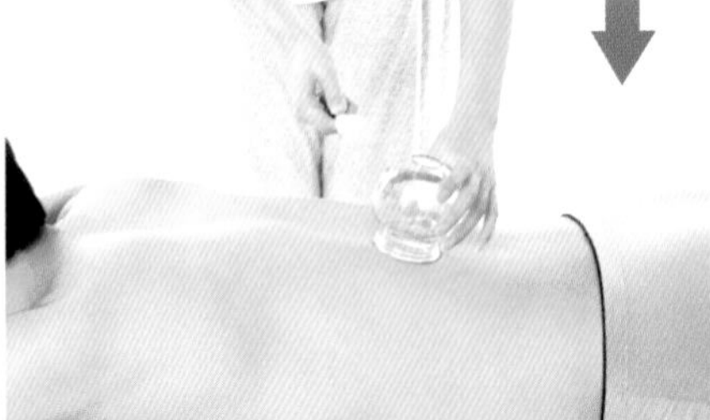

### 2. Shenshu Point

**Location:** 1.5 cun horizontally from the second lumbar spinal process.

**Method:** Use the moving cupping method. Move the cup on the bladder meridian on the back by segment along the meridian, and move it several times mainly on the Shenshu point. Repeatedly push and pull on the point back and forth, until the skin becomes red. The cup may be retained on the abovementioned point for 10–15 minutes after the moving cupping. With the cup removed, perform moxibustion with a moxa stick for 3–5 minutes until warmth is felt.

### 3. Pangguangshu Point

**Location:** In the sacral area, at the same level as the second posterior sacral foramen, 1.5 cun lateral to the median sacral crest.

**Method:** Use the moving cupping method. Move the cup on the bladder meridian on the back by segment along the meridian, and move it several times mainly on the Pangguangshu point. Repeatedly push and pull on the point back and forth, until the skin becomes red. The cup may be retained on the abovementioned point for 10–15 minutes until warmth is felt.

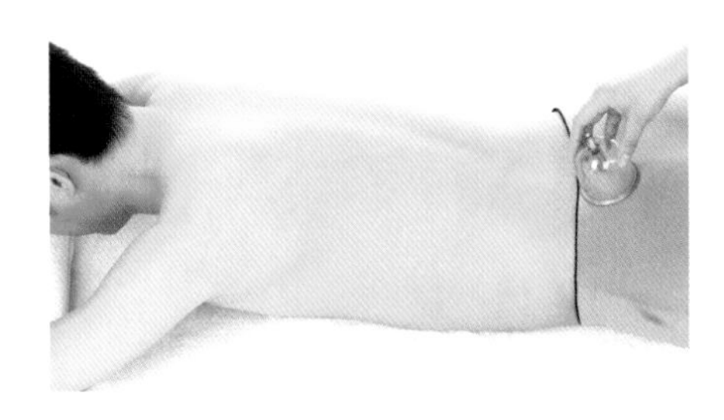

### 4. Guanyuan Point

**Location:** About 3 cun below the navel.

**Method:** Select and apply a cup of appropriate size to the point, retaining the cup for 10–15 minutes. With the cup removed, perform moxibustion with a moxa box for 3–5 minutes until warmth is felt.

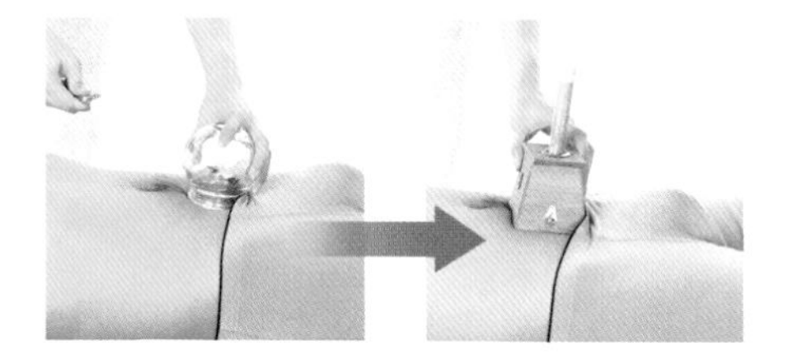

### 5. Zusanli Point

**Location:** About 3 cun below the knee on the outer side of the tibia.

**Method:** First knead Zusanli point with the thumb pulp for 2–3 minutes, and then select a cup of appropriate size and apply it to the point, retaining the cup for 10–15 minutes. With the cup removed, perform moxibustion with a moxa stick for 3–5 minutes until warmth is felt.

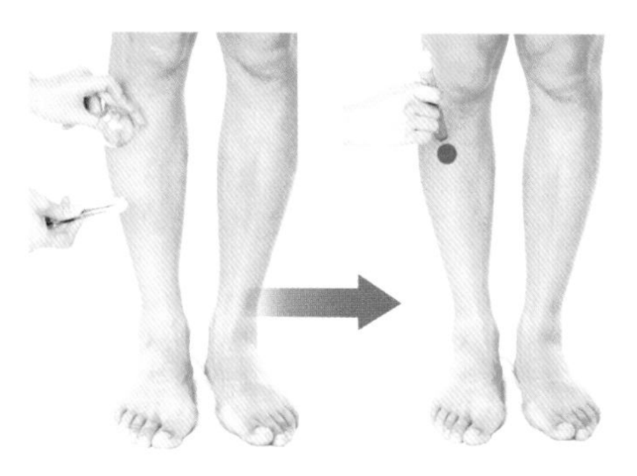

### 6. Taixi Point

**Location:** In a cavity between the medial malleolus and Achilles tendon.

**Method:** Select a cup of appropriate size and apply it to the point, retaining the cup for 10–15 minutes. With the cup removed, perform moxibustion with a moxa stick for 3–5 minutes until warmth is felt.

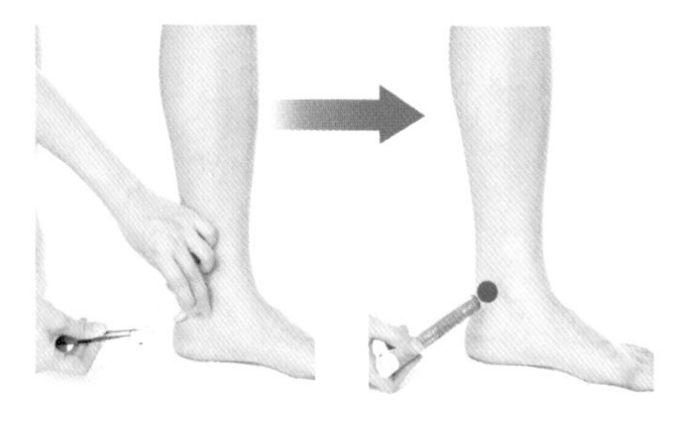

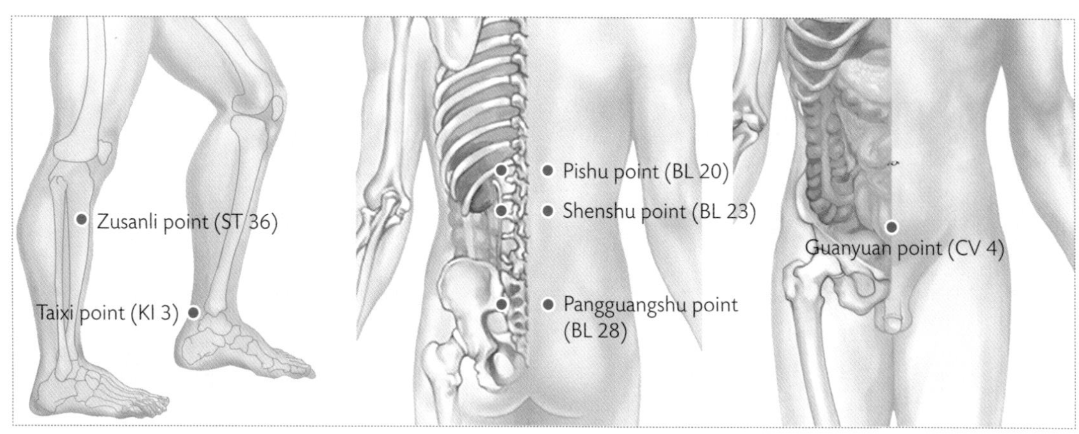

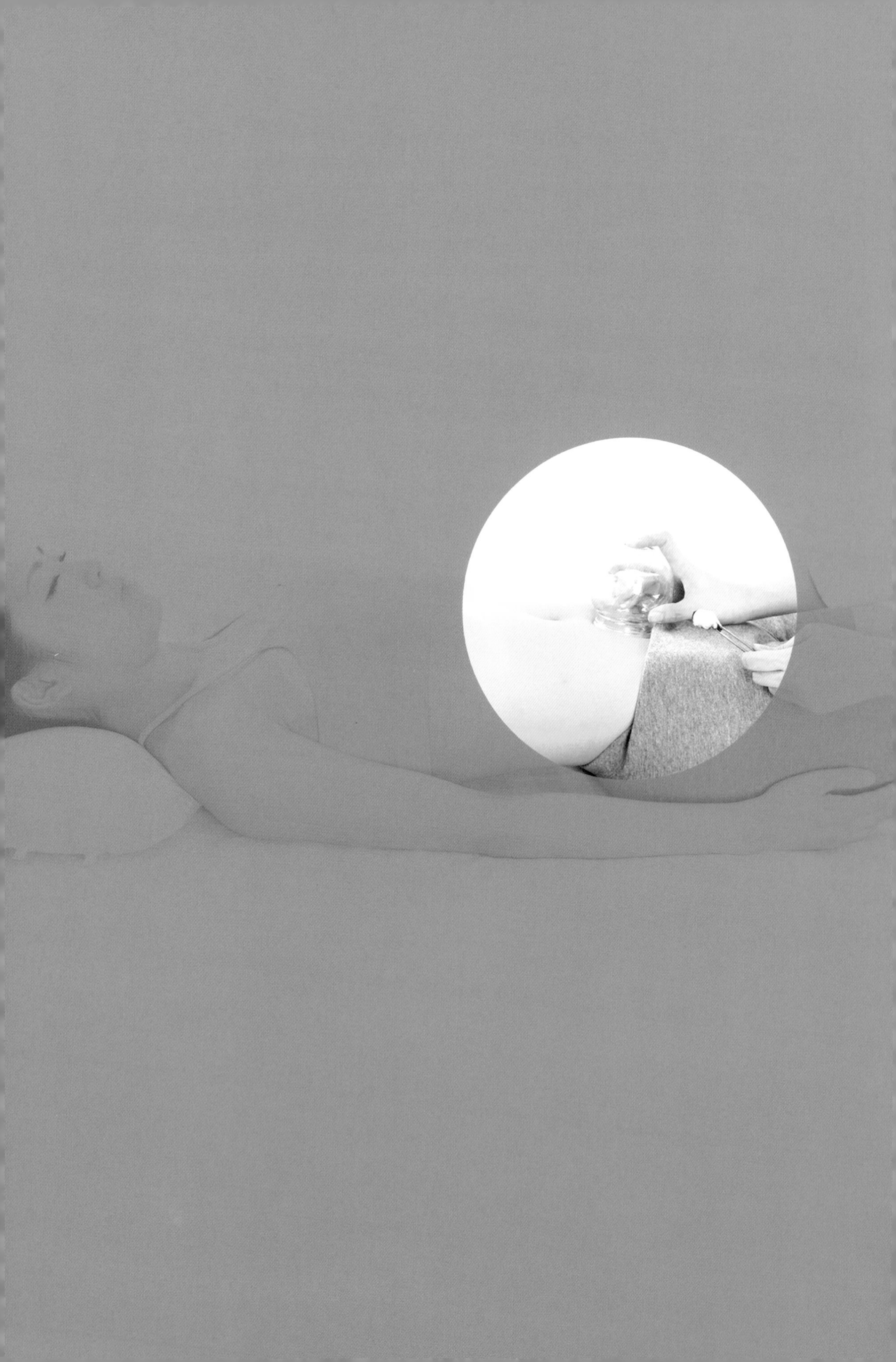

# Chapter Ten
## Gynecological Diseases

Women always have a few days of physical discomfort each month, and sometimes they can feel unbearable pain in the stomach, especially after middle age when all kinds of problems come about, making them upset and weary. In fact, these symptoms can be effectively alleviated through the correct cupping method. Let's see how to operate specifically.

## 1 Postpartum Depression

This symptom means the depression of a woman due to physical and psychological factors after childbirth, with symptoms including nervousness, doubt, guilt, fear, and so on.

The parturient needs to quit smoking and alcohol and eat less irritating food, maintain a balanced diet, engage in exercise, and participate in some beneficial physical and mental activities, which helps emotional stability. Husband and family should take care of the parturient in daily life, for example by comforting her, cooking a rich supper, or doing housework for her, so that the mother feels the care and love from her family.

The cupping should be performed on Ganshu, Xinshu, Taichong, Yinlingquan, and Shenmen points.

### Cupping Methods

**1. Ganshu Point**

**Location:** 1.5 cun away from the ninth thoracic spinal process on the inner side of the scapula.

**Method:** Use the moving cupping method by moving the cup on the bladder meridian on the back by segment along the meridian. Move the cup several times mainly on Ganshu point, and repeatedly push and pull on the point back and forth, until the skin becomes red. The cup may be retained on the abovementioned point for 10–15 minutes after the moving cupping.

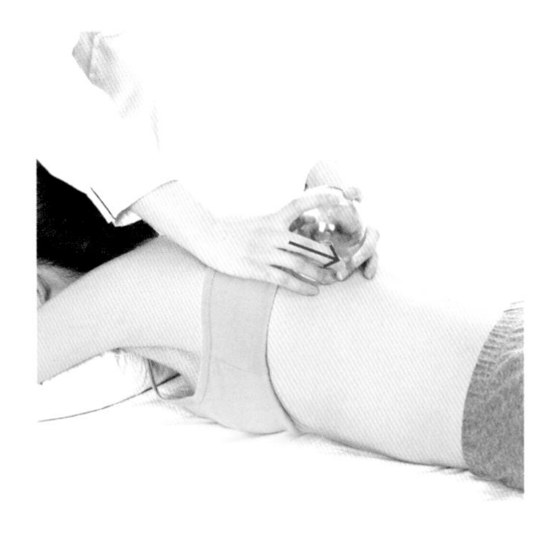

### 2. Xinshu Point

**Location:** Under the fifth thoracic vertebra on the inner side of the scapula, 1.5 cun horizontally away.

**Method:** Use the moving cupping method. Move the cup on the bladder meridian on the back by segment along the meridian, and move the cup several times mainly on the Xinshu point. Repeatedly push and pull on the point back and forth, until the skin becomes red. The cup may be retained on the abovementioned point for 10–15 minutes after the moving cupping.

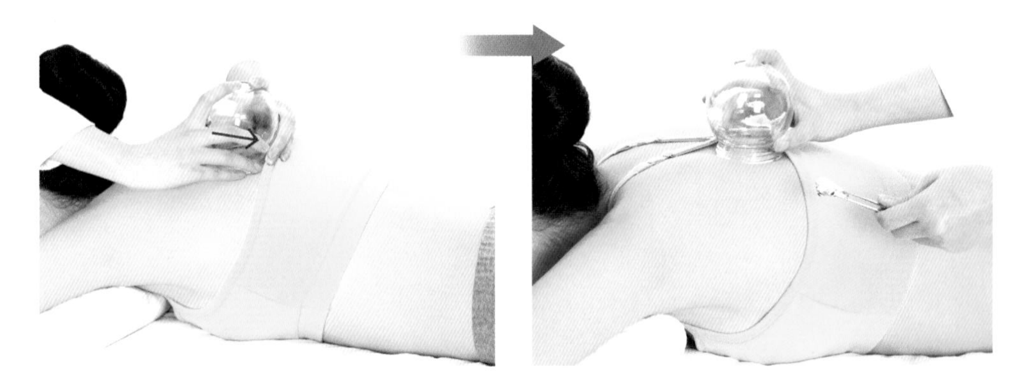

### 3. Taichong Point

**Location:** On the foot in a notch between the first and second metatarsal bones.

**Method:** First knead Taichong point with the thumb pulp for 2–3 minutes until soreness and swelling is felt, and then select and apply a cup of appropriate size to the point, retaining the cup for 10–15 minutes.

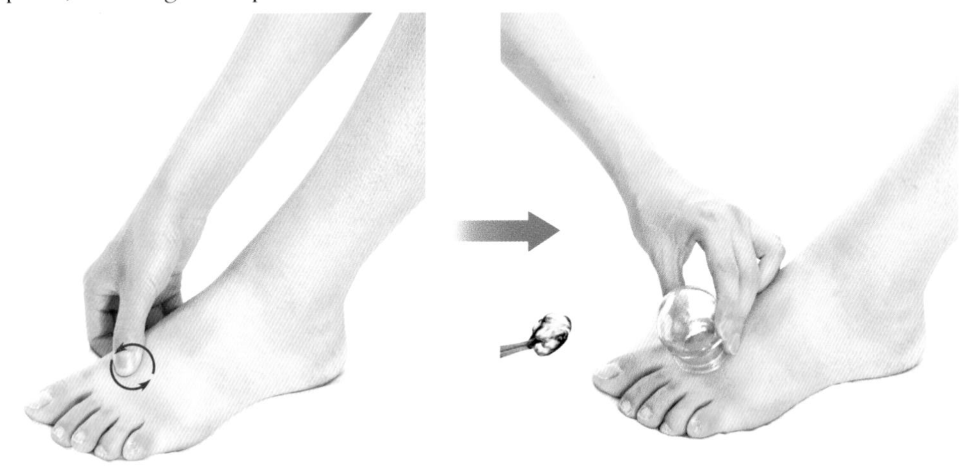

### 4. Yinlingquan Point

**Location:** In the depression on the inner edge of the shinbone below the knee.

**Method:** First knead Yinlingquan point with the thumb pulp for 2–3 minutes, and then cup this point, retaining the cup for 10–15 minutes. With the cup removed, perform moxibustion with a moxa stick for 3–5 minutes until warmth is felt.

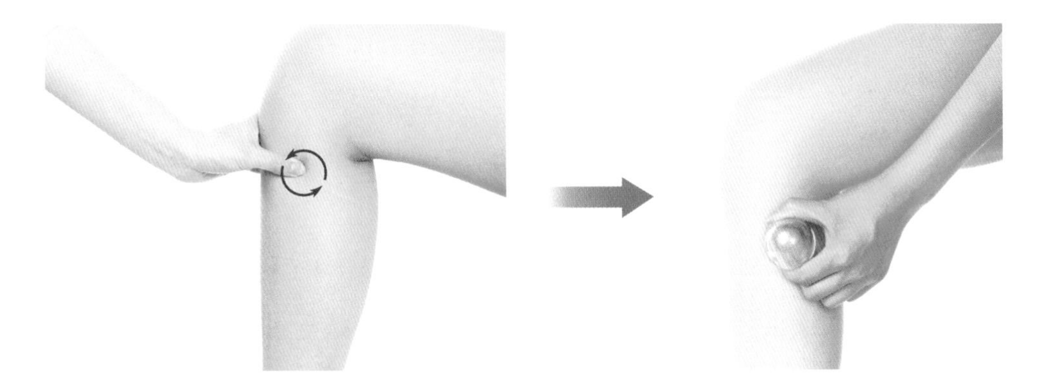

### 5. Shenmen Point

**Location:** On the inner wrist near the small finger when the palm is turned upward.

**Method:** First knead Shenmen point with the thumb pulp for 2–3 minutes, and then select and apply a small cup to the point, retaining the cup for 5–10 minutes.

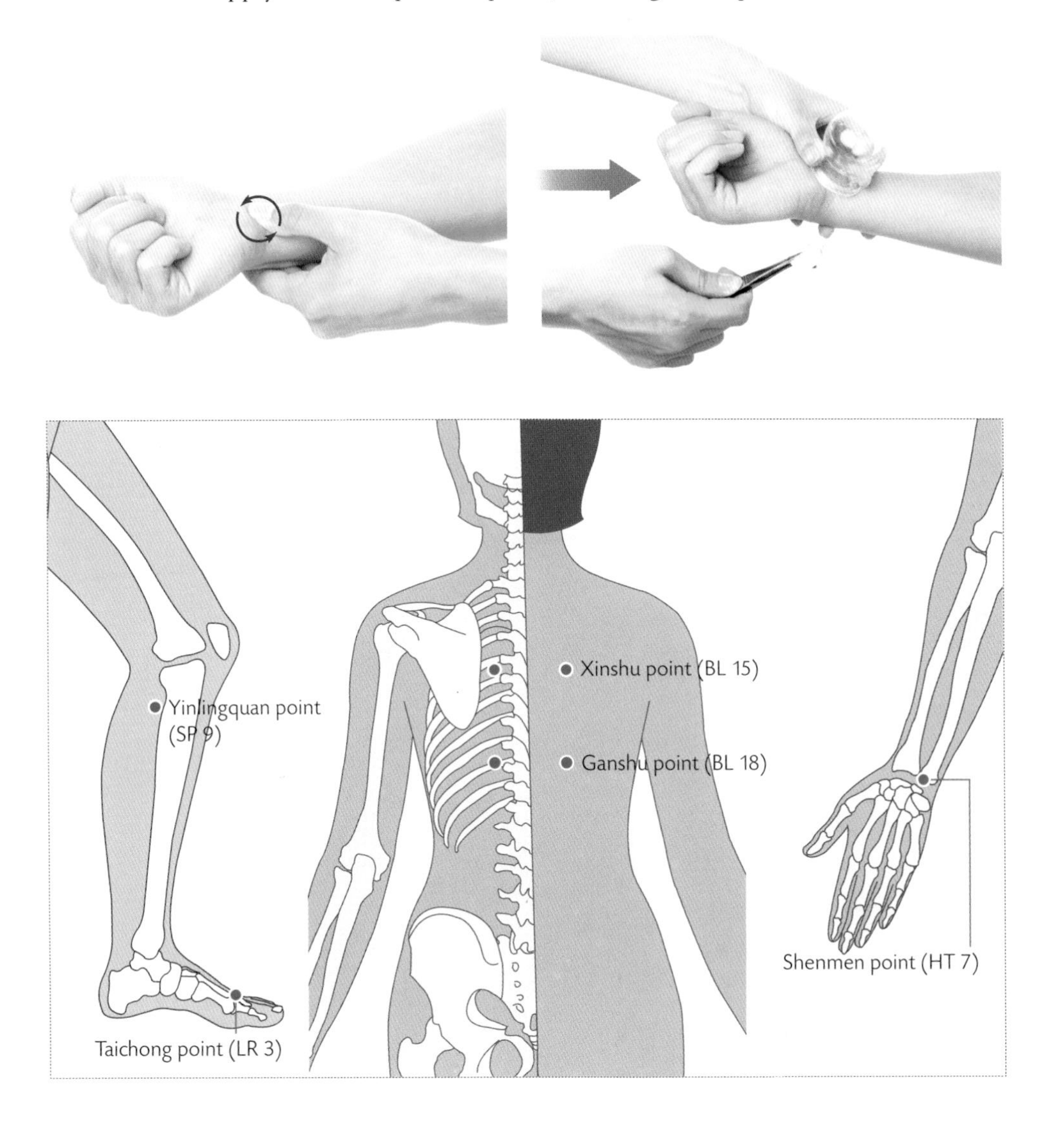

# 2 Dysmenorrhea

Patients suffer periodic abdominal pain, radiating to lumbosacral region, and even syncope due to severe pain before, during or after menstruation. It happens every month with the menstrual cycle, accompanied by nausea and vomiting, dripping cold sweat, cold hands and feet, and even fainting.

Women with dysmenorrhea, especially those who need long-term regulation, can drink more liquids with tonifying qi and blood, such as red ginger tea. Eating more donkey-hide gelatin and longan can also supplement qi and blood. Pay attention to menstrual health, avoid fatigue and cold, avoid swimming and bath, and do not exercise strenuously or have a sexual life during menstruation. The primary disease should be treated actively for secondary dysmenorrhea, and see a doctor when necessary.

Generally, the cupping should be performed 3–5 days before menstruation, until 2 days after menstruation. Two groups may be cupped, one group a day, and two groups in turn. The first group includes Diji, Shiqizhui, and Guanyuan points, and the second group includes Ganshu, Pishu, Geshu, Zhishi, and Guilai points.

## Cupping Methods

### The First Group of Points

#### 1. Diji Point

**Location:** 3 cun below the Yinlingquan point, on the line connecting the Yinlingquan point and the medial malleolus.

**Method:** First knead Diji point with the thumb pulp for 2–3 minutes until soreness and swelling is felt, and then select and apply a cup of appropriate size to the point, retaining the cup for 10–15 minutes. With the cup removed, perform moxibustion with a moxa stick for 3–5 minutes until warmth is felt.

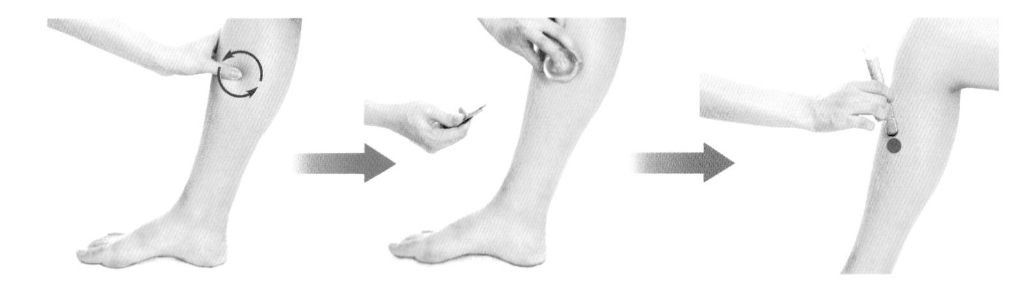

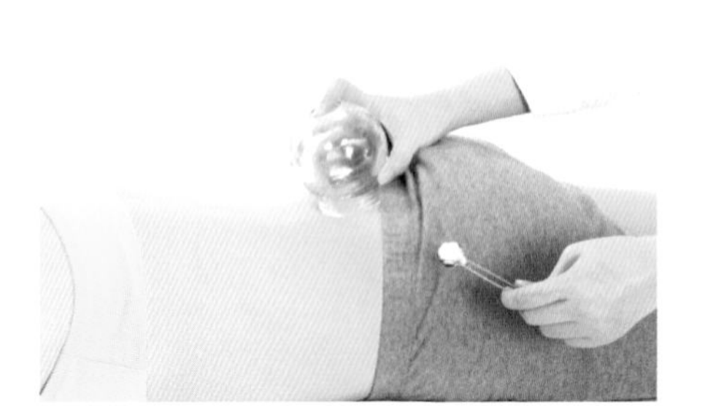

#### 2. Shiqizhui Point

**Location:** On the waist, on the posterior midline, in the depression below the spinous process of the fifth lumbar vertebra.

**Method:** Select and apply a cup of appropriate size to the point, retaining the cup for 10–15 minutes. With the cup removed, perform moxibustion with a moxa stick for 3–5 minutes until warmth is felt.

### 3. Guanyuan Point

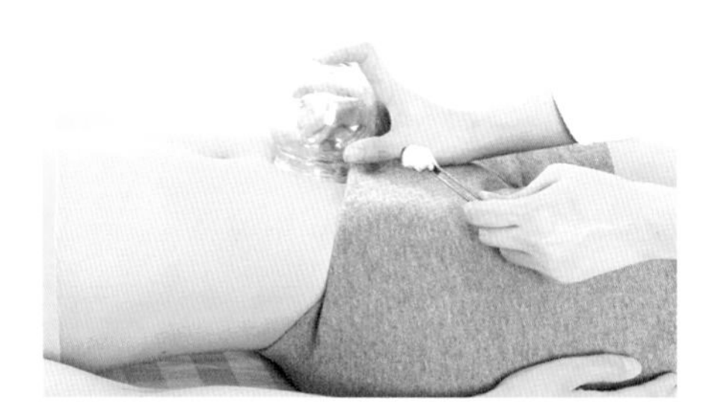

**Location:** About 3 cun below the navel.

**Method:** First knead Guanyuan point with the thumb pulp for 2–3 minutes, and then select and apply a cup of appropriate size to the point, retaining the cup for 10–15 minutes. With the cup removed, perform moxibustion with a moxa stick for 3–5 minutes until warmth is felt.

## The Second Group of Points

### 1. Ganshu, Pishu, Geshu and Zhishi Points

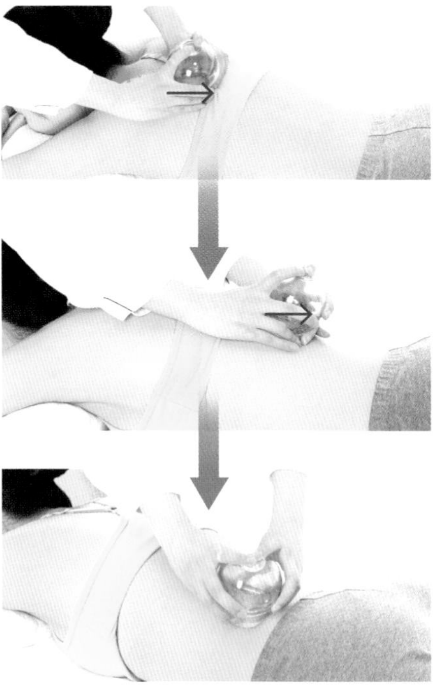

**Location:** Ganshu point is 1.5 cun away from the ninth thoracic spinal process on the inner side of the scapula; Pishu point is 1.5 cun away horizontally from the eleventh thoracic vertebra; Geshu point is 1.5 cun away from the spinous process of the seventh thoracic vertebra; Zhishi point is 3 cun away from the spinous process of the second lumbar vertebra.

**Method:** Use the moving cupping method. Move the cup on the bladder meridian on the back by segment along the meridian, and move it several times mainly on the four points. Repeatedly push and pull on the points back and forth, until the skin becomes red. The cup may be retained on the points for 10–15 minutes after the moving cupping. With the cup removed, perform moxibustion with a moxa stick for 3–5 minutes until warmth is felt.

### 2. Guilai Point

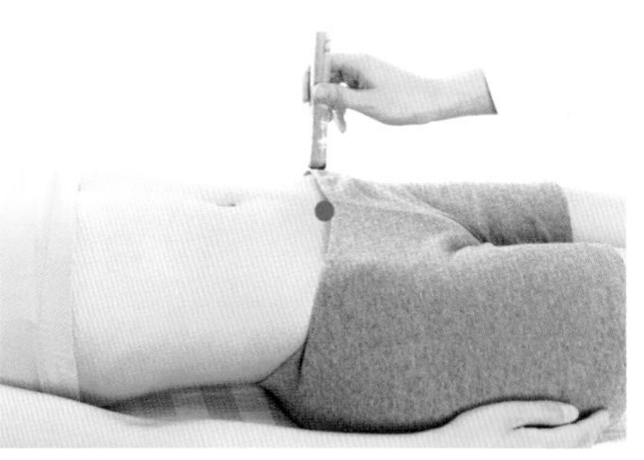

**Location:** 4 cun below the navel and two cun away from the frontal middle line.

**Method:** Select and apply a cup of appropriate size to the point, retaining the cup for 10–15 minutes. With the cup removed, perform moxibustion with a moxa stick for 3–5 minutes until warmth is felt.

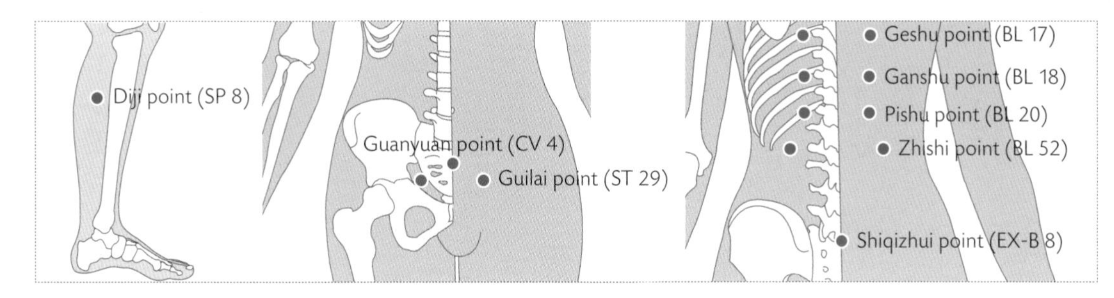

# 3 Hyperplasia of Mammary Glands

Patients feel breast pains which are often distending pain or stabbing pain, and can involve one or both sides of the breast, with a single or multiple lumps. A small number of patients may appear nipple discharge, mostly in light yellow or light milky white color.

To prevent this disease, one should have self-examination and regular re-examination, and should see a doctor for treatment if the lump continues to increase. Patients are prohibited from the abuse of contraceptives and estrogen-containing cosmetic products or food. Keep a comfortable and optimistic mood. Patients should change the diet structure, prevent obesity, eat less fried foods, animal fats, and sweets, and do not eat too much tonic food, but eat more vegetables and fruits, whole grains, walnuts, black sesame seeds, fungus, mushrooms and so on.

The cupping should be performed mainly on Danzhong, Hegu, Taichong, Ganshu, Pishu, Shenshu, Zusanli, and Sanyinjiao points.

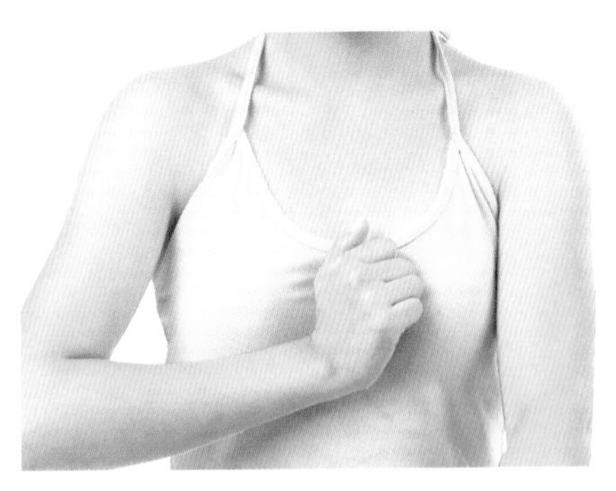

## Cupping Methods

### 1. Danzhong Point

**Location:** Directly in the middle of the chest between the nipples.

**Method:** First, knead from Danzhong point towards the affected side with the thenar muscle at palm heel for 3–5 minutes, and then select and apply a cup of appropriate size to Danzhong point, retaining the cup for 10–15 minutes.

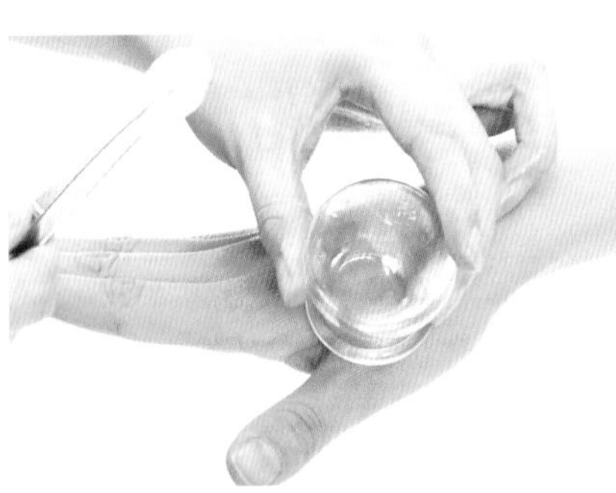

### 2. Hegu Point

**Location:** In the highest point on the back of the hand between the thumb base and the base of the index finger (in the webbing between these two fingers).

**Method:** First knead Hegu point with the thumb pulp for 2–3 minutes, and then select and apply a cup of appropriate size to the point, retaining the cup for 5–10 minutes.

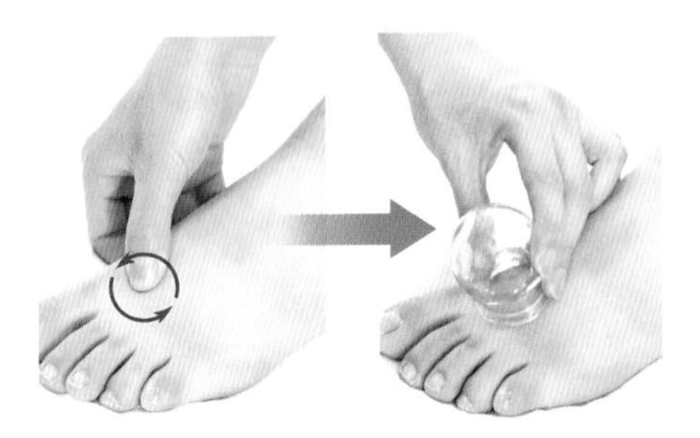

### 3. Taichong Point

**Location:** On the foot in a notch between the first and second metatarsal bones.

**Method:** First knead Taichong point with the thumb pulp for 2–3 minutes, and then apply a small cup to the point, retaining the cup for 5–10 minutes.

### 4. Ganshu, Pishu and Shenshu Points

**Location:** Ganshu point is 1.5 cun away from the ninth thoracic spinal process on the inner side of the scapula; Pishu point is 1.5 cun away horizontally from the eleventh thoracic vertebra; Shenshu point is 1.5 cun horizontally from the second lumbar spinal process.

**Method:** Use the moving cupping method. Move the cup on the bladder meridian on the back by segment along the meridian, and move the cup several times mainly on Ganshu, Pishu and Shenshu points. Repeatedly push and pull on the points back and forth, until the skin becomes red. The cup may be retained on the abovementioned points for 10–15 minutes after the moving cupping.

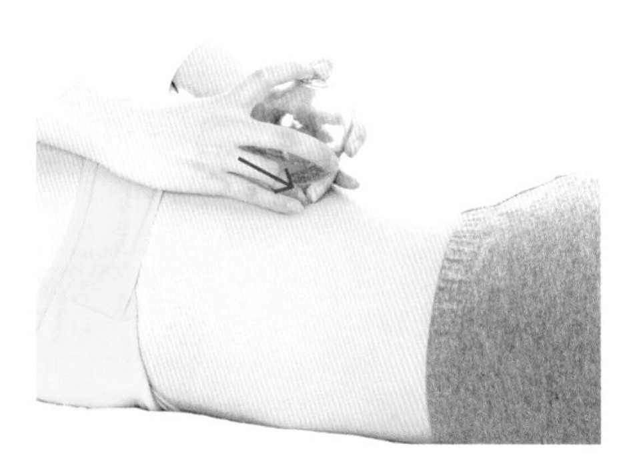

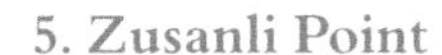

### 5. Zusanli Point

**Location:** About 3 cun below the knee on the outer side of the tibia.

**Method:** Select a cup of appropriate size and apply it to the point, retaining it for 10–15 minutes.

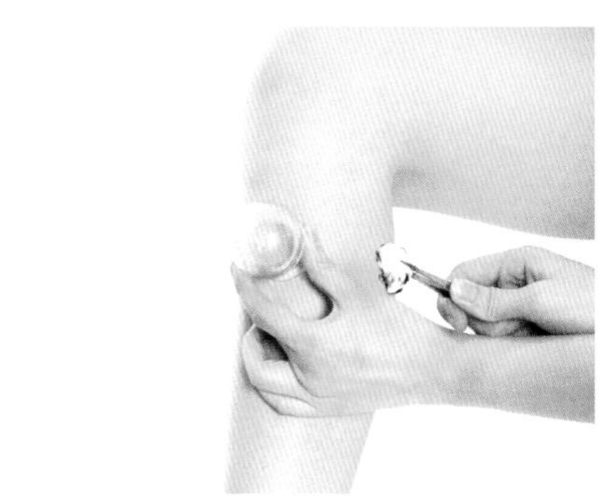

### 6. Sanyinjiao Point

**Location:** At the rear edge of the shinbone, 3 cun above the ankle.

**Method:** First knead Sanyinjiao point with the thumb pulp for 2–3 minutes, and then select and apply a cup of appropriate size to the point, retaining the cup for 10–15 minutes.

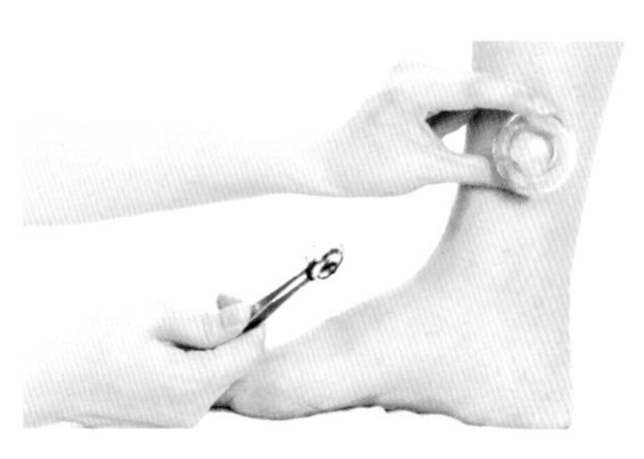

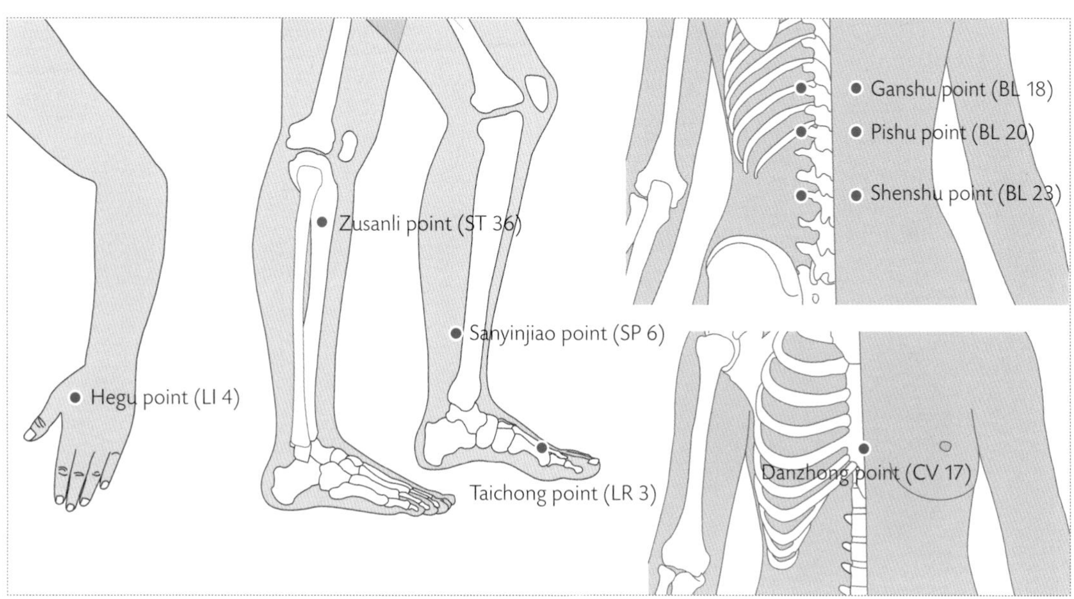

# 4 Female Infertility

Female infertility refers to a woman who is not pregnant after the couple has cohabited for two years after marriage, with a normal sex life, and without contraception, and the man's reproductive function is normal.

Women can drink more brown sugar tea and ginger tea, but less coffee, and avoid eating roast beef and mutton. The cupping treatment of infertility is only an adjunctive therapy, but cannot completely replace other therapies. The primary disease should be treated actively for infertility of other causes.

The cupping should be applied to Zigong, Zhongji, Guanyuan, Sanyinjiao, Xuehai, Zusanli, and Guilai points.

## Cupping Methods

### 1. Zigong Point

**Location:** 4 cun below the navel and three cun away from the frontal middle line.

**Method:** Select and apply a cup of appropriate size to the point, retaining the cup for 10–15 minutes.

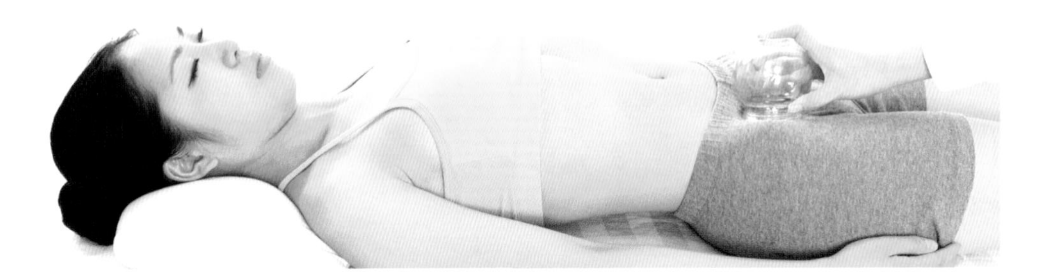

### 2. Zhongji Point

**Location:** On the lower abdomen, 4 cun below the center of the umbilicus, on the anterior midline.

**Method:** Select and apply a cup of appropriate size to the point, retaining the cup for 10–15 minutes.

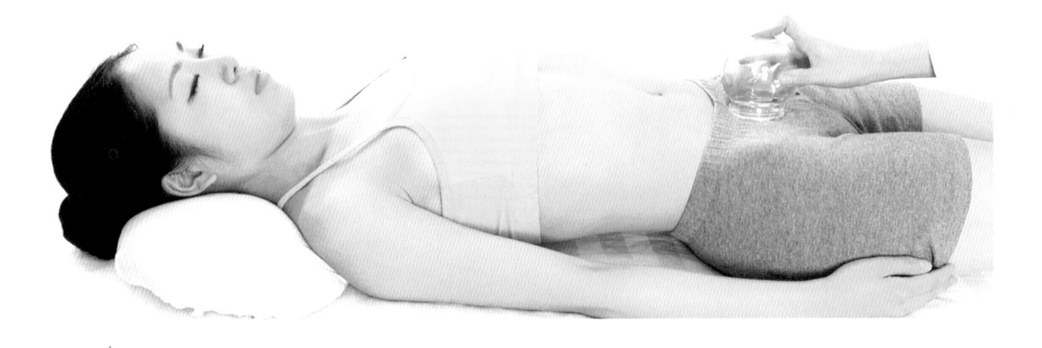

### 3. Guanyuan Point

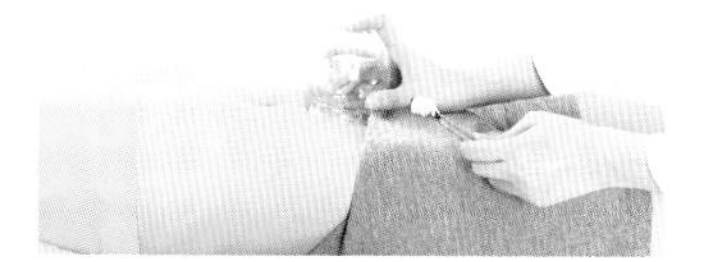

**Location:** About 3 cun below the navel.

**Method:** Select and apply a cup of appropriate size to the point, retaining the cup for 10–15 minutes.

### 4. Sanyinjiao Point

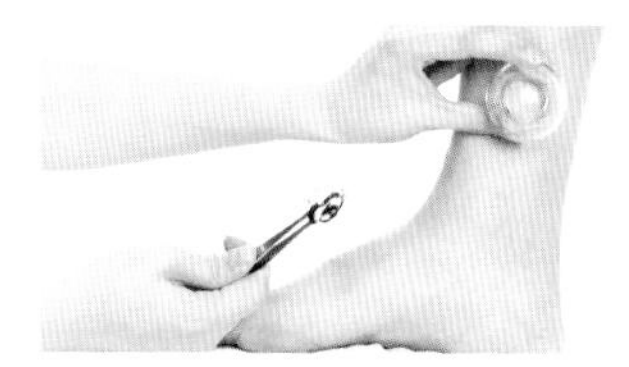

**Location:** At the rear edge of the shinbone, 3 cun above the ankle.

**Method:** Select and apply a cup of appropriate size to the point, retaining the cup for 10–15 minutes.

### 5. Xuehai Point

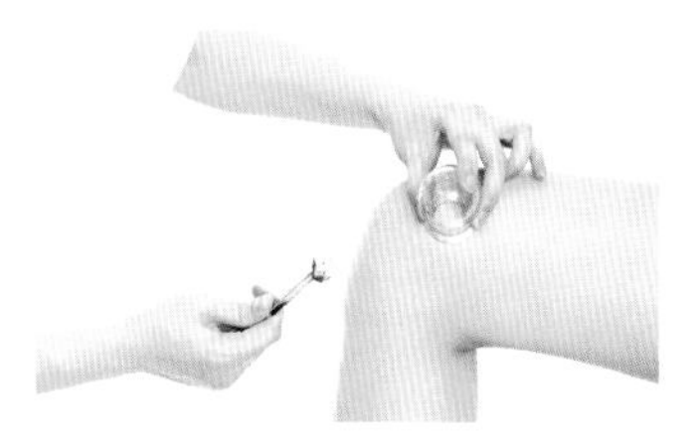

**Location:** In a cavity about 2 cun away from the inner upper corner of the patella, when the knee is bent.

**Method:** Select and apply a cup of appropriate size to the point, retaining the cup for 10–15 minutes.

### 6. Zusanli Point

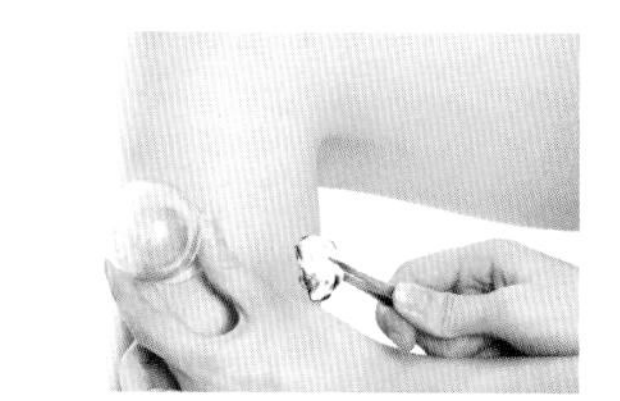

**Location:** About 3 cun below the knee on the outer side of the tibia.

**Method:** Select and apply a cup of appropriate size to the point, retaining the cup for 10–15 minutes.

### 7. Guilai Point

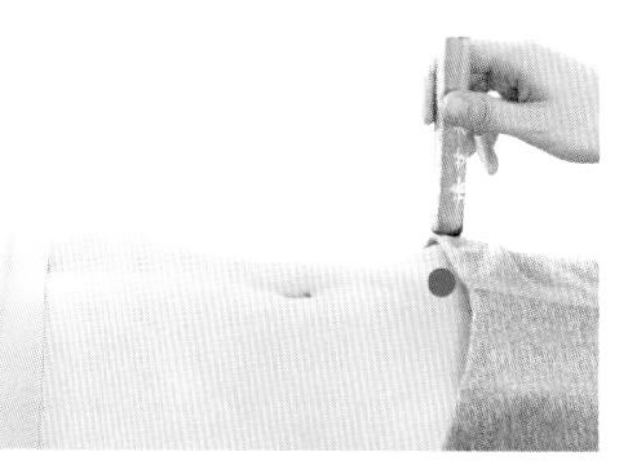

**Location:** 4 cun below the navel and two cun away from the frontal middle line.

**Method:** Select and apply a cup of appropriate size to the point, retaining the cup for 10–15 minutes. With the cup removed, perform moxibustion with a moxa stick for 3–5 minutes until warmth is felt.

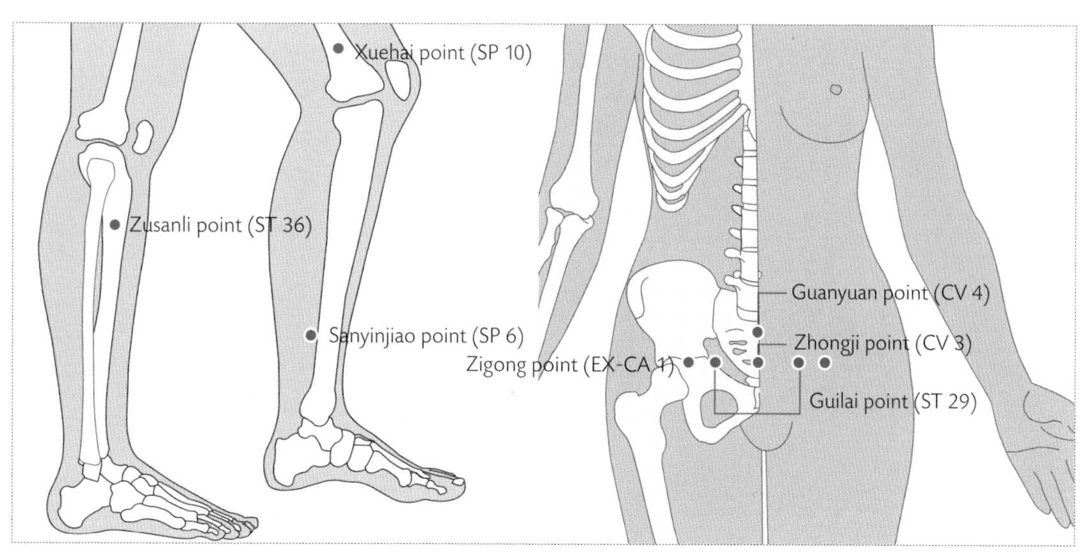

# 5 Chronic Pelvic Inflammation

The patients suffer from the aching pain on the lower abdomen and lumbosacral region, often intensified after being tired or sexual intercourse, before and after menstruation. Some may have low-grade fever and are prone to fatigue. Some can lead to secondary infertility.

To prevent the disease, women should pay attention to menstrual health, and avoid fatigue, cold, swimming and bath. As the course of the disease is long, women should diagnose and treat early, adhere to long-term cupping, and cooperate actively with medication.

The cupping can be applied to two groups of points, one group a day and two groups in turn, until the symptoms are alleviated or disappear. The first group mainly includes Ciliao, Baihuanshu, Guanyuan, Zhongji, and Shuidao points, and the second group includes Yinlingquan, Sanyinjiao, Dazhui, Shiqizhui, and Yaoyan points.

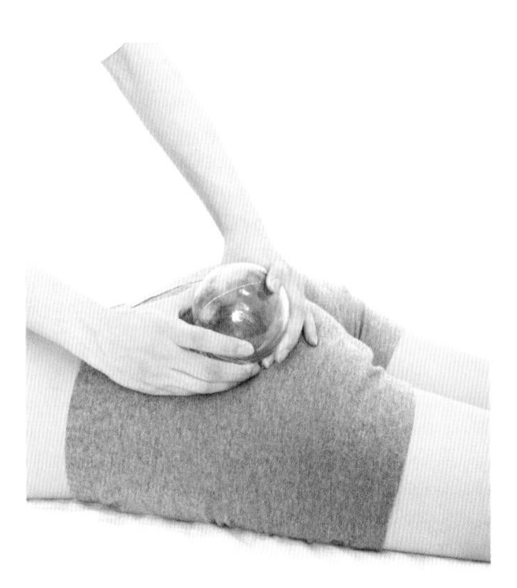

## Cupping Methods

### The First Group of Points

#### 1. Ciliao and Baihuanshu Points

**Location:** Ciliao point is in the sacral region, in the second posterior sacral foramen; Bihuanshu point is in the sacral region, at the same level as the fourth posterior sacral foramen, 1.5 cun lateral to the median sacral crest.

**Method:** Move the cup continuously on the lumbosacral region, focusing on Ciliao and Baihuanshu points, until the skin becomes red. Cup on Ciliao point, and retain the cup for 10–15 minutes. After the cup is removed, perform moxibustion with a moxa stick for 3–5 minutes until warmth is felt.

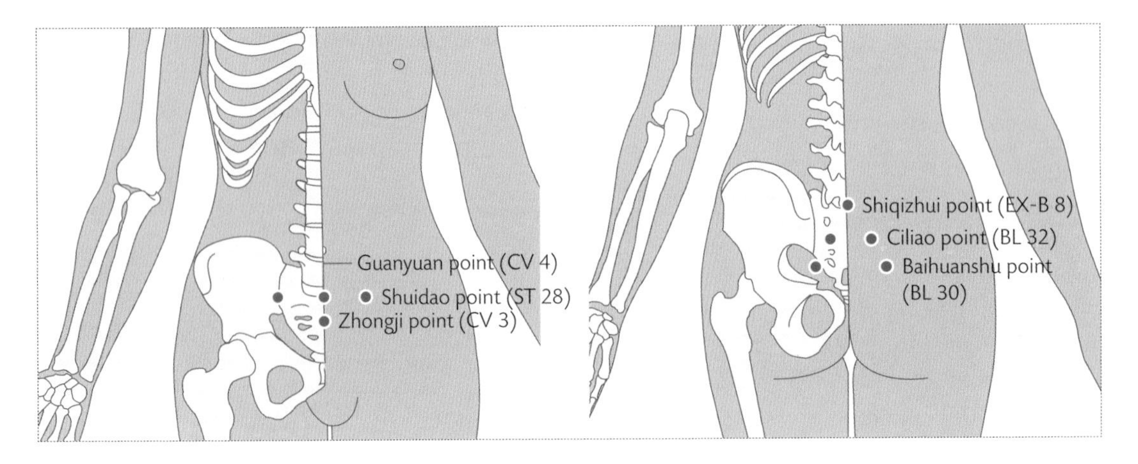

### 2. Guanyuan Point

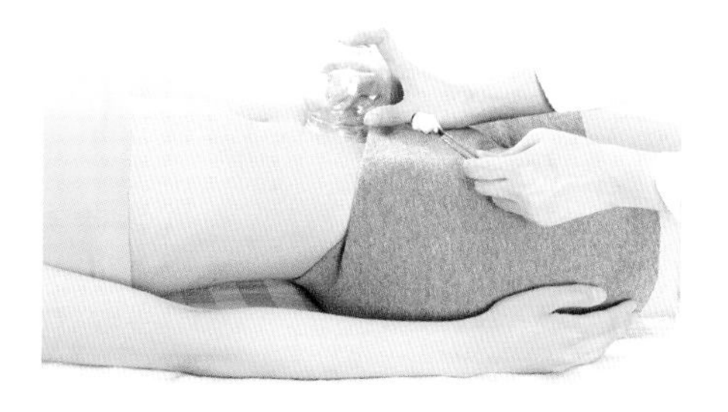

**Location:** About 3 cun below the navel.

**Method:** First knead Guanyuan point with the thumb pulp for 2–3 minutes, and then select and apply a cup of appropriate size to the point, retaining the cup for 10–15 minutes. With the cup removed, perform moxibustion with a moxa stick for 3–5 minutes until warmth is felt.

### 3. Zhongji Point

**Location:** On the lower abdomen, 4 cun below the center of the umbilicus, on the anterior midline.

**Method:** First knead Zhongji point with the thumb pulp for 2–3 minutes, and then select and apply a cup of appropriate size to the point, retaining the cup for 10–15 minutes. With the cup removed, perform moxibustion with a moxa stick for 3–5 minutes until warmth is felt.

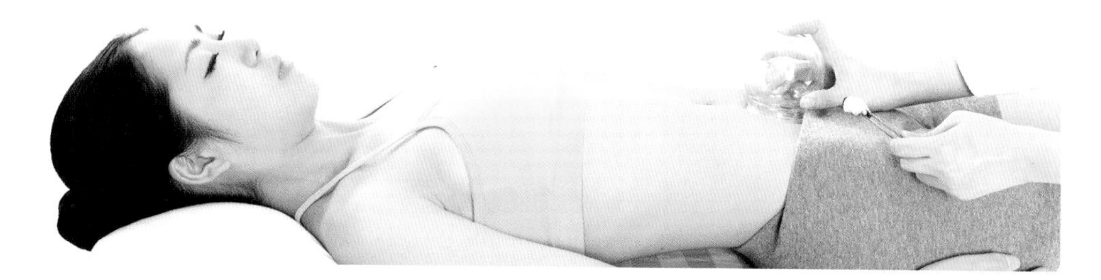

### 4. Shuidao Point

**Location:** 3 cun below the navel and two cun from the frontal middle line.

**Method:** Select and apply a cup of appropriate size to the point, retaining the cup for 10–15 minutes.

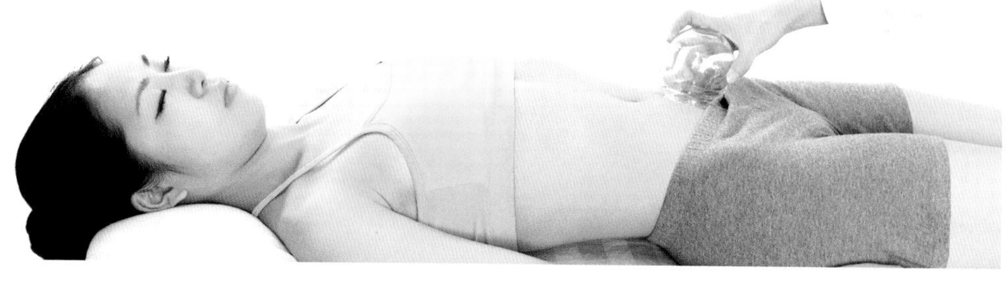

## The Second Group of Points

### 1. Shiqizhui Point

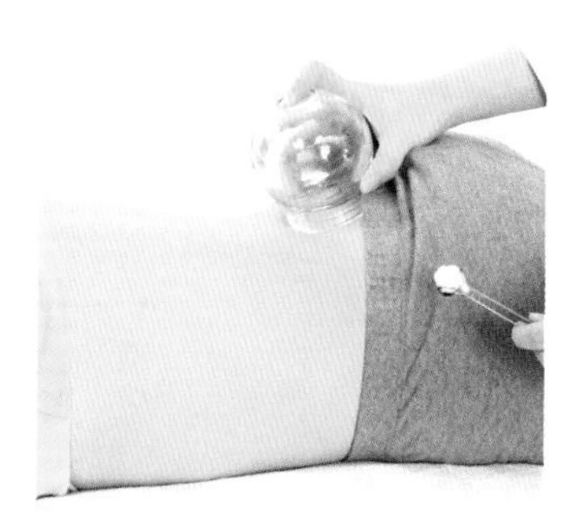

**Location:** On the waist, on the posterior midline, in the depression below the spinous process of the fifth lumbar vertebra.

**Method:** Apply a cup to the point, retaining the cup for 10–15 minutes. With the cup removed, perform moxibustion with a moxa stick for 3–5 minutes until warmth is felt.

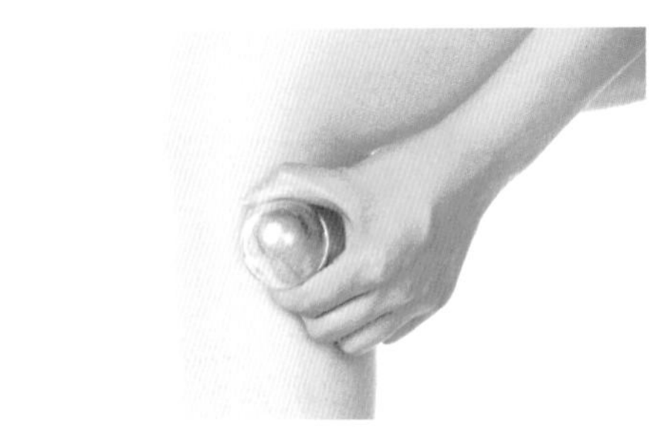

### 2. Yinlingquan Point

**Location:** In the depression on the inner edge of the shinbone below the knee.

**Method:** First knead Yinlingquan point with the thumb pulp for 2–3 minutes, and then cup this point, retaining the cup for 10–15 minutes. With the cup removed, perform moxibustion with a moxa stick for 3–5 minutes.

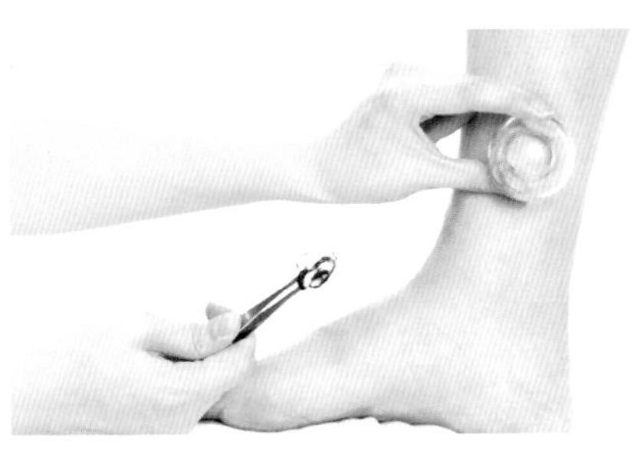

### 3. Sanyinjiao Point

**Location:** At the rear edge of the shinbone, 3 cun above the ankle.

**Method:** First knead Sanyinjiao point with the thumb pulp for 2–3 minutes, and then select and apply a cup of appropriate size to the point, retaining the cup for 10–15 minutes. Then perform moxibustion with a moxa stick for 3–5 minutes until warmth is felt.

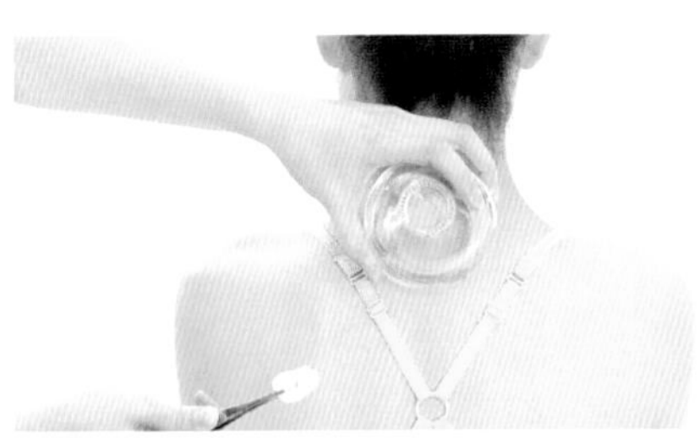

### 4. Dazhui Point

**Location:** Under the spinous process of the seventh cervical vertebrae.

**Method:** Select a cup of appropriate size and apply it to Dazhui point. Retain the cup for 10–15 minutes.

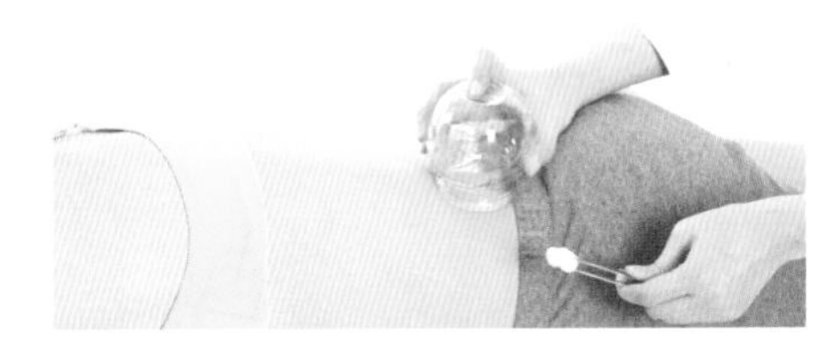

### 5. Yaoyan Point

**Location:** 3.5 cun away from the spinous process of the fourth lumbar vertebra.

**Method:** Select a cup of appropriate size and apply it to Yaoyan point. Retain the cup for 10–15 minutes.

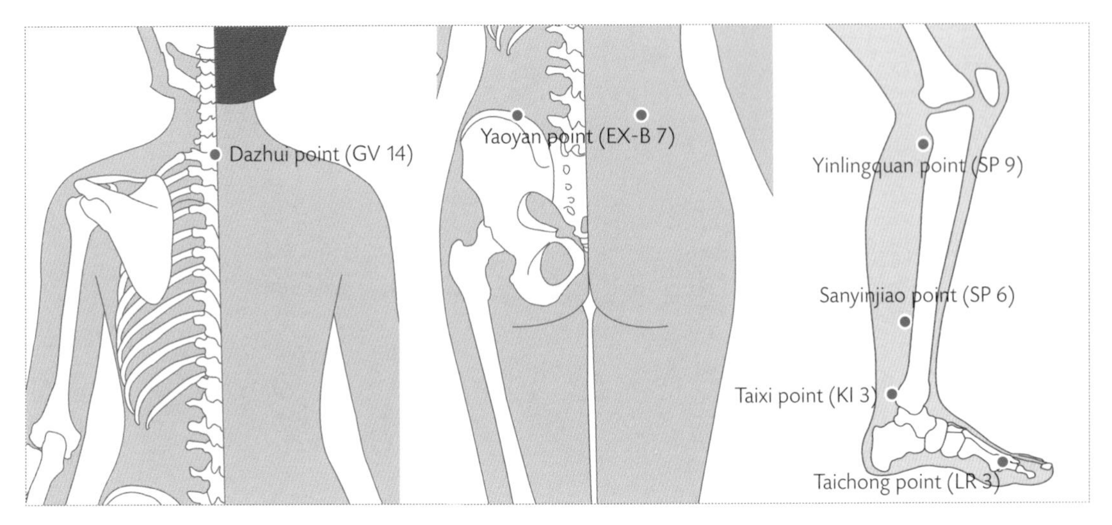

# 6 Menopausal Syndrome

The patient with this disease suffer from menstrual disorders, accompanied by dizziness, palpitations, insomnia, dream-disturbed sleep, irritability, inattention, memory loss, and even frequent urination, urgency of urination, blood pressure increase, and so on.

The patient should always keep ease of the mind, and have a correct attitude towards the menopausal syndromes. Appropriately participate in physical exercise to enhance physical fitness and improve resistance. For diet, they can often eat coix seeds, red dates, corns, angelica, black sesame seeds, and other foods that tonify the qi and blood.

The cupping should be performed on Sanyinjiao, Taixi, and Taichong points, in conjunction with Ganshu, Shenshu, and Qihai points for deficiency in the liver and the kidney, and Pishu, Zusanli, and Yinlingquan points for liver depression and blood deficiency.

## Cupping Methods

### 1. Sanyinjiao Point

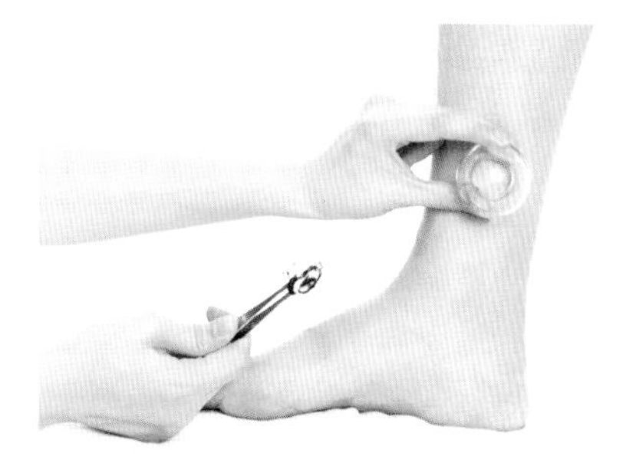

**Location:** At the rear edge of the shinbone, 3 cun above the ankle.

**Method:** Knead Sanyinjiao point with the thumb pulp for 2–3 minutes, and then cup this point, retaining the cup for 10–15 minutes.

### 2. Taixi Point

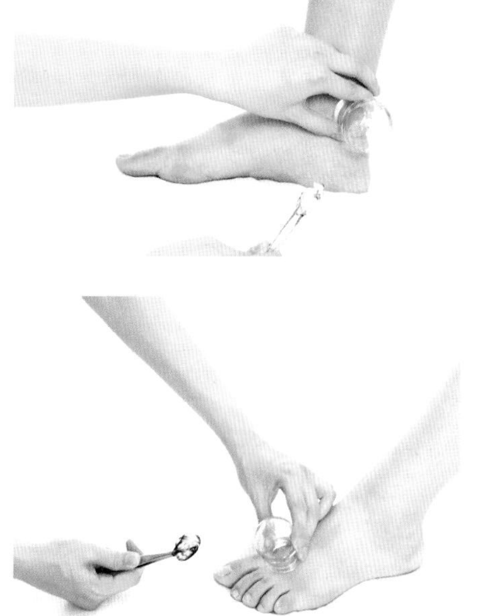

**Location:** In a cavity between the medial malleolus and Achilles tendon.

**Method:** First knead Taixi point with the thumb pulp for 2–3 minutes, and then select a cup of appropriate size and apply it to the point, retaining the cup for 10–15 minutes.

### 3. Taichong Point

**Location:** On the foot in a notch between the first and second metatarsal bones.

**Method:** First knead Taichong point with the thumb pulp for 2–3 minutes, and then select and apply a cup of appropriate size to the point, retaining the cup for 10–15 minutes.

### 4. Ganshu and Shenshu Points

**Location:** Ganshu point is 1.5 cun away from the ninth thoracic spinal process on the inner side of the scapula; Shenshu point is 1.5 cun horizontally from the second lumbar spinal process.

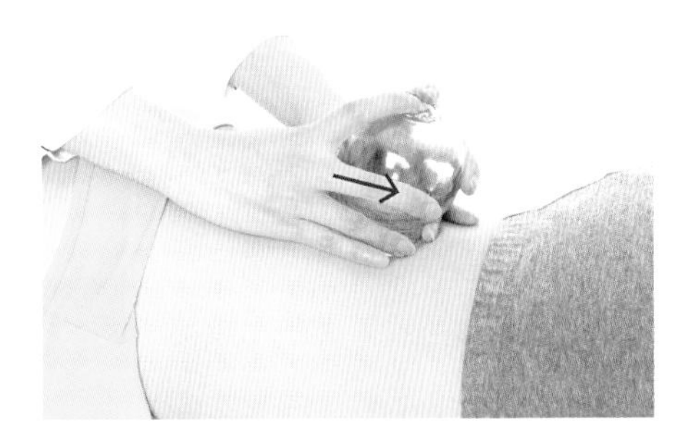

**Method:** Use the moving cupping method by moving the cup on the bladder meridian on the back by segment along the meridian. Move the cup several times mainly on Ganshu and Shenshu points, and repeatedly push and pull on the points back and forth, until the skin becomes red. The cup may be retained on the abovementioned points for 10–15 minutes after the moving cupping.

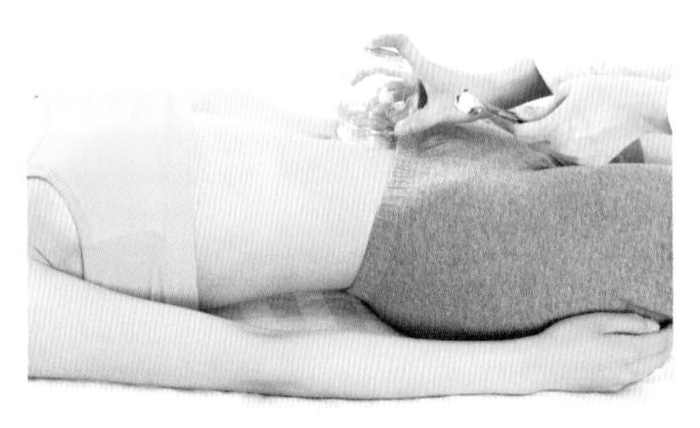

### 5. Qihai Point

**Location:** About 1.5 cun below the navel.

**Method:** First knead Qihai point with the thumb pulp for 2–3 minutes, and then select and apply a cup of appropriate size to the point, retaining the cup for 10–15 minutes. With the cup removed, perform moxibustion with a moxa stick for 3–5 minutes until warmth is felt.

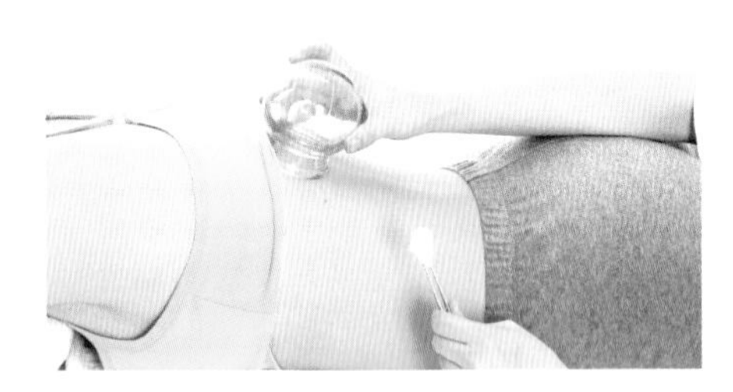

### 6. Pishu Point

**Location:** 1.5 cun away horizontally from the eleventh thoracic vertebra.

**Method:** Select and apply a cup of appropriate size to the point, retaining the cup for 10–15 minutes.

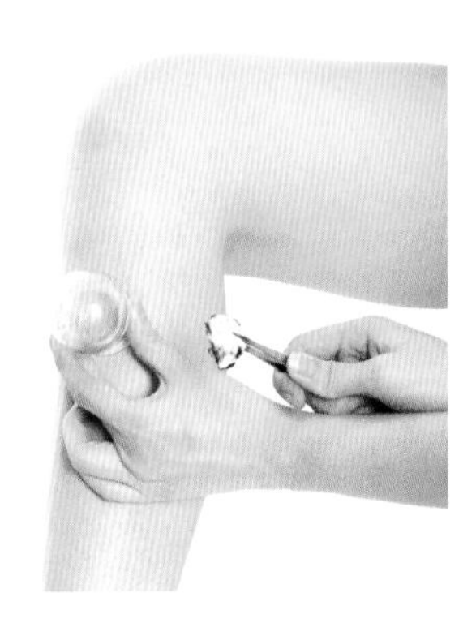

### 7. Zusanli Point

**Location:** About 3 cun below the knee on the outer side of the tibia.

**Method:** First knead Zusanli point with the thumb pulp for 2–3 minutes, and then select a cup of appropriate size and apply it to the point, retaining the cup for 10–15 minutes. With the cup removed, perform moxibustion with a moxa stick for 3–5 minutes until warmth is felt.

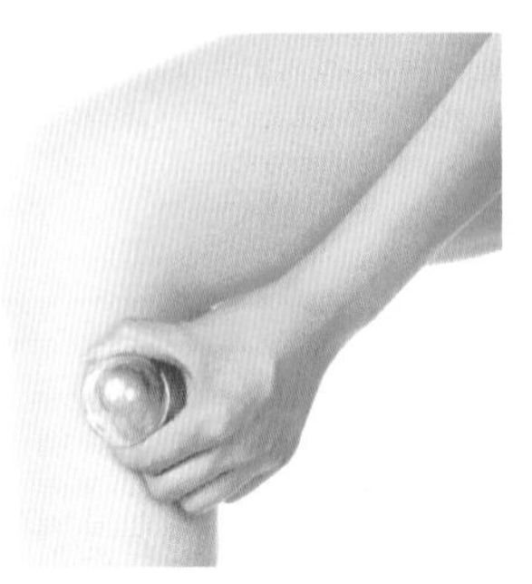

### 8. Yinlingquan Point

**Location:** In the depression on the inner edge of the shinbone below the knee.

**Method:** First knead Yinlingquan point with the thumb pulp for 2–3 minutes, and then select a cup of appropriate size and apply it to the point, retaining the cup for 10–15 minutes. With the cup removed, perform moxibustion with a moxa stick for 3–5 minutes until warmth is felt.

# 7 Postpartum Hypogalactia

The symptoms of this disease are insufficient or no milk, and during lactation, milk drops after being squeezed and is thin, or the breast is big with pieces of mammary gland, and milk is thick and difficult to drip when squeezed with pain, or no milk at all.

If the amount of breast milk is indeed little, some Chinese medicine may be used for promoting lactation, for example, cowherb seed, pith of rice-paper plant, ligusticum wallichii, angelica and astragalus. For diet, increase the mother's nutrition, eat foods rich in protein, carbohydrates, vitamins and minerals, like milk, eggs, fish, vegetables, fruits, drink more ham carp soup and soy trotter soup. Mothers should develop good breast-feeding habits, and feed as needed and frequently. In general, suck another side after one side is sucked empty. If the breasts are not emptied, the extra milk should be squeezed out.

The cupping should be applied to Danzhong, Shaoze, Ruzhong, Rugen, Ganshu, and Pishu points.

## Cupping Methods

### 1. Danzhong Point

**Location:** Directly in the middle of the chest between the nipples.

**Method:** First, knead from Danzhong point towards the breast with the thenar muscle at the palm feel for 3–5 minutes, and then select and apply a cup of appropriate size to Danzhong point, retain the cup for 10–15 minutes. Then perform moxibustion with a moxa stick for 3–5 minutes until warmth is felt.

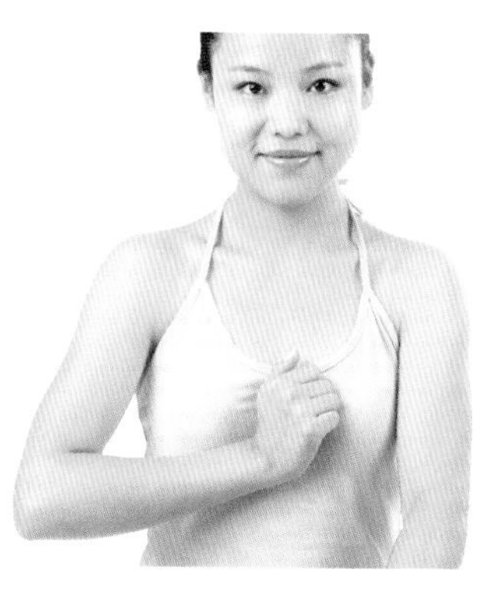

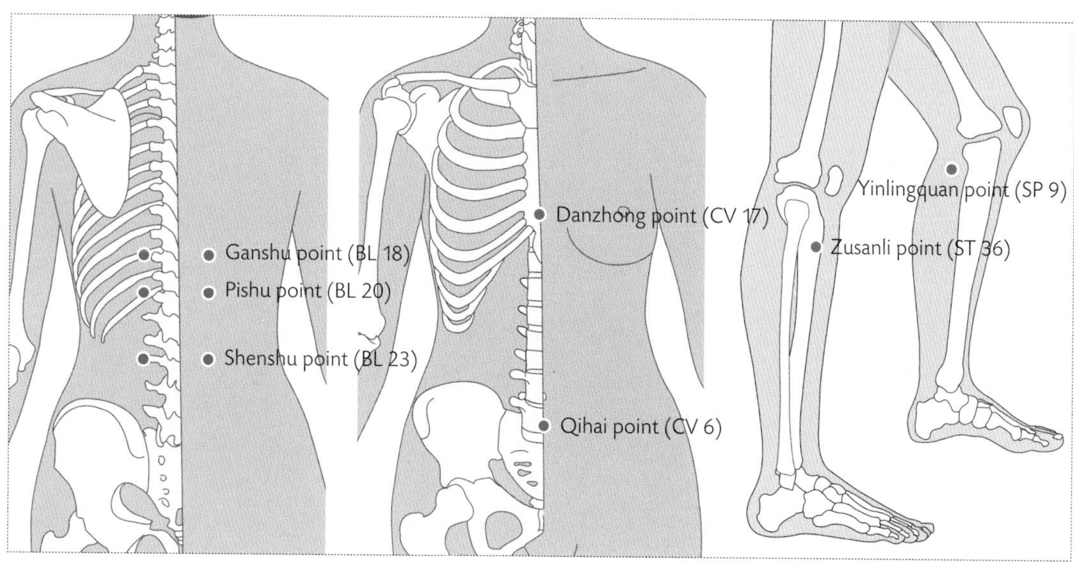

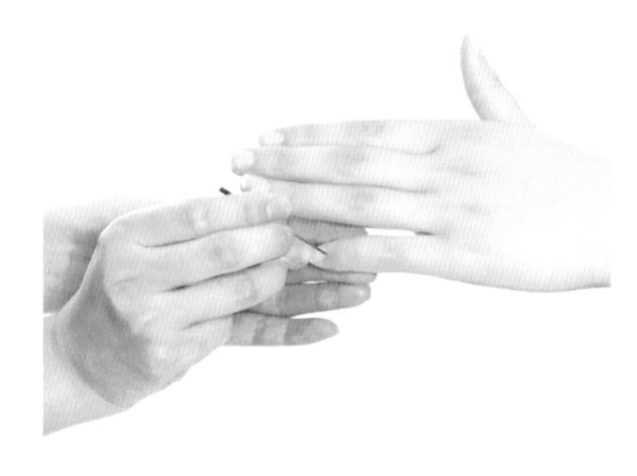

## 2. Shaoze and Ruzhong Points

**Location:** Shaoze point is at the bottom corner of the nail bed on the outer side of the small finger; Ruzhong point is at the center of the nipple.

**Method:** Ask a professional to first pierce Shaoze point to bleed 5–10 drops, and then knead the breast. If there is a white or yellow rice-like substance blocking the nipple, it can be picked with a disinfected lancet, or wash with white vinegar and salt. Then select a cup of appropriate size to cup Ruzhong point, retain the cup for 3–5 minutes until milk is discharged.

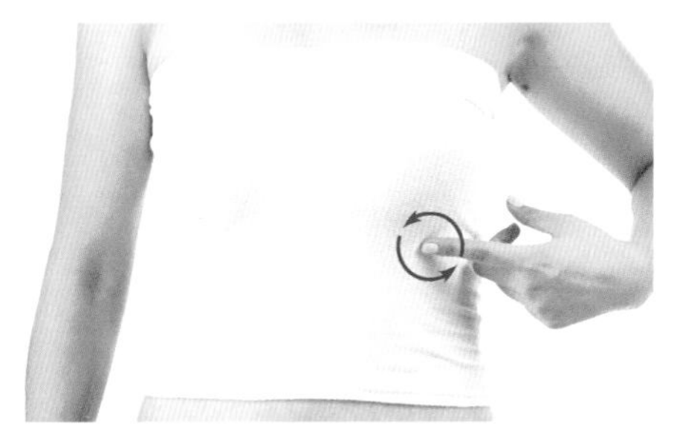

## 3. Rugen Point

**Location:** In the fifth intercostal space at the base of the breast, directly under the nipple.

**Method:** First knead Rugen point with the index finger for 2–3 minutes, and then select a cup of appropriate size and apply it to the point, retaining the cup for 3–5 minutes.

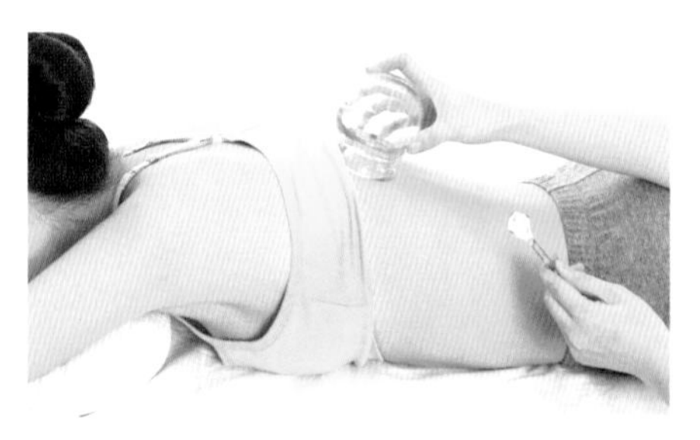

## 4. Ganshu Point

**Location:** 1.5 cun away from the ninth thoracic spinal process on the inner side of the scapula.

**Method:** Select a cup of appropriate size and apply it to the point, retaining the cup for 10–15 minutes.

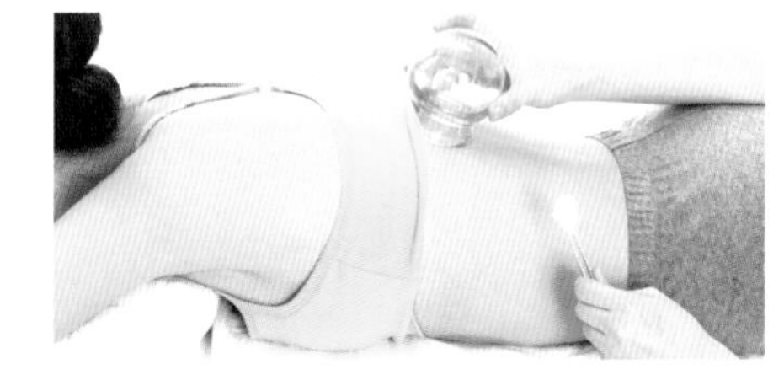

## 5. Pishu Point

**Location:** 1.5 cun away horizontally from the eleventh thoracic vertebra.

**Method:** Select a cup of appropriate size and apply it to the point, retaining the cup for 10–15 minutes.

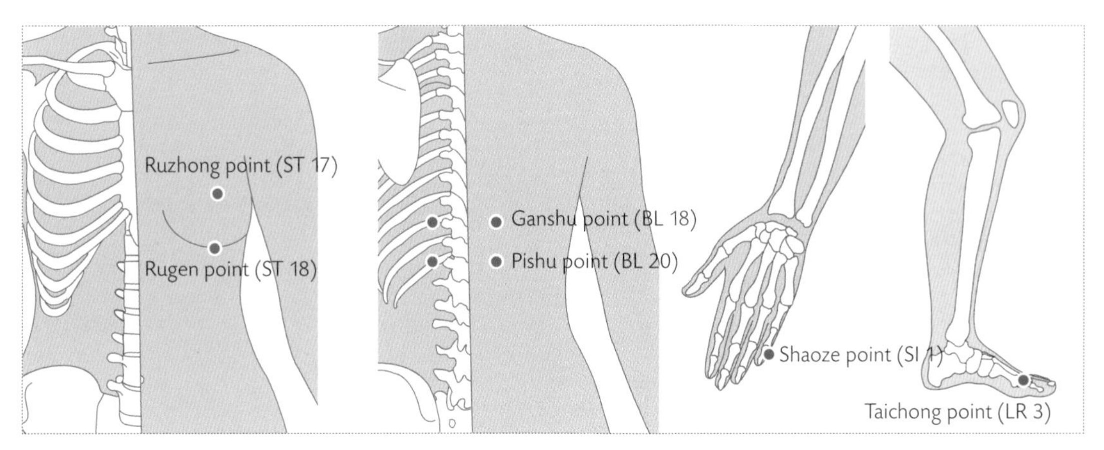

# 8 Irregular Menstruation

The symptoms of this disease include abnormal menstrual cycle or bleeding, abdominal pain and general symptoms all over the body before and during menstruation, advanced menstruation, delayed menstruation, irregular and intermittent bleeding between periods, and so on.

The patients may eat more black-bone chicken, mutton, roe, freshwater shrimp, prawns, red dates, mussels, black beans, sea cucumber, walnuts, and any other food supplementing qi and nourishing blood and food with higher iron content. They should pay attention to their menstrual health, and eat less raw, cold, spicy, and irritating food during or before menstruation. If necessary, one needs to go to the hospital for examination.

Generally, the cupping should be performed 3–5 days before menstruation, until 2 days after menstruation, and may be performed in two groups, one group a day, with two groups in turn. The first group includes Taichong, Diji, Xuehai, and Ciliao points, and the second group includes Sanyinjiao, Yinlingquan, Taixi, Ganshu, Pishu, and Shenshu points.

## Cupping Methods

### The First Group of Points

#### 1. Taichong Point

**Location:** On the foot in a notch between the first and second metatarsal bones.

**Method:** First knead Taichong point with the thumb pulp for 2–3 minutes until soreness and swelling is felt, and then select and apply a cup of appropriate size to the point, retaining the cup for 10–15 minutes.

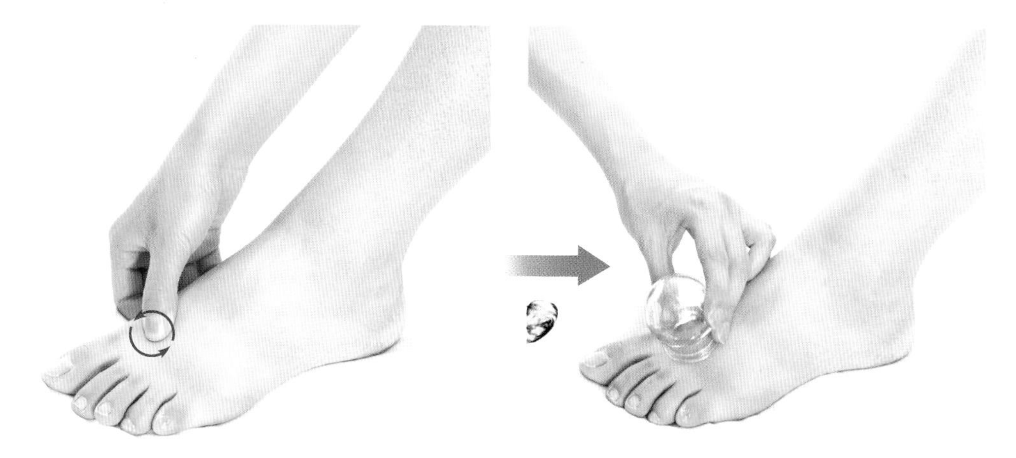

#### 2. Diji Point

**Location:** 3 cun below the Yinlingquan point, on the line connecting the Yinlingquan point and the medial malleolus.

**Method:** First knead Diji point with the thumb pulp for 2–3 minutes until soreness and swelling is felt, and then select and apply a cup of appropriate size to the point, retaining the cup for 10–15 minutes. With the cup removed, perform moxibustion with a moxa stick for 3–5 minutes until warmth is felt.

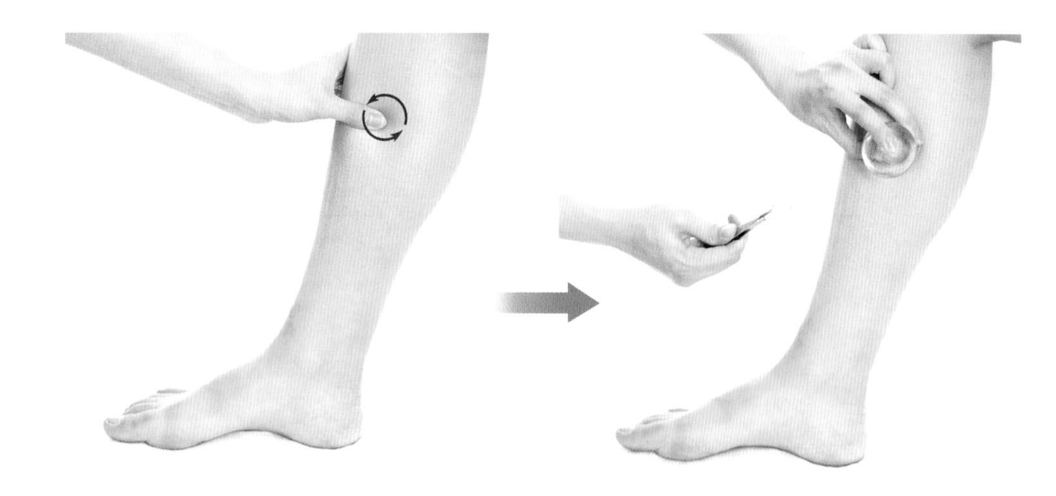

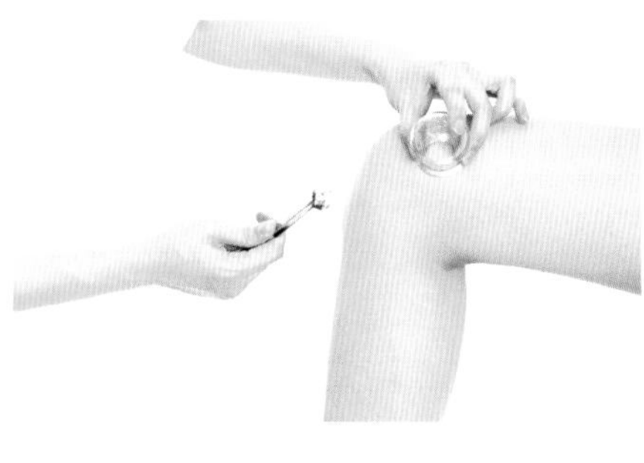

### 3. Xuehai Point

**Location:** In a cavity about 2 cun away from the inner upper corner of the patella, when the knee is bent.

**Method:** Select and apply a cup of appropriate size to the point, retaining the cup for 10–15 minutes. With the cup removed, perform moxibustion with a moxa stick for 3–5 minutes until warmth is felt.

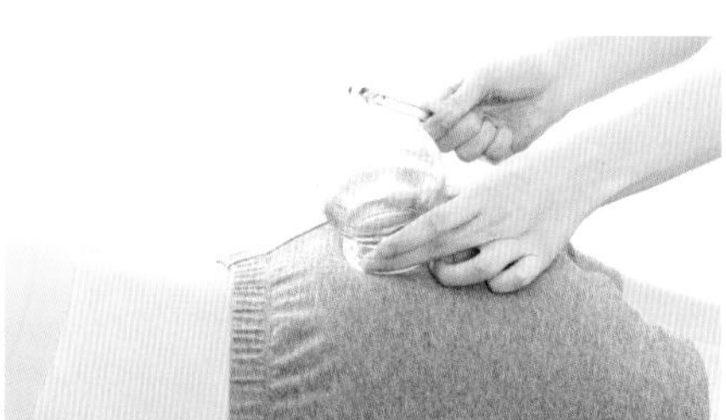

### 4. Ciliao Point

**Location:** In the sacral region, in the second posterior sacral foramen.

**Method:** Apply a cup of appropriate size to the point, retaining the cup for 10–15 minutes. With the cup removed, perform moxibustion with a moxa stick for 3–5 minutes until warmth is felt.

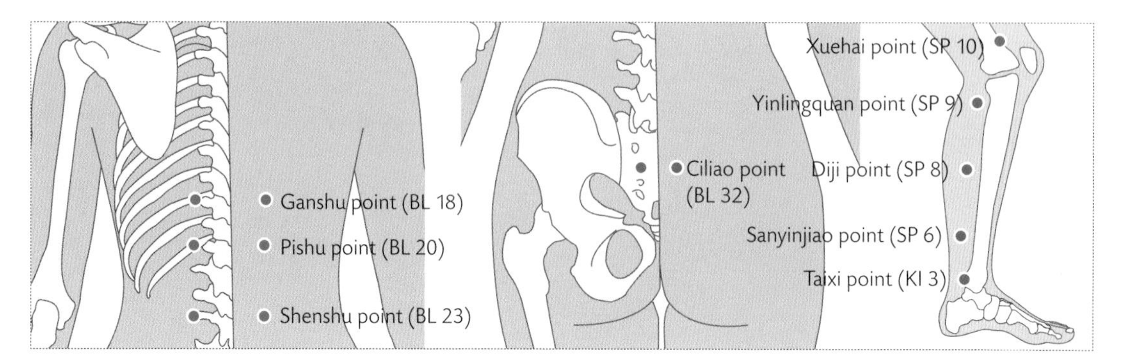

### The Second Group of Points

#### 1. Sanyinjiao Point

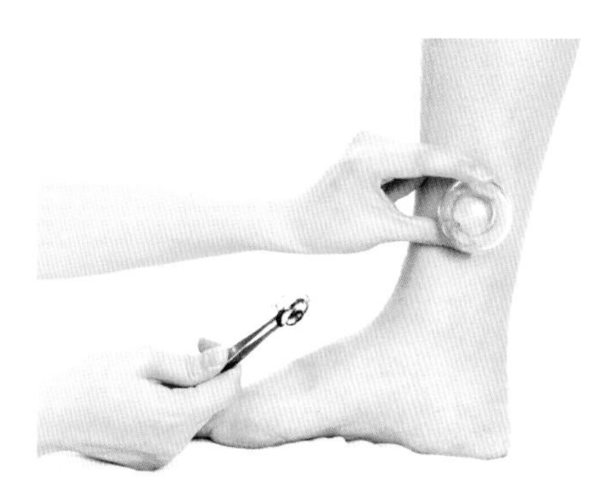

**Location:** At the rear edge of the shinbone, 3 cun above the ankle.

**Method:** First knead Sanyinjiao point with the thumb pulp for 2–3 minutes and then apply a cup to the point, retaining the cup for 10–15 minutes. With the cup removed, perform moxibustion with a moxa stick for 3–5 minutes, until warmth is felt.

#### 2. Yinlingquan Point

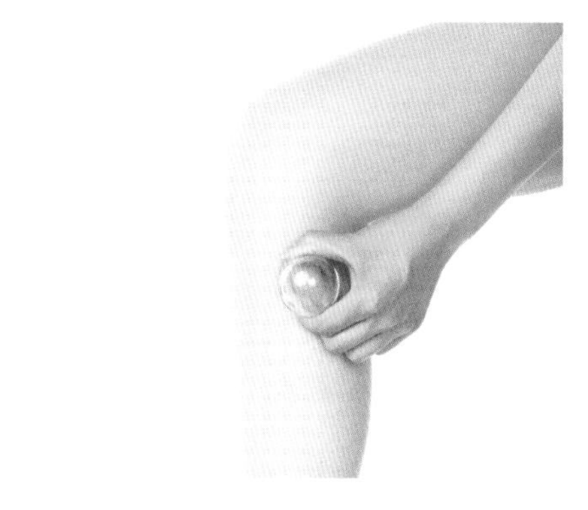

**Location:** In the depression on the inner edge of the shinbone below the knee.

**Method:** First knead Yinlingquan point with the thumb pulp for 2–3 minutes, and then cup this point, retaining the cup for 10–15 minutes. With the cup removed, perform moxibustion with a moxa stick for 3–5 minutes until warmth is felt.

#### 3. Taixi Point

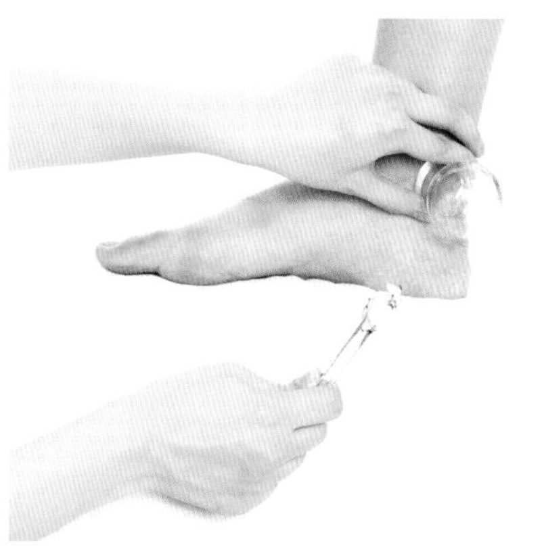

**Location:** In a cavity between the medial malleolus and Achilles tendon.

**Method:** Apply a cup to the point, retaining the cup for 10–15 minutes. With the cup removed, perform moxibustion with a moxa stick for 3–5 minutes until warmth is felt.

#### 4. Ganshu, Pishu and Shenshu Points

**Location:** Ganshu point is 1.5 cun away from the ninth thoracic spinal process on the inner side of the scapula; Pishu point is 1.5 cun away horizontally from the eleventh thoracic vertebra; Shenshu point is 1.5 cun horizontally from the second lumbar spinal process.

**Method:** Use the moving cupping method. Move the cup on the bladder meridian on the back by segment along the meridian, and move it several times mainly on Ganshu, Pishu and Shenshu Points. Repeatedly push and pull on the points back and forth, until the skin becomes red. The cup may be retained on the abovementioned points for 10–15 minutes after the moving cupping. With the cup removed, perform moxibustion with a moxa stick for 3–5 minutes until warmth is felt.

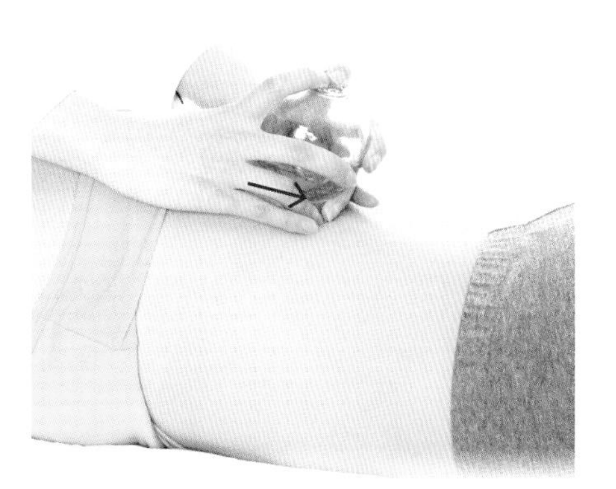

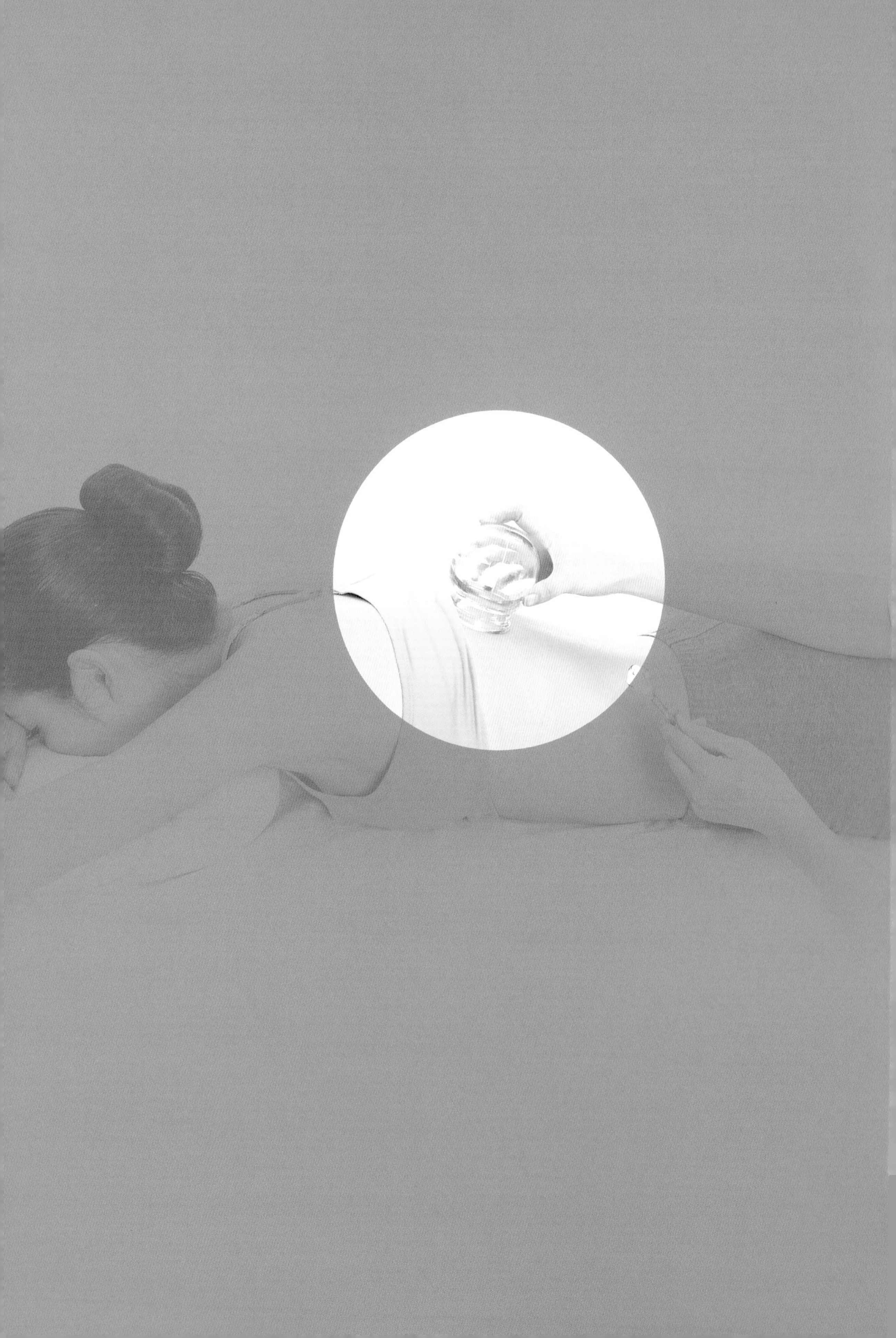

# Chapter Eleven
# Physical Attractiveness

Everyone wants to be attractive and have a graceful figure, but not everyone is a born beauty. If one is not satisfied with his or her appearance, then he or she can constantly improve it through cupping. It can help one lose weight, improve the skin, and shape the body to make one more beautiful and younger!

## 1 Slimming

Overweight people are those whose actual weight is 20% more than the standard weight, often accompanied by a variety of other diseases, such as diabetes, high blood pressure and cardiovascular disease caused by obesity.

This type of people should control and have a reasonable diet, reduce the intake of high-fat food and avoid fried food. Drink less coffee, and quit smoking and alcohol consumption. Eat more kelp, red beans, white gourds, and hawthorns as they are conducive to weight loss. In addition, they should strengthen physical exercise to reduce weight and promote consumption of excess energy.

The cupping should focus on around the local fat areas, and may plus Zhongwan, Sanyinjiao, Pishu, Fenglong, Tianshu, Shangjuxu, Zusanli, and Jimen points.

### Cupping Methods

**Local Fat Areas**

**Method:** Select a cup of appropriate size and apply it to the fat areas, retaining the cup for 15–20 minutes.

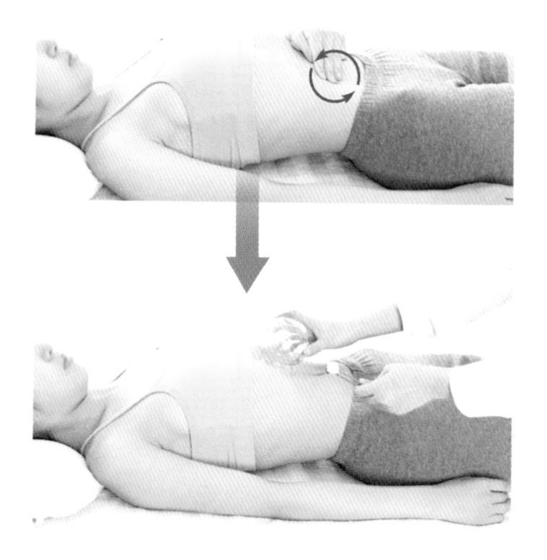

**1. Zhongwan Point**

**Location:** On the upper abdomen, 4 cun above the center of the umbilicus, on the anterior midline.

**Method:** First massage the abdomen above the bellybutton for about ten circles with the palm or corporately the index finger, the middle finger, and the ring finger. Then select a cup of appropriate size, and apply it to Zhongwan point, retaining the cup for 10–15 minutes.

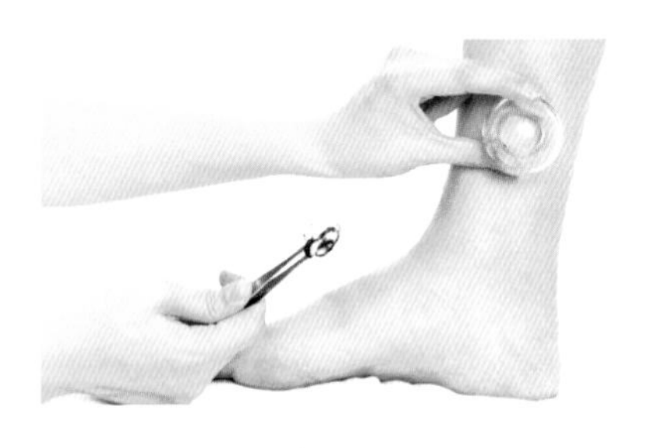

### 2. Sanyinjiao Point

**Location:** At the rear edge of the shinbone, 3 cun above the ankle.

**Method:** First knead Sanyinjiao point with the thumb pulp for 2–3 minutes, and then select and apply a cup of appropriate size to the point, retaining the cup for 10–15 minutes.

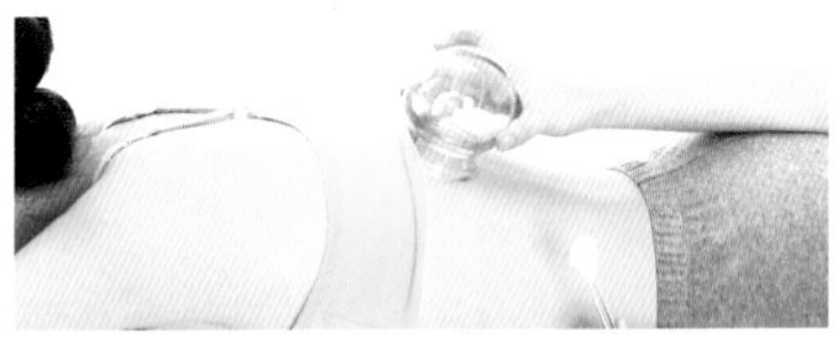

### 3. Pishu Point

**Location:** 1.5 cun away horizontally from the eleventh thoracic vertebra.

**Method:** Select and apply a cup of appropriate size to the point, retaining the cup for 10–15 minutes.

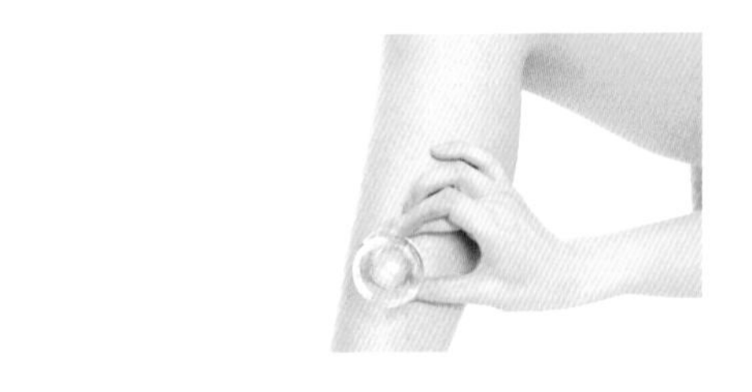

### 4. Fenglong Point

**Location:** 8 cun above the ankle tip.

**Method:** First knead Fenglong point with the thumb pulp for 2–3 minutes, and then select and apply a cup of appropriate size to the point, retaining the cup for 10–15 minutes.

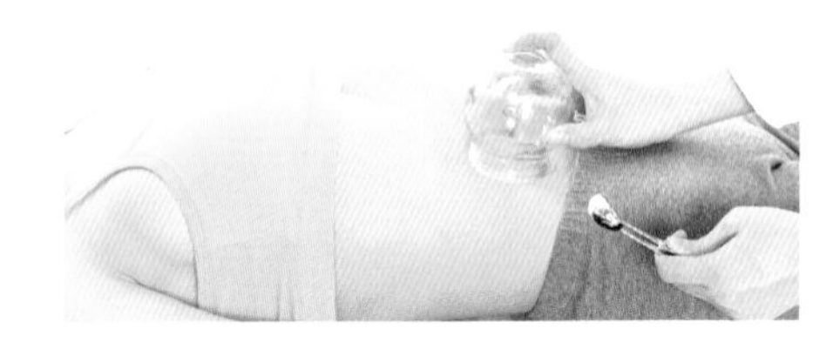

### 5. Tianshu Point

**Location:** About 2 cun horizontally away from the navel.

**Method:** Select a cup of appropriate size and apply it to the point, retaining the cup for 10–15 minutes.

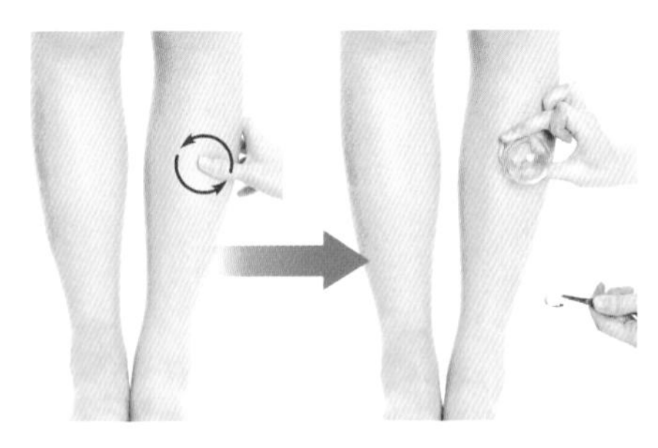

### 6. Shangjuxu Point

**Location:** One middle finger cun (the length of the second section of the middle finger) on the outside of the tibial crest, 3 cun below the Zusanli point.

**Method:** First knead Shangjuxu point with the thumb pulp for 2–3 minutes, and then select and apply a cup of appropriate size to the point, retaining the cup for 10–15 minutes.

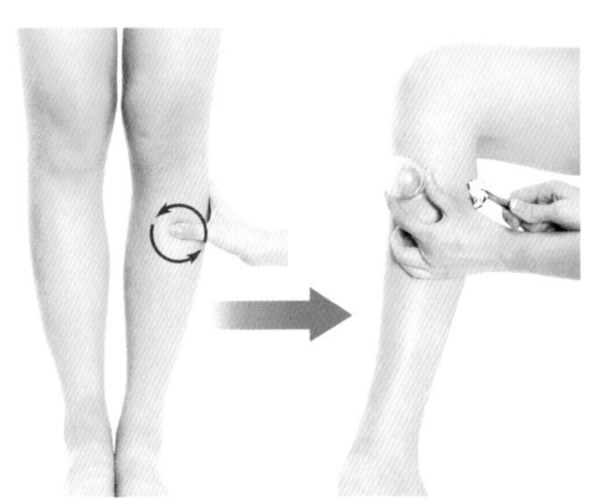

### 7. Zusanli Point

**Location:** About 3 cun below the knee on the outer side of the tibia.

**Method:** First knead Zusanli point with the thumb pulp for 2–3 minutes, and then select a cup of appropriate size and apply it to the point, retaining the cup for 10–15 minutes.

### 8. Jimen Point

**Location:** On the medial aspect of the thigh, at the

junction of the upper one third and lower two thirds of the line connecting the medial end of the base of the patella and the Chongmen point, at the femoral artery between the adductor longus muscle and the sartorius muscle.

**Method:** Select a cup of appropriate size and apply it to the point, retaining the cup for 10–15 minutes.

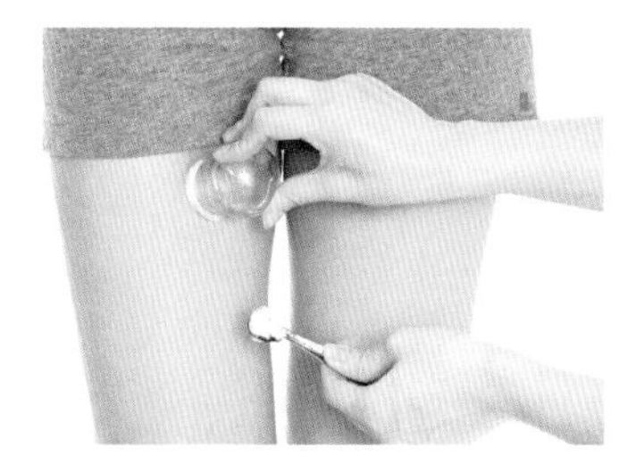

**Standard Body Weight**

Standard Body Mass Index (BMI) = weight (lb) / [height (in)] $^2$ × 703 or BMI = weight (kg) / [height (m)]$^2$. Ideal BMI score for women is 20-21, and that for men is 22. 24 or higher number means overweight, and below 18.5 is underweight.

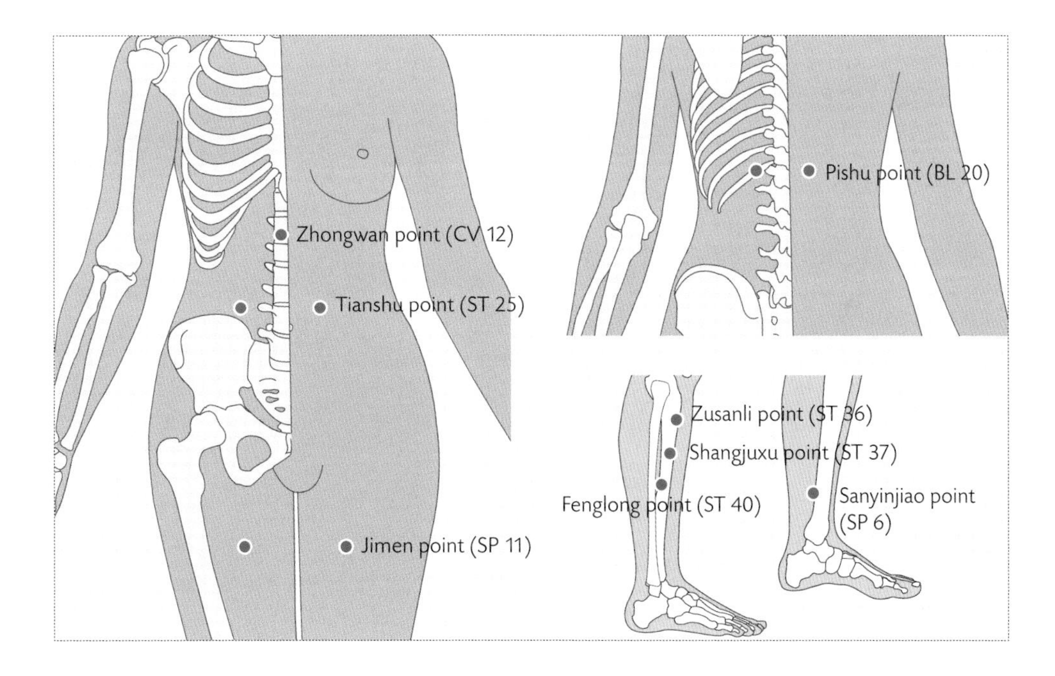


# 2 Get Rid of Freckles

Freckles are light brown small spots in the size ranging from a needle tip to a grain appearing on the forehead, nose, cheeks and other parts, and sometimes on the neck, shoulders and the back of the hands, without itching or other abnormal feelings.

During treatment, people with freckles should get lots of rest, avoid prolonged outdoor activities, and avoid exposure to the sun. In addition, they should eat less or do not eat irritating food, such as pepper, strong tea, wine, soda, and so on.

The cupping should be performed on Ganshu, Shenshu, Qihai, Zusanli, and Sanyinjiao points.

## Cupping Methods

### 1. Ganshu Point

**Location:** 1.5 cun away from the ninth thoracic spinal process on the inner side of the scapula.

**Method:** Use the moving cupping method by moving the cup on the bladder meridian on the back by segment along the meridian. Move the cup several times mainly on Ganshu point, and repeatedly push and pull on the point back and forth, until the skin becomes red. The cup may be retained on the abovementioned point for 5 minutes after the moving cupping.

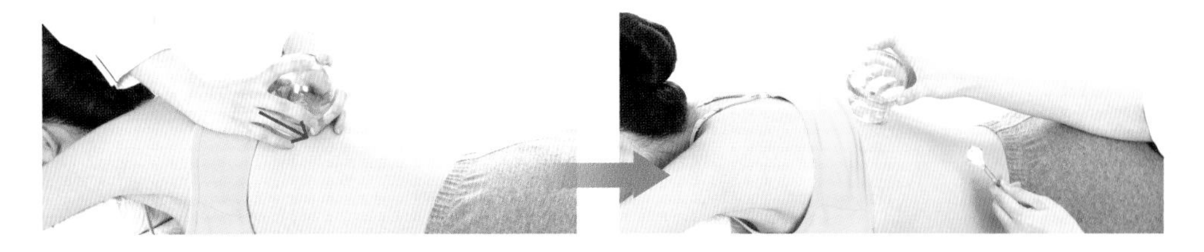

### 2. Shenshu Point

**Location:** 1.5 cun horizontally from the second lumbar spinal process.

**Method:** Use the moving cupping method by moving the cup on the bladder meridian on the back by segment along the meridian. Move the cup several times mainly on Shenshu point, and repeatedly push and pull on the point back and forth, until the skin becomes red. The cup may be retained on the abovementioned point for 5 minutes after the moving cupping.

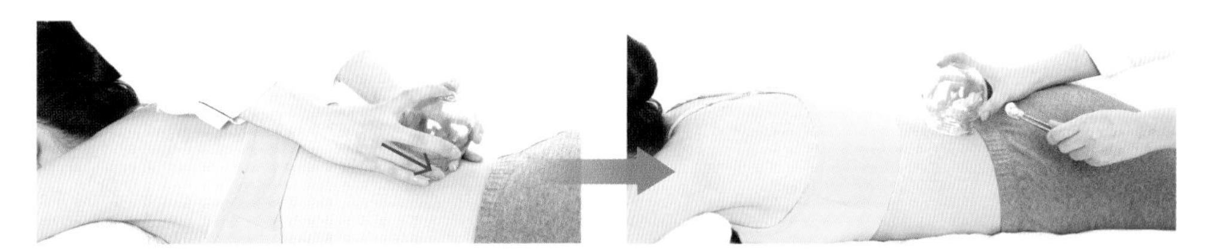

### 3. Qihai Point

**Location:** About 1.5 cun below the navel.

**Method:** First knead Qihai point with the thumb pulp for 2–3 minutes, and then apply a cup to the point, retaining the cup for 10–15 minutes. With the cup removed, perform moxibustion with a moxa stick for 3–5 minutes until warmth is felt.

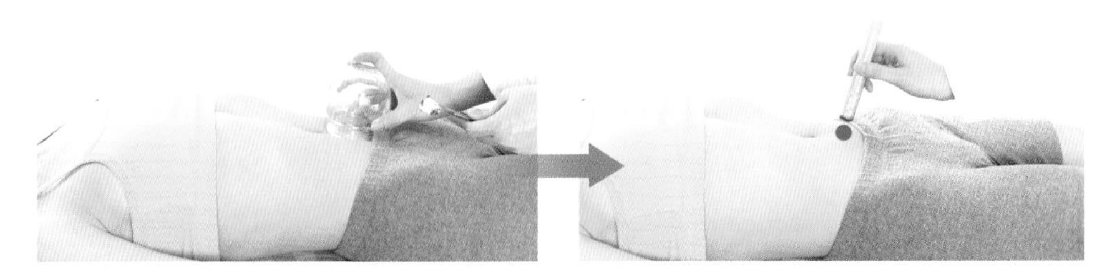

### 4. Zusanli Point

**Location:** About 3 cun below the knee on the outer side of the tibia.

**Method:** First knead Zusanli point with the thumb pulp for 2–3 minutes, and then select a cup of appropriate size and apply it to the point, retaining the cup for 10–15 minutes. With the cup removed, perform moxibustion with a moxa stick for 3–5 minutes until warmth is felt.

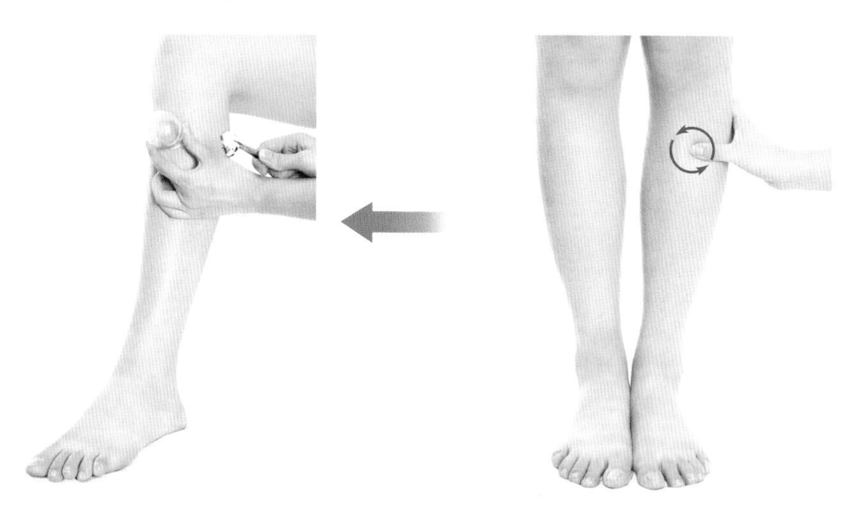

### 5. Sanyinjiao Point

**Location:** At the rear edge of the shinbone, 3 cun above the ankle.

**Method:** First knead Sanyinjiao point with the thumb pulp for 2–3 minutes, and then select and apply a cup of appropriate size to the point, retaining the cup for 10–15 minutes. With the cup removed, perform moxibustion with a moxa stick for 3–5 minutes until warmth is felt.

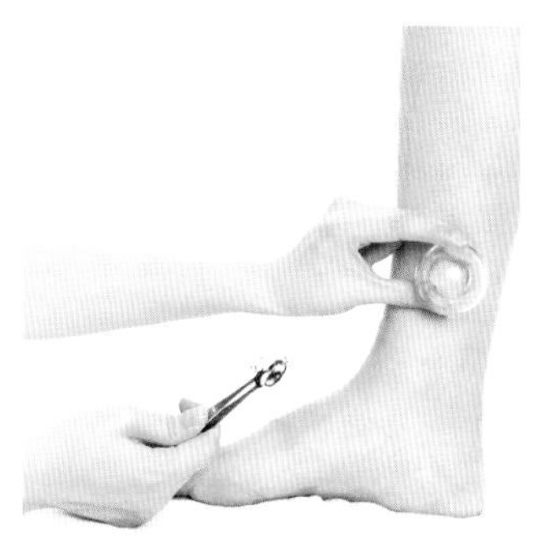

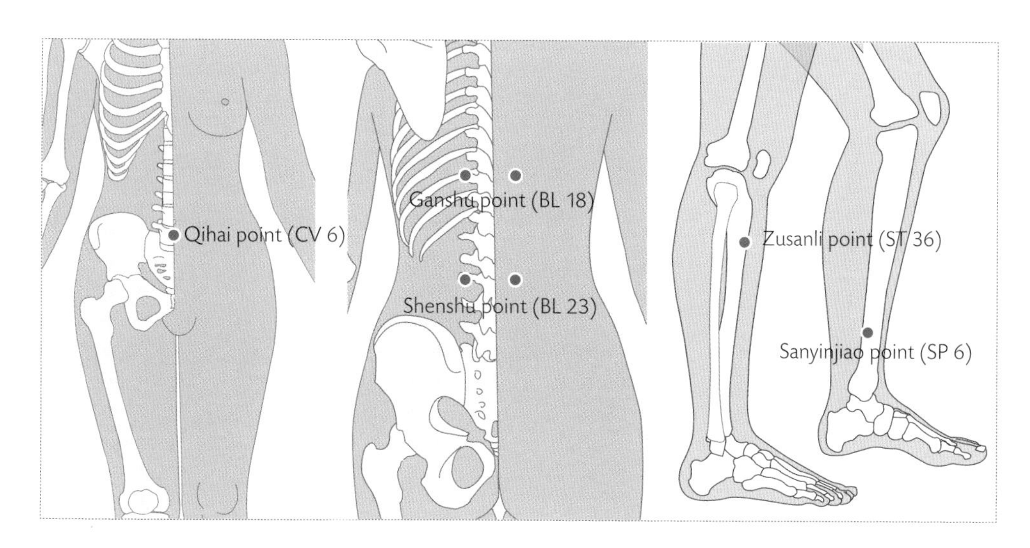

# 3 Brighten the Skin Color

Dull and gloomy skin is mostly caused by a lack of nutrition in the local skin, excessive exposure to the sun, lack of water, mental factors, long-term lack of sleep, etc.

To improve dull skin, one should drink less coffee and strong tea, instead, drink medlar and American ginseng tea every day, eat more fruits and red dates, donkey-hide gelatin, and other blood-tonifying food, and drink plenty of water. Prevent sunlight, and apply sunscreen when the light is strong. In addition, maintaining a normal weight, doing exercise, and keeping adequate sleep are helpful for brightening the skin color.

The cupping should be applied to Zusanli, Guanyuan, Xuehai, Sanyinjiao, and associated back-shu points.

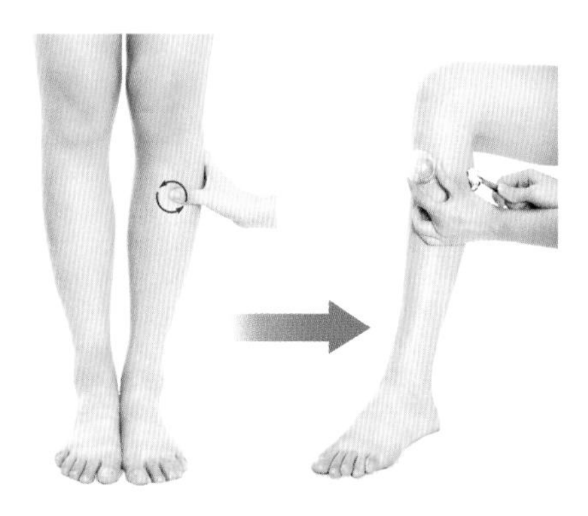

## Cupping Methods

### 1. Zusanli Point

**Location:** About 3 cun below the knee on the outer side of the tibia.

**Method:** First knead Zusanli point with the thumb pulp for 2–3 minutes, and then select a cup of appropriate size and apply it to the point, retaining the cup for 10–15 minutes. With the cup removed, perform moxibustion with a moxa stick for 3–5 minutes until warmth is felt.

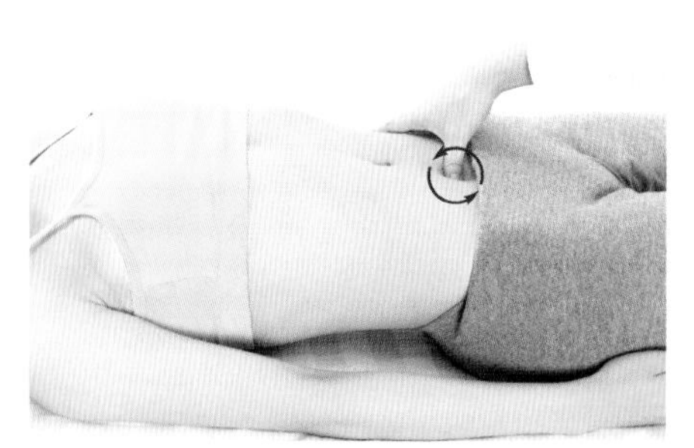

### 2. Guanyuan Point

**Location:** About 3 cun below the navel.

**Method:** First knead Guanyuan point with the thumb pulp for 2–3 minutes, and then select and apply a cup of appropriate size to the point, retaining the cup for 10–15 minutes. With the cup removed, perform moxibustion with a moxa stick for 3–5 minutes until warmth is felt.

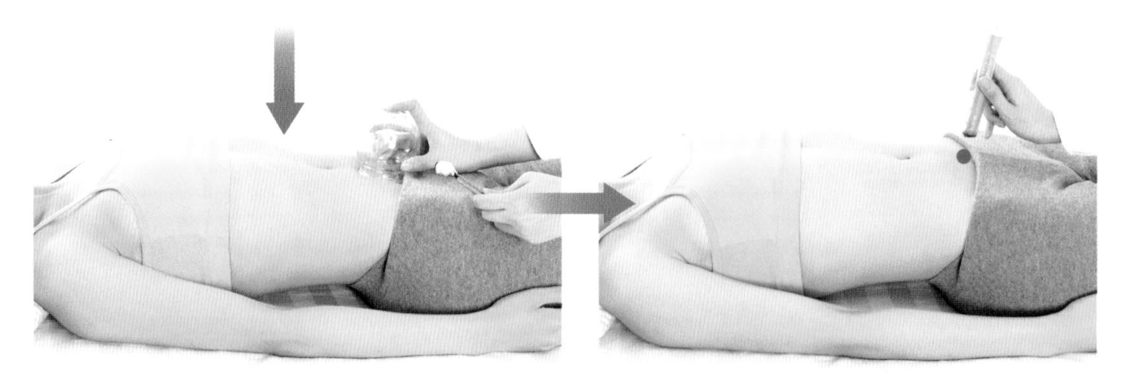

### 3. Xuehai Point

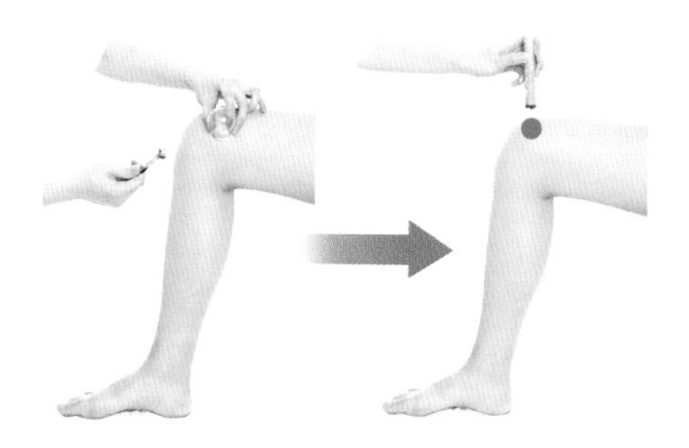

**Location:** In a cavity about 2 cun away from the inner upper corner of the patella, when the knee is bent.

**Method:** First knead Xuehai point with the thumb pulp for 2–3 minutes, and then select and apply a cup of appropriate size to the point, retaining the cup for 10–15 minutes. With the cup removed, perform moxibustion with a moxa stick for 3–5 minutes until warmth is felt.

### 4. Sanyinjiao Point

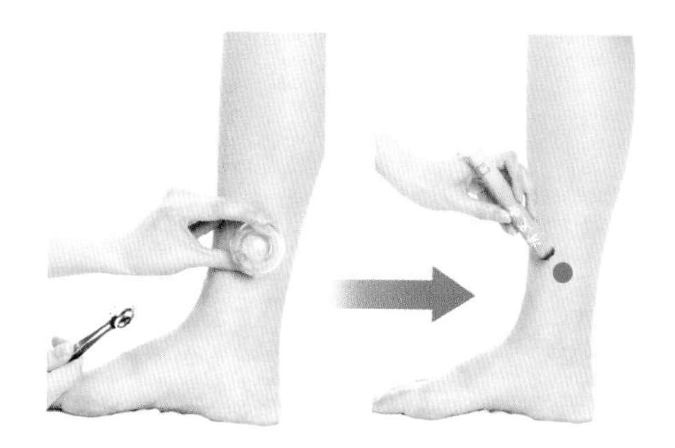

**Location:** At the rear edge of the shinbone, 3 cun above the ankle.

**Method:** First knead Sanyinjiao point with the thumb pulp for 2–3 minutes, and then select and apply a cup of appropriate size to the point, retaining the cup for 10–15 minutes. With the cup removed, perform moxibustion with a moxa stick for 3–5 minutes until warmth is felt.

### 5. Associated Back-Shu Points

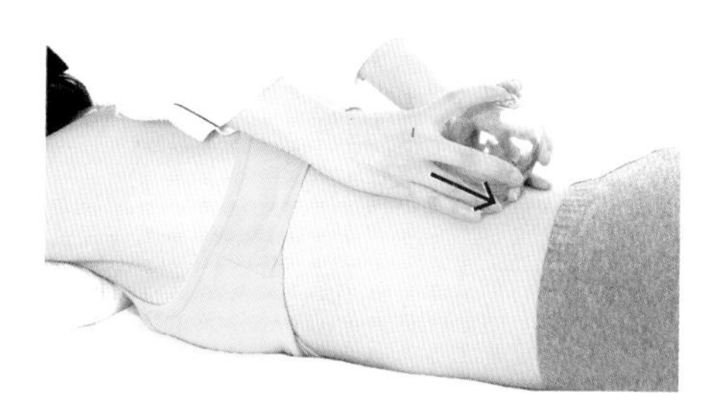

**Method:** Use the moving cupping method. Move the cup on the bladder meridian on the back by segment along the meridian, and move several times mainly on back-shu points, and repeatedly push and pull on the points back and forth until the skin becomes red. The cup may be retained on the abovementioned points for 10–15 minutes after the moving cupping.

**Associated Back-Shu Points**

Associated back-shu points mean the points on the bladder meridian. They are points on the back where qi of the five viscera and six bowels are infused, totaling 12 points, i.e. Feishu, Jueyinshu, Xinshu, Ganshu, Danshu, Pishu, Weishu, Sanjiaoshu, Shenshu, Dachangshu, Xiaochangshu, and Pangguangshu points.

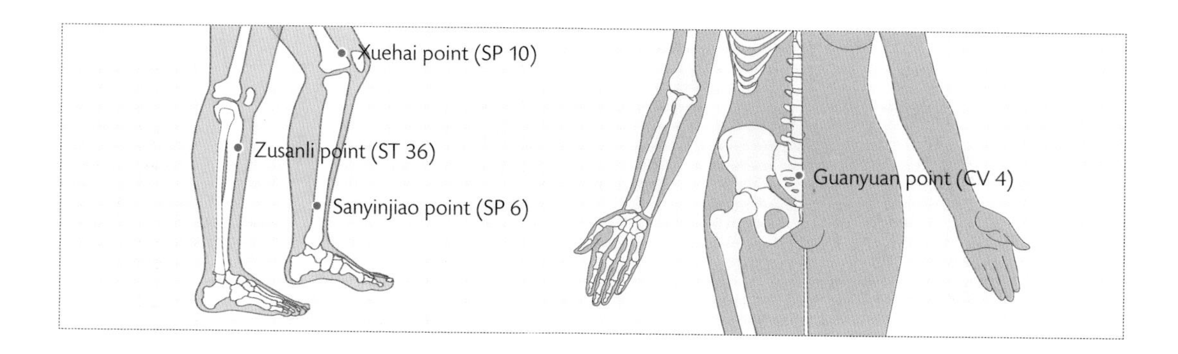

# 4 Eliminate Wrinkles

Wrinkles are the small fine lines appearing on the forehead, upper and lower eyelids, paropia, area before ears, cheeks, neck, chin, mouth, and other parts.

To reduce wrinkles, it is necessary to maintain adequate sleep, eat more sunflower seeds and tomatoes, cucumbers and other fruits and vegetables. In addition, do not use too much cosmetics, and remove makeup before going to bed. Some facial massage techniques can be used in the process of eliminating wrinkles, by gently pressing and massaging with finger pulps in the wrinkle area along a straight line, repeating five times, or by gently massaging the temples with fingertips five times. Both sides of the head and muscles around the eyes have obvious relaxed effects.

The cupping should be performed on local wrinkled skin, and Sibai, Yangbai, Taiyang, Quanliao, and Dicang points.

## Cupping Methods

### 1. Affected Parts

**Method:** First, massage the face lightly with the finger pulp or the thenar muscle of the palm heel, and then select a cup of appropriate size and move it lightly on local skin back and forth for 3–5 minutes. The movement should be gentle and slow, with moderate pressure. Do not retain the cup.

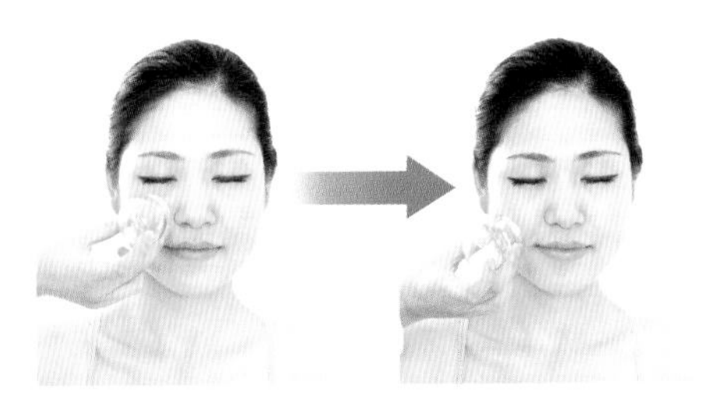

### 2. Sibai Point

**Location:** Directly below the pupil, in a cavity below the orbit.

**Method:** Select a cup of appropriate size and move it from Sibai point towards both sides of the cheeks for 3–5 minutes. The movement should be gentle and slow, with moderate pressure. Do not retain the cup.

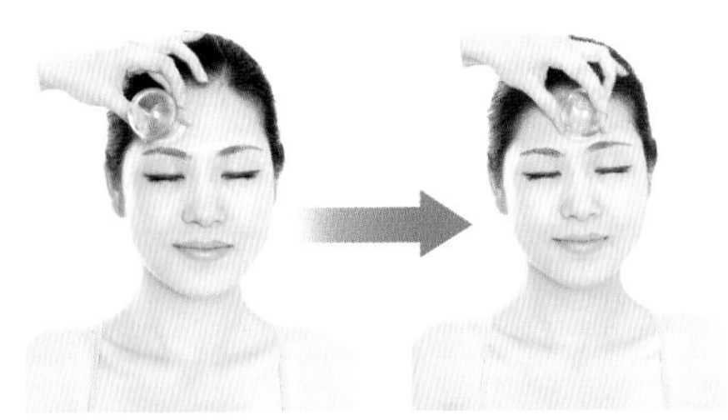

### 3. Yangbai Point

**Location:** Directly in line with the pupil, 1 cun above the eyebrow on the forehead.

**Method:** Select a cup of appropriate size and move it from Yangbai point towards the frontal part for 3–5 minutes. The movement should be gentle and slow, with moderate pressure. Do not retain the cup.

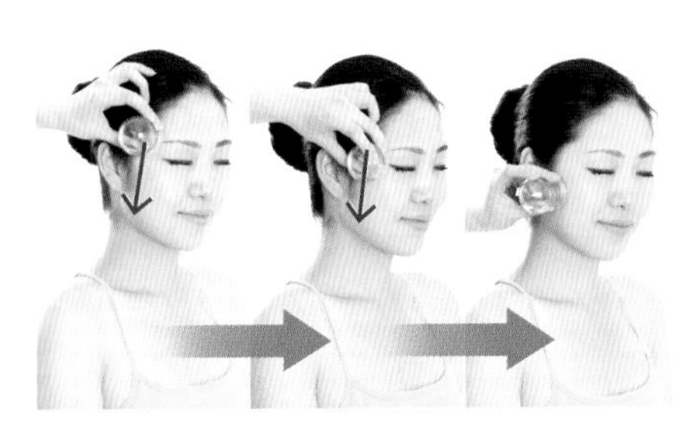

### 4. Taiyang Point

**Location:** In the depression about 1 cun behind the space between the outer tip of the brow and outer eye corner.

**Method:** Select a cup of appropriate size and move it from Taiyang point towards the temporal regions and two ears for 3–5 minutes. The movement should be gentle and slow, with moderate pressure. Do not retain the cup.

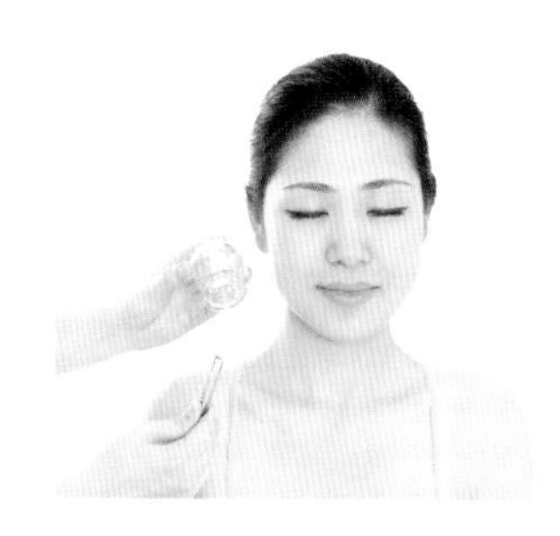

### 5. Quanliao Point

**Location:** Directly in the lower part of the outer canthus, in a cavity of the lower margin of the cheekbone.

**Method:** Select a cup of appropriate size and apply it to Quanliao point by using the flash cupping method. Retain the cup for less than 10 minutes.

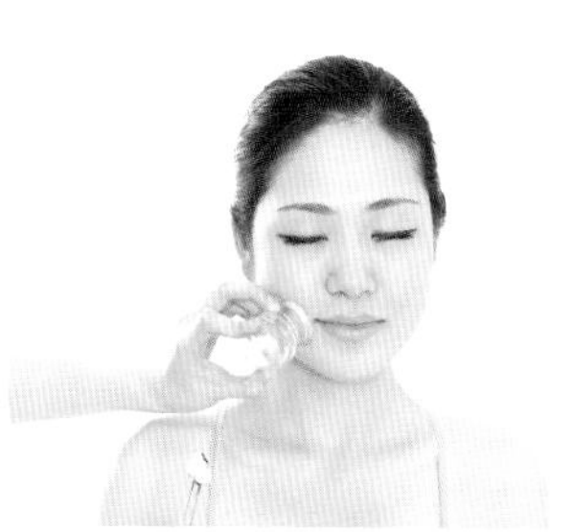

### 6. Dicang Point

**Location:** About 0.4 cun away from the mouth corner, directly in line with the pupil.

**Method:** Select a cup of appropriate size and apply it to Dicang point by using the flash cupping method. Retain the cup for less than 10 minutes.

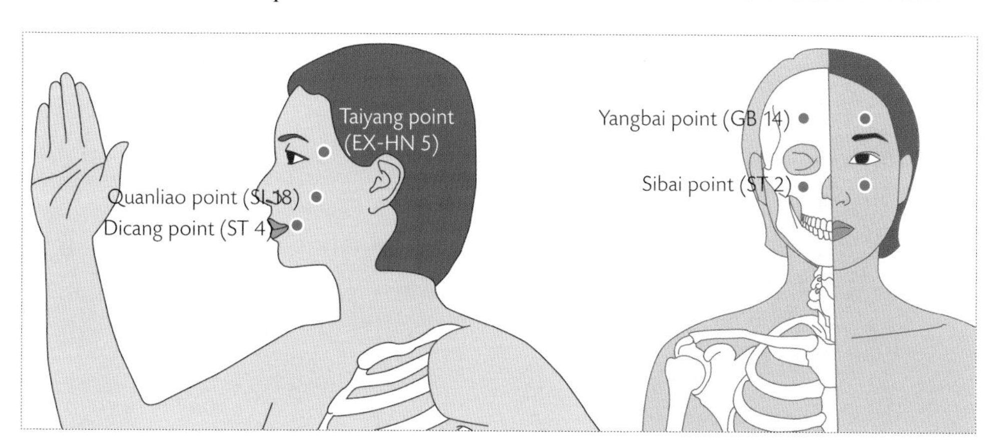


## 5 Improve Hair Quality

People with bad hair quality can suffer constant shedding, with hair that lacks luster, and are dry, yellow with bifurcation or easy to break.

To improve hair quality, one may eat more black sesame seeds, angelica, mulberries, walnuts, and other food tonifying blood and brightening the hair. Often massaging the scalp and combing the hair 300 times a day can effectively prevent white hair and hair loss. In addition, one should also maintain adequate sleep and a good mood.

The cupping should be performed on Yongquan, Taixi, Xuehai, Geshu, and Sanyinjiao points.

## Cupping Methods

### 1. Yongquan Point

**Location:** In a depression in the front of the sole of the foot, about one-third of the way down from the toes.

**Method:** First knead Yongquan point with the palm for 2–3 minutes, until a feeling of heat is present. Then select a cup of appropriate size and apply it to the point, retaining the cup for 10–15 minutes. With the cup removed, perform moxibustion with a moxa stick for 3–5 minutes until warmth is felt.

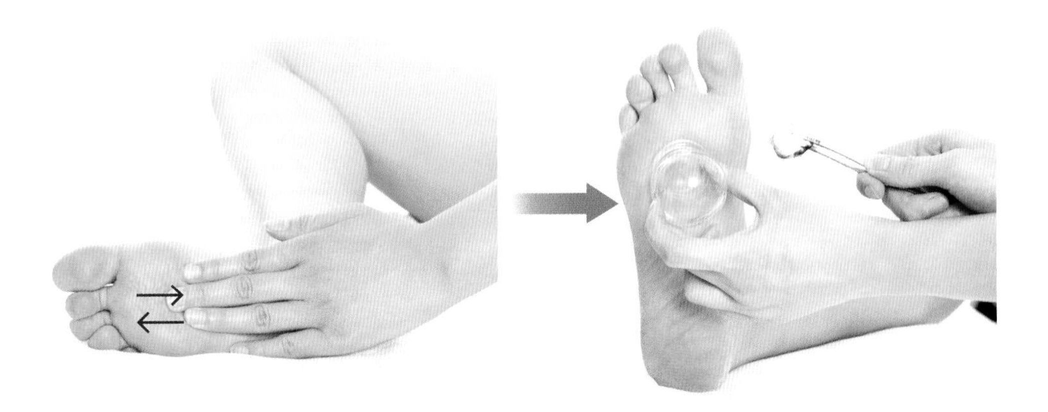

### 2. Xuehai Point

**Location:** In a cavity about 2 cun away from the inner upper corner of the patella, when the knee is bent.

**Method:** First knead Xuehai point with the thumb pulp for 2–3 minutes, and then select and apply a cup of appropriate size to the point, retaining the cup for 10–15 minutes. With the cup removed, perform moxibustion with a moxa stick for 3–5 minutes until warmth is felt.

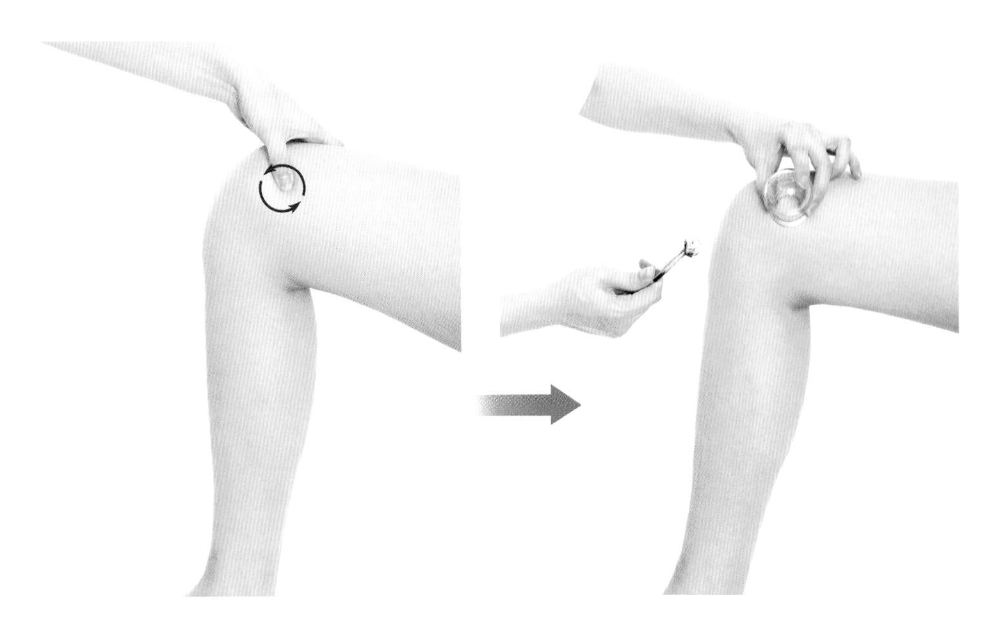

### 3. Taixi Point

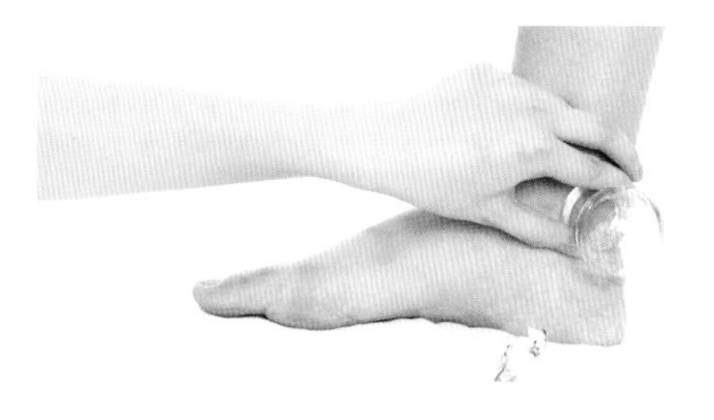

**Location:** In a cavity between the medial malleolus and Achilles tendon.

**Method:** First knead Taixi point with the thumb pulp for 2–3 minutes, and then select a cup of appropriate size and apply it to the point, retaining the cup for 10–15 minutes.

### 4. Geshu Point

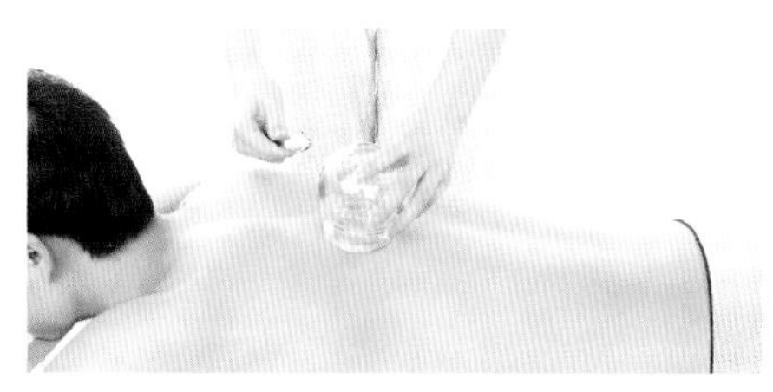

**Location:** 1.5 cun away from the spinous process of the seventh thoracic vertebra.

**Method:** Select a cup of appropriate size and apply it to Geshu point. Retain the cup for 10–15 minutes.

### 5. Sanyinjiao Point

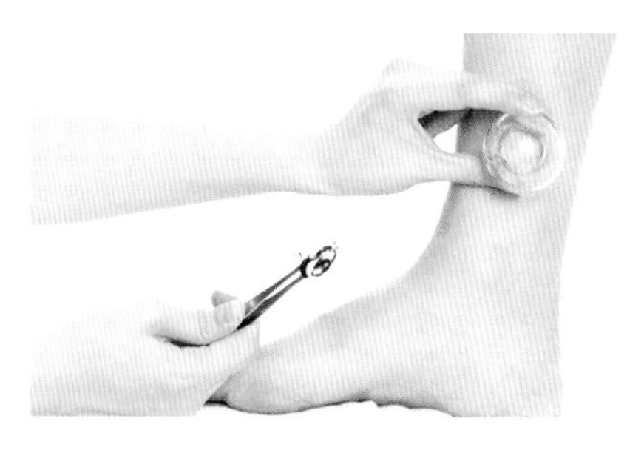

**Location:** At the rear edge of the shinbone, 3 cun above the ankle.

**Method:** Knead Sanyinjiao point with the thumb pulp for 2–3 minutes, and then cup this point, retaining the cup for 10–15 minutes. With the cup removed, perform moxibustion with a moxa stick for 3–5 minutes until warmth is felt.

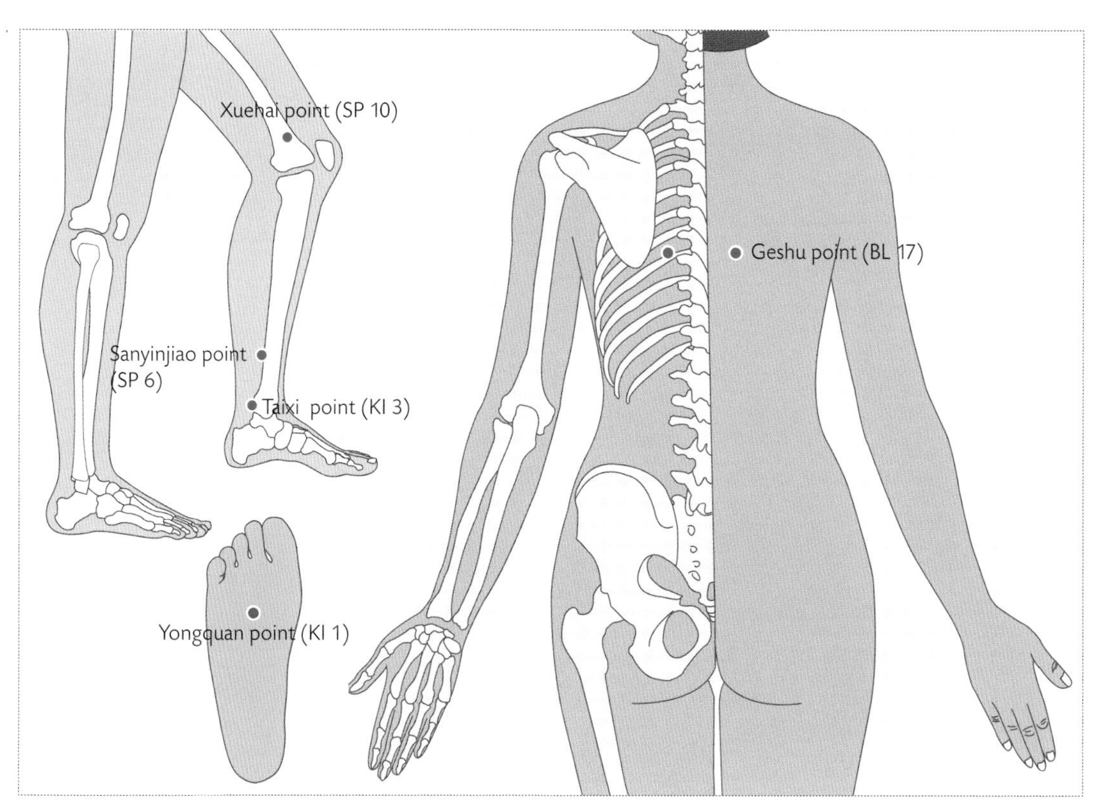

# 6 Chest Fitness

Men who do not have a strong chest need to exercise the chest often, and women who have too small breasts with poor flexibility or flat chest need to exercise their chest often.

Women should pay attention to taking off bra during sleep, so as to avoid constraining the chest or hindering the normal discharge of lymph. This not only allows a healthy development of the chest, but also prevents chest diseases.

The cupping should be performed on Danzhong, Rugen, Dabao, and Qimen points.

## Cupping Methods

### 1. Danzhong Point

**Location:** Directly in the middle of the chest between the nipples.

**Method:** First, knead from Danzhong point towards both sides of the chest with the thenar muscle of the palm heel for 3–5 minutes, and then select a cup of appropriate size and move it lightly around the chest back and forth for 3–5 minutes. The movement should be gentle and slow, with moderate pressure.

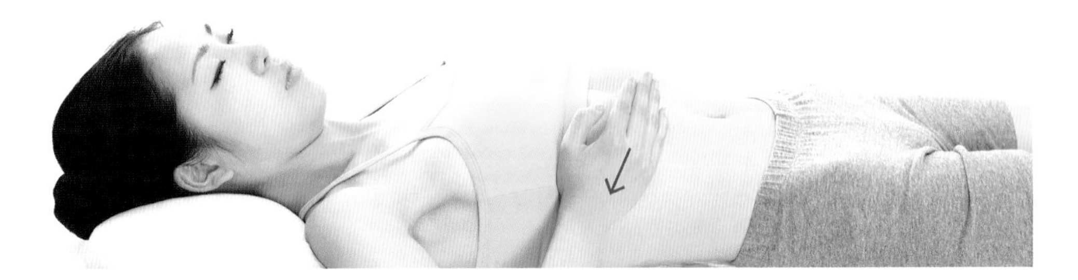

### 2. Rugen Point

**Location:** In the fifth intercostal space at the base of the breast, directly under the nipple.

**Method:** First, knead from Rugen point upwards with the thenar muscle of the palm heel for 3–5 minutes, and then select a cup of appropriate size and move it lightly around the chest back and forth for 3–5 minutes. The movement should be gentle and slow, with moderate pressure.

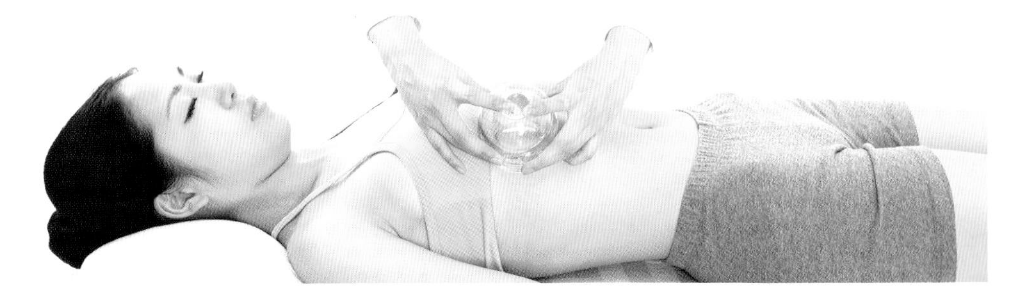

### 3. Dabao Point

**Location:** In the lateral thoracic region, and on the midaxillary line in the sixth intercostal space.

**Method:** First, knead from Dabao point towards the center of the chest with the palm heel for 3–5 minutes, and then select a cup of appropriate size and move it lightly around the chest back and forth for 3–5 minutes. The movement should be gentle and slow, with moderate pressure.

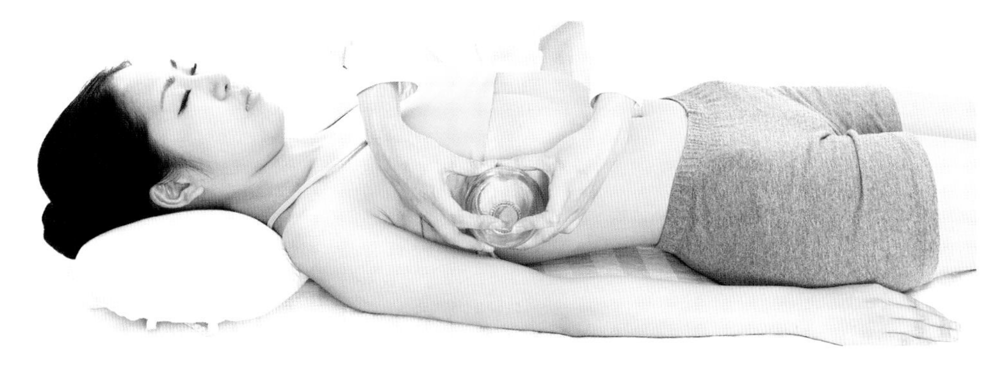

### 4. Qimen Point

**Location:** In the sixth intercostal space directly below the nipple.

**Method:** First, knead around Qimen point with the palm, or corporately the index finger, the middle finger, and the ring finger for 3–5 minutes, and then select and apply a cup of appropriate size to the point, retaining the cup for 3–5 minutes.

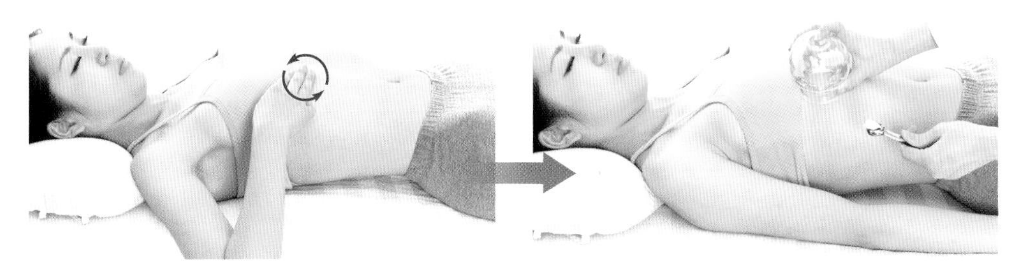

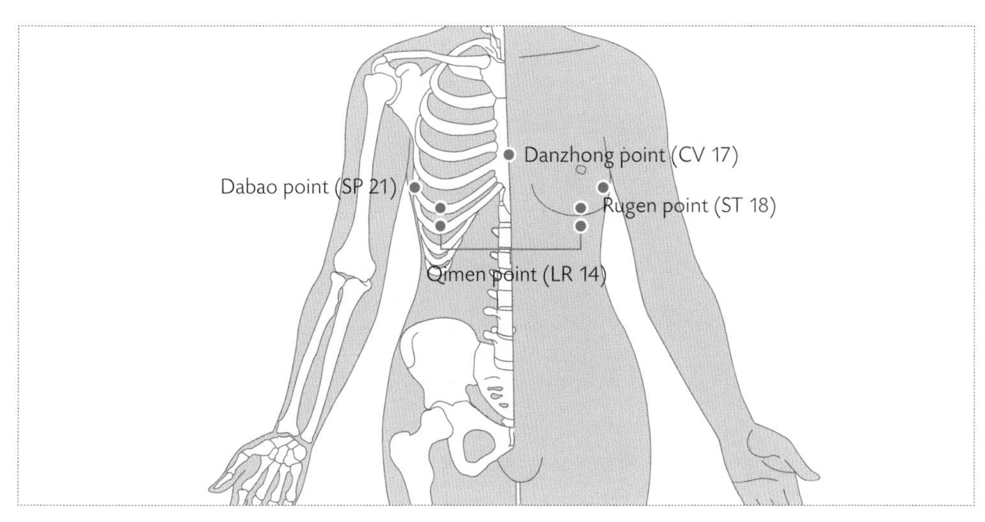

# 7 Waist Fitness

People in modern times, especially office workers, after having sat in the office for a long time, are always prone to waist stiffness, lack of flexibility, easiness to sprain, or fat accumulation in the waist, which affect appearance.

To avoid waist disease and improve the esthetics of the waist, people must ensure appropriate amount of exercise and avoid sitting for a long time. People who need to sit for a long time should stand up and exercise between intervals. In addition, they should have more light diets, and eat less high-fat food.

The cupping should be performed on Shenque, Tianshu, Zhangmen, Daimai, and Mingmen points.

## Cupping Methods

### 1. Shenque Point

**Location:** At the center of the navel.

**Method:** First, massage the abdomen centering on Shenque point with the palm heel, or corporately the index finger, the middle finger, and the ring finger for 3–5 minutes, with an appropriately large force. Then apply a cup to the point, retaining it for 10–15 minutes.

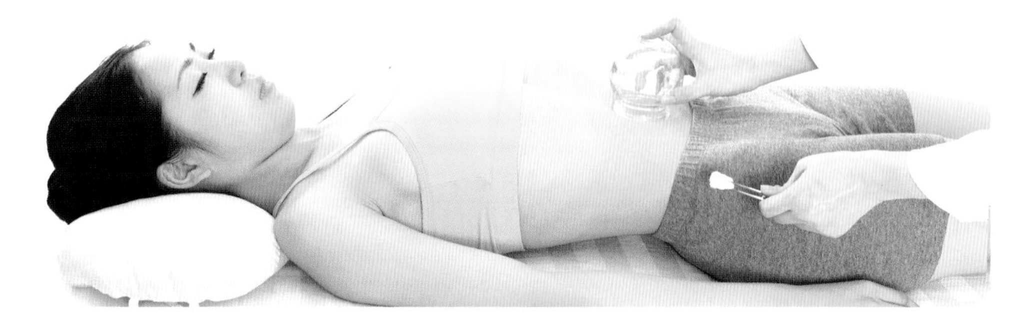

### 2. Tianshu Point

**Location:** About 2 cun horizontally away from the navel.

**Method:** Select a cup of appropriate size and apply it to the point, retaining the cup for 10–15 minutes.

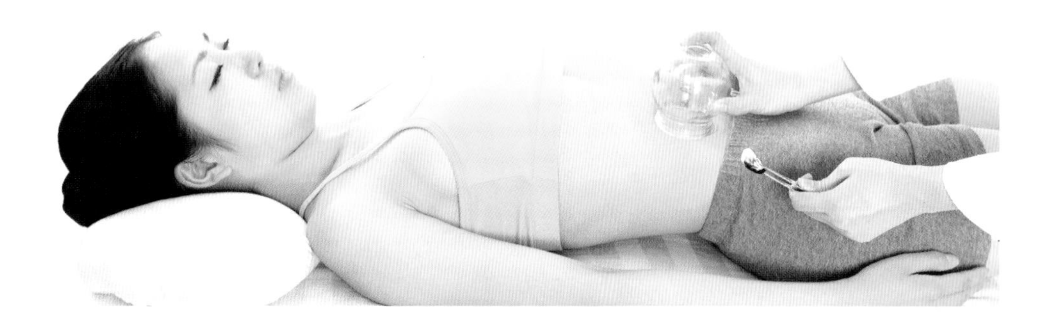

### 3. Zhangmen Point

**Location:** On the lateral abdomen, below the free extremity of the eleventh rib.

**Method:** First, knead from Zhangmen point downwards both sides of the waist with the palm heel with an appropriately large force. Then select a cup of appropriate size and apply it to the point, retaining the cup for 10–15 minutes.

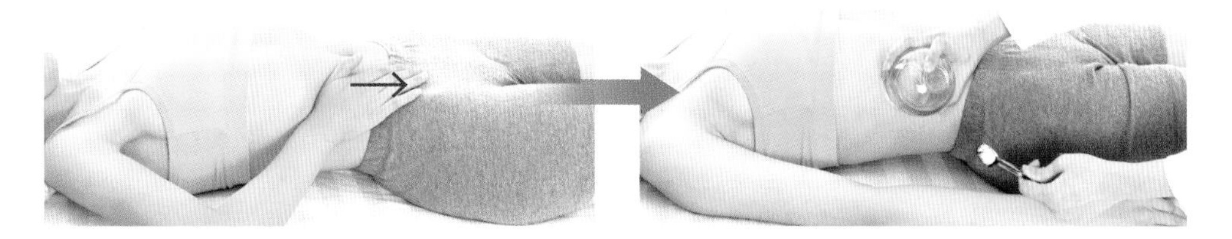

### 4. Daimai Point

**Location:** On the lateral abdomen below the free extremity of the eleventh rib and at the same level as the center of the umbilicus.

**Method:** First, knead Daimai point circularly with the palm heel with an appropriately large force. Then select a cup of appropriate size and apply it to the point, retaining the cup for 10–15 minutes.

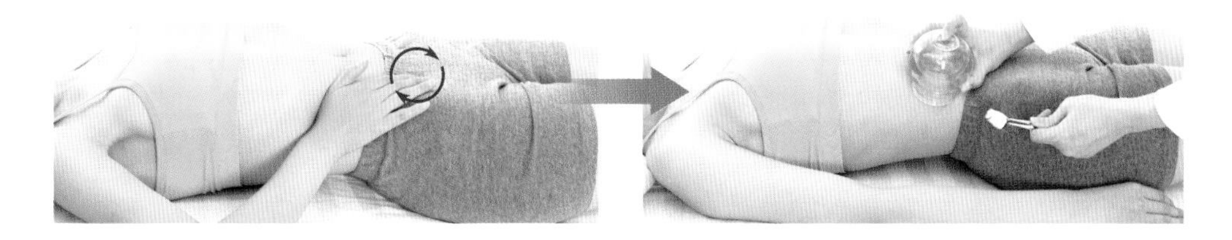

### 5. Mingmen Point

**Location:** In a cavity below the spinous process of the second cervical vertebra.

**Method:** First, knead from Mingmen point towards both sides of the waist with the palm heel, with an appropriately large force. Then select a cup of appropriate size and apply it to the point, retaining the cup for 10–15 minutes.

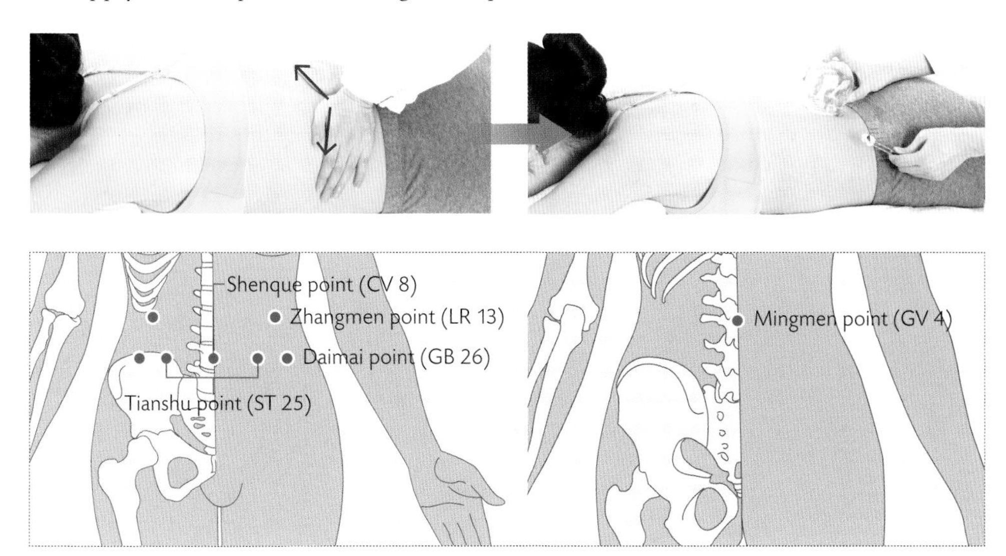

# 8 Anti-Aging

With the passage of time, many parts of the body will show signs of aging, featuring skin wrinkles, decreased immunity, slow response, slow metabolism, and so on.

To delay aging, one should pay attention to healthcare, and maintain a proper balance of work and rest to avoid overstrain. For the diet, one should pay attention to nutritional balance.

The cupping should be applied to Yongquan, Guanyuan, Zusanli, and Mingmen points.

## Cupping Methods

### 1. Yongquan Point

**Location:** In a depression in the front of the sole of the foot, about one-third of the way down from the toes.

**Method:** First knead Yongquan point with the palm for 2–3 minutes, until a feeling of heat is present. Then select a cup of appropriate size and apply it to the point, retaining the cup for 10–15 minutes. With the cup removed, perform moxibustion with a moxa stick for 3–5 minutes until warmth is felt.

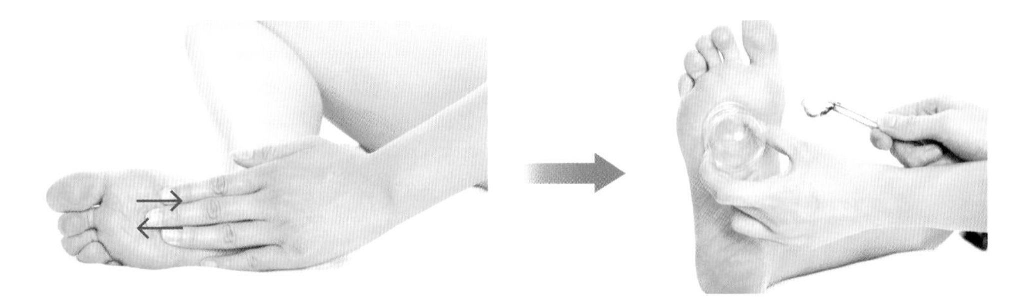

### 2. Guanyuan Point

**Location:** About 3 cun below the navel.

**Method:** First knead Guanyuan point with the thumb pulp for 2–3 minutes, and then apply a cup to Guanyuan point, retaining the cup for 10–15 minutes. With the cup removed, perform moxibustion with a moxa stick for 3–5 minutes until warmth is felt.

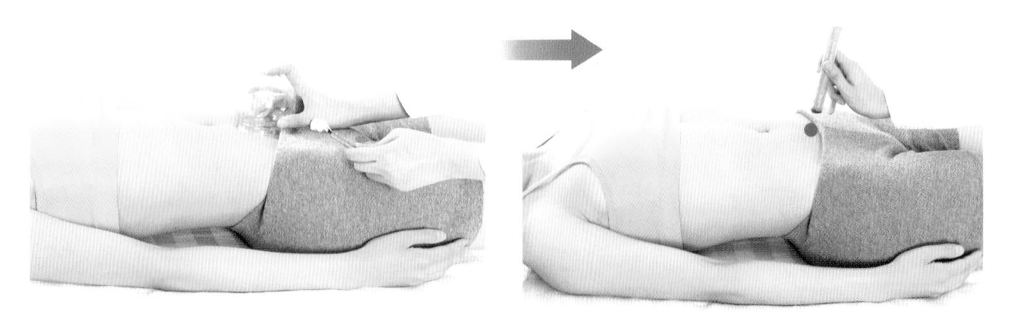

### 3. Zusanli Point

**Location:** About 3 cun below the knee on the outer side of the tibia.

**Method:** First knead Zusanli point with the thumb pulp for 2–3 minutes, and then apply a cup to Zusanli point, retaining the cup for 10–15 minutes. With the cup removed, perform moxibustion with a moxa stick for 3–5 minutes until warmth is felt.

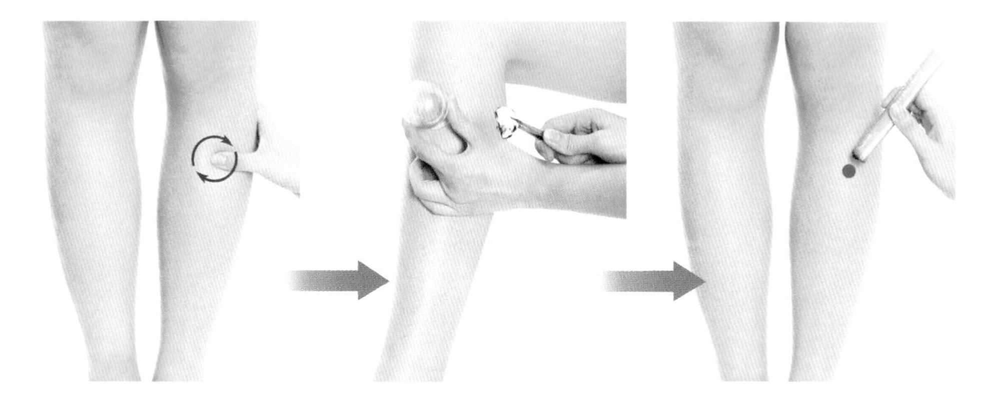

### 4. Mingmen Point

**Location:** In a cavity below the spinous process of the second cervical vertebra.

**Method:** Select and apply a cup of appropriate size to Mingmen point, retaining the cup for 10–15 minutes. With the cup removed, perform moxibustion with a moxa stick for 3–5 minutes until warmth is felt.

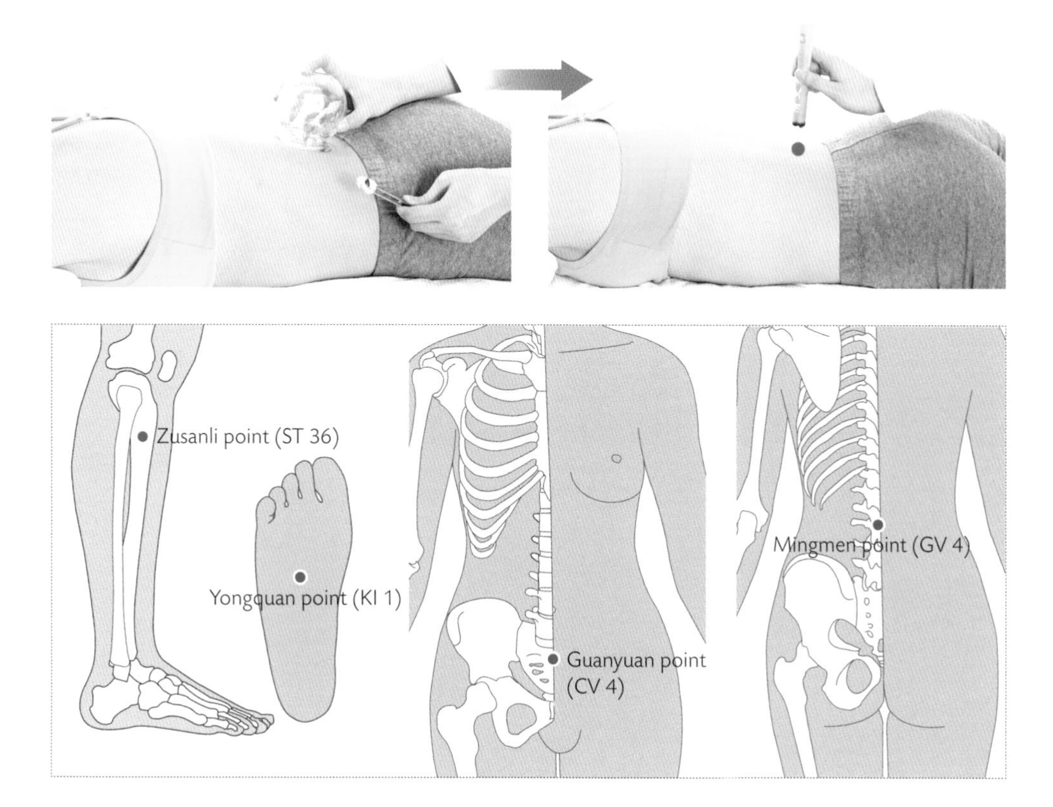

# Appendix

# Index

## G



## H



## I



## J



## K



## L



## M



## N

## P



## Q



## R



## S



## T

## U



## V



## W



## X



## Y



## Z